Oncology for Palliative Medicine

SECOND EDITION

Peter Hoskin

Reader in Oncology
Mount Vernon Hospital
Northwood, Middlesex

and

Wendy Makin

Consultant in Oncology and Palliative Care
Christie Hospital, Manchester

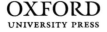

OXFORD
UNIVERSITY PRESS

*This book has been printed digitally and produced in a standard specification
in order to ensure its continuing availability*

OXFORD
UNIVERSITY PRESS

Great Clarendon Street, Oxford OX2 6DP

Oxford University Press is a department of the University of Oxford.
It furthers the University's objective of excellence in research, scholarship,
and education by publishing worldwide in

Oxford New York

Auckland   Cape Town Dar es Salaam Hong Kong   Karachi
Kuala Lumpur Madrid Melbourne Mexico City   Nairobi
New Delhi Shanghai Taipei Toronto
With offices in
Argentina Austria Brazil Chile Czech Republic France Greece
Guatemala Hungary Italy Japan South Korea Poland Portugal
Singapore Switzerland Thailand Turkey Ukraine Vietnam

Oxford is a registered trade mark of Oxford University Press
in the UK and in certain other countries

Published in the United States
by Oxford University Press Inc., New York

ISBN-10: 0-19-262811-9
ISBN-13: 978-0-19-262811-4

gy for Palliative Medicine

Preface

The care of patients with cancer, and their families, continues to be the main source of work for most palliative care professionals. As cancer management becomes increasingly complex, there is more to be offered to those who have recurrent and progressive disease. Whereas in the past, palliative care was frequently signalled by the acknowledgement that "there's nothing more that can be done", there is now much earlier access to support and symptom control measures alongside active anti-tumour therapies.

The mix of patients who attend hospices now includes those who are still receiving chemotherapy, and those who may require further surgery or radiotherapy. As well as understanding the patient experience from diagnosis, those who care for them in palliative care services must also be able to recognize and manage any treatment-related side-effects and complications.

The aim of the first edition of this book was to provide the doctors and nurses who specialize in palliative care with primary knowledge of different types of cancer, their patterns of behaviour, and the disease processes which underlie clinical problems. It sets out to explain the bases upon which clinical decisions are made by oncologists, with particular emphasis on the place of palliative treatment.

For this second edition the core content has been updated to include examples of the patient journey through investigations and treatment, and clinical scenarios that relate to frequently encountered symptom control problems. It is hoped that this volume will enable earlier recognition of those opportunities for further treatment, which could make a difference to the quality of life that remains, and encourage discussion with oncology colleagues.

Our patients are our best textbook and stimulus for learning. What we are taught in our striving to improve the situation for one individual may well improve our efforts to help others in the future.

Middlesex and Manchester P.H.
June 2003 W.M.

Contents

Chapter 1

Palliative oncology

Principles of palliation

The most obvious aim of palliation is to improve quality of life: to relieve tumour-related symptoms and, at best, to prevent their return in the remaining life span of the person. This sometimes includes treatments that aim to prevent an anticipated problem such as a pathological fracture. Palliative interventions used in radiotherapy usually treat localized, symptomatic disease that may be only one of many sites of tumour in the individual; surgeons may leave some, or even all, of the tumour *in situ*, but use techniques to relieve obstruction of the bowel or urinary tracts where the cancer itself is inoperable. Therefore such treatments would not be expected to influence the progression of the malignancy as a whole nor prolong survival unless a life-threatening development is averted or delayed.

If we are clear that a specific palliative treatment will not influence survival, it may be reasonable to keep this in reserve until significant symptoms arise. An example here is an elderly person with an advanced lung cancer discovered as an incidental finding on a chest X-ray. However this may not be acceptable to some patients who are now aware of their diagnosis and would prefer for some treatment to be given.

Gains from effective palliation have to be balanced against whatever the treatment itself entails, in terms of hospital attendance, side effects and period of recovery or rehabilitation in someone whose life expectancy is already limited. In radiotherapy, regimens are used which can be planned quickly, given over a relatively short period of time, and with less troublesome acute side effects compared with those of schedules given with the aim of cure.

For most situations with widespread secondary cancer at presentation, palliation or no treatment is the only option, with the exception of some cancers that are highly responsive to chemotherapy. The situation is less clear-cut for patients without distant spread but who have locally advanced primary tumours. For them, major surgery, radical radiotherapy and/or chemotherapy are proposed in the hope of curing a proportion, while achieving remission and useful control of the cancer for a period of time in others. Examples here include later stage head and neck and cervical cancers; up to 40 per cent of women with stage III cervical cancers will be cured. Among the rest, some will have inexorable progression of their pelvic disease but there will also be an additional group in whom the pelvic tumour remains under control although they eventually succumb to disease elsewhere.

The distinction between curative and palliative intentions may be less clear-cut when chemotherapy is used. Haematological malignancies, for which chemotherapy is the main treatment modality, warrant an intensive and rather aggressive management from diagnosis in most patients. These include those with high-grade lymphoma, of whom less than 40 per cent will be cured – but none unless such an approach is adopted. This may also apply to those with recurrence, although there may be a tendency to move to gentler regimens in terms of side effects when control of the disease rather than cure is all that can be achieved.

The patient with inoperable upper gastrointestinal cancer, or small cell lung cancer, will see chemotherapy as the only lifeline that is offered. For these individuals, the chance of cure is very small but it is hard to not accept any treatment. Clearly there must be other gains including prolongation of survival.

There is good evidence that chemotherapy can produce good tumour regression, relief of symptoms and increased survival (compared with untreated patients) for a number of solid tumours – breast, lung, ovary and colorectal cancers. However a significant number of people go through treatment with little or no benefit and may also experience or even die from, chemotherapy-associated problems. For some, they continue on one regimen or another for most of their remaining lives. It is this that often raises concerns among the other, non-oncological professionals who are also supporting these patients and their families outside the hospital setting: is treatment embarked upon too readily; how were the decisions made and does the patient have enough information and understanding to make a fully informed decision?

The essential requirement is for everyone to be clear and realistic about the possible outcomes from any treatment; while influenced by tumour size, stage and other prognostic factors, ultimately we can only talk in terms of the recorded result in well-defined groups and extrapolate these to suggest the chances of achieving these in the next patient. The type of cancer, stage and prognostic factors, general condition and presence of other medical problems in the individual (rather than chronological age) will influence a decision on the treatment to be recommended. However most patients are willing to undergo major procedures if these offer even a small chance of cure.

Outcomes and end-points in palliation and their evaluation

The two fundamental outcomes of any cancer therapy are prolongation of survival and quality of life, the latter being a complex and individual value judgement that weighs benefits against costs. One of the challenges of palliation is that we do not expect to achieve cure, nor necessarily complete resolution of all cancer-associated symptoms; so how much benefit is enough to justify a particular treatment? The oncologist has to define some means by which to measure and compare different interventions; without doing so it would be difficult to know which are superior and for progress to be made in treatments for patients. It is also important to know if potentially expensive therapies are really cost effective and offer the best use of available resources. The person with cancer will be hoping to live for as long as possible and for the best that can be achieved.

To be sure of a genuine effect of a cancer treatment, the new therapy must be compared with either none at all or with the previously used gold standard in a randomized, controlled trial. Recruitment may be difficult if the comparison is between 'treatment now, or treatment later if you need it'. Such a non-treatment arm is sometimes described as offering 'best supportive care'; certainly patients in trials do often benefit from closer on-going contact and support from the research team so that worries and symptoms may be picked up promptly. However the frequency of assessment by a palliative care specialist professional is not usually documented! There is ongoing work to agree on standardisation of best supportive care for use in future studies.

To evaluate survival, patients of similar age, performance status, tumour stage and prognostic factors should be grouped together for comparison. They are followed up through to death and the median survival for the group is determined as well as the range of minimum to maximum survivals. In patients with recurrent or metastatic colorectal cancer given chemotherapy, the possible survival benefit compared with no treatment can be 6–10 months. In advanced non-small cell lung cancer, the survival benefit for those on chemotherapy is 6–8 weeks. This may still be deemed to be worthwhile by patients but professionals may be more sceptical unless there is also evidence of an overall benefit in quality of life.

Quality of life is of course a value judgement made by an individual. A simple method to obtain a global assessment could be a patient rating of 'how good are you feeling today', as marked on a visual analogue scale. Categorisation of performance status, such as the Karnofsky scale, is a functional assessment used since 1949. This uses a descriptive score from 100 (normal function) through to 0 (dead); 50 describes someone who needs considerable assistance and frequent medical care; 30 would be represented by the severely disabled person who has to be cared for in hospital and so on. It has been useful to define subsets of patients for comparison within trials and is an indicator of prognosis, but this is a rating by the professional, not the patient. In terms of quality of life, there are those who can find personal fulfilment in emotional and social terms, in spite of what might be regarded as intolerable physical constraints and this is not an uncommon finding in palliative care.

Other tools attempt to score across a range of physical, emotional and social domains. The EORTC QLQ-C 30 is an example of a complex questionnaire that was designed for use in clinical trials in oncology. The 30 questions include an overall rating of health and quality of life, as well as questions that ask about the impact of specific symptoms on that person during the previous week (rated from 'not at all' to 'very much'). This and other tools have been modified further and validated for use with specific types of cancer; in head and neck cancer for example, there would be more detailed assessment of feeding, speech and communication. The FACT questionnaire has been used as a part of the evaluation of treatments for lung cancer. However in a trial setting, the answers given by patients are usually confidential and used subsequently in the analysis of the trial results; thus there is no assurance that the involved professionals are aware of the concerns that seriously affect the quality of life of that patient. As such tools are refined, there would appear to be a role for their routine use in follow-up of all patients on cancer treatment but in practice this is not usually the case.

It is important that these questionnaires are answered by the patients themselves and not by carers or professionals on their behalf. They are used in conjunction with standardized ratings of treatment toxicity or morbidity for the type of treatment modality being used.

Oncologists also try to objectively document tumour response as part of the evaluation of some, but not all, palliative treatments. This might include clinical or radiological measurement tumour size, or levels of tumour markers if available. Even outside a clinical trial setting, these are important to determine the benefit of completed or on-going therapies. They also enable the doctor and patient together to decide whether or not to continue with more chemotherapy and this makes it easier to stop if there is clearly no longer benefit. However there are some patients whose individual tumour response is poor, e.g. 30–50 per cent reduction in tumour size, yet they may still have some symptomatic benefit. It may also be true that the psychological benefit of receiving some form of treatment may positively affect quality of life; nevertheless this would not justify the use of chemotherapy to provide an expensive and potentially dangerous placebo effect.

Where research does demonstrate measurable benefit, there is continuing responsibility among oncologists to ensure that these can be demonstrated in the wider population, which may include the elderly and others who may have been too frail to include in the original trials.

New, unproven cancer treatments are first evaluated among patients with advanced or recurrent disease, as these individuals may have no other useful option to be offered. Many would have received standard available therapies in the past, so the chances of a useful response to an experimental therapy may be very small. Their willingness to participate underlines the importance, for some patients, to continue with something at all costs. For others there is undoubtedly altruism in wishing to contribute to advances for the sake of future patients and this may give some meaning to their own difficult experience.

When not to treat

Many situations encountered in oncology are grey areas where what might be appropriate treatment for one patient is not for another. It is important that patients are enabled to accept 'no treatment' when no benefit is likely. The most obvious of these is the person who is symptom-free despite evidence of extensive disease: it is difficult to make this person feel any better with active treatment. For many types of solid tumours, systemic treatment when the situation is no longer curable will have minimal impact on survival and may reduce quality of life at a time when they are still able to enjoy it.

The other consideration is whether or not the individual is likely to survive long enough to gain benefit: it is rarely justifiable to embark on surgery, radiotherapy or chemotherapy in the last days of life. It is however important not to deny patients active treatment of symptoms because they are thought to have a short prognosis. A single radiotherapy treatment to a painful bone metastasis is reasonable in someone who is expected to live 4–6 weeks or more, but not if this entails a lengthy and difficult journey to a distant radiotherapy centre.

It is seen therefore that 'when not to treat' with specific anti-tumour therapy is a decision which has to be individualised for any patient and the circumstances in which they are to be managed. Increasingly, cost effectiveness is encroaching on healthcare decisions. There must therefore be clear evidence that benefit may accrue from a given treatment but equally it is important that patients should not be denied treatment simply because there is no expectation of cure. It should also be emphasised that active symptom management and care will continue despite a decision not to continue with surgery, radiotherapy or chemotherapy.

Table 1.1 outlines common clinical areas where active treatment is available but where it may not always be appropriate to offer this.

Table 1.1 Considerations in selection of patients for oncological treatments

	Indications for treatment	**Contraindications**
Liver metastases	Chemocurable tumour, e.g. lymphoma, germ cell tumour Hormone sensitive, e.g. breast, prostate	Asymptomatic in incurable tumours, e.g. non-small cell lung cancer NSCLC, bladder
Painful hepatomegaly	Consider RT or chemotherapy for sensitive tumours, e.g. small cell lung cancer SCLC, breast, colorectal, bladder	
Brain metastases	Good performance status Limited disease outside central nervous system (CNS)	Major neurological damage Progression outside CNS
Lung metastases	Chemocurable or hormone sensitive tumour as above	Asymptomatic disease in incurable tumour
Small bowel obstruction	Non-malignant causes	Multi-level obstruction Disseminated disease
Spinal cord compression	Good performance status Early diagnosis	Established complete paraplegia
Haemorrhage	Almost all cases, e.g. haematuria, haemoptysis rectal or vaginal bleeding	Minor bleeding in final days of life

The evolving relationship between oncology and palliative care

At the start of the 20th century, the embryonic cancer services established cancer pavilions for incurables and these were the foundations for some of the first cancer specialist centres. Although it was possible to cure some patients with surgery and the new radium treatment, there were few second line options when these had failed. Support, symptom control and terminal care were always part of the role of the oncologist and remain so. The endeavours directed to improve cancer cure rates have also brought benefits to those who will ultimately die from their malignancy, in terms of better and longer control of the disease and significant increases in survival for many.

As a consequence of this progress and the increasing range of potentially useful treatments even for incurable disease, there are an increasing number of patients who continue with some form of active treatment and often chemotherapy into a late stage of their illness. The point of transition into the pre-terminal phase is harder to define – and possibly harder for patients to accept. There is a real concern that palliative care is considered only when treatment stops: kept, like morphine, for the end. While this is a disadvantage experienced by some, we are also seeing the opposite: through effective collaboration and integration between oncology and palliative care specialists, there are more referrals made at an earlier point in the cancer journey. This has implications for services, as patients are admitted to hospices in between courses of chemotherapy for respite or management of difficult symptoms. The patients and families who accept hospice care have not necessarily let go of the fight against the cancer and may have high expectations for interventions in the event of deterioration. It is essential that palliative care professionals have a good knowledge of oncology and are able to identify both cancer and treatment related problems.

In a hospital setting there is merging of supportive and palliative care. Palliative care teams may become involved because of distressing problems from diagnosis onwards. They may continue to support a patient who is thought to be cured of the cancer, but who struggles with difficult sequelae of the disease and the treatment itself. While contributing to the co-ordination of services including access to those provided by hospice and community teams, there is a specialist clinical role in palliative care for those patients and families who present extremely difficult and complex problems to oncology and primary care teams.

Chapter 2

Cancer biology

The malignant cell differs from the normal tissue by a number of fundamental properties which results in proliferation, invasion and metastasis. This behaviour results from changes in the genetic material of the cell – the genes – and indeed cancer can be considered a genetic disease. Oncogenes are sequences of DNA which because of a change in its structure resulting in amplification of its protein production are causally related to the development and maintenance of malignant growth (the 'malignant phenotype'); over 200 such genes have been identified.

The causes of cancer are often unknown for an individual patient although a number of aetiological factors have been identified. This chapter will seek to explore these issues to give a background for the reader to understand the processes by which a malignant growth can cause symptoms from both the local and metastatic sites, ultimately leading to death.

Malignancy arises from changes in cell regulation and tissue growth. In order to understand the process it is important to have a background in the normal mechanisms by which growth is controlled in human tissues. There is a complex system of control pathways which ensures that cell replacement occurs at an appropriate rate to maintain and where necessary repair the complement of cells in normal tissue, without the production of an excess or disorder to the normal balance between cells of different types within a given tissue. This is the result of the interplay between growth stimulant and suppressor function within the cell. A number of specific growth factors have been identified together with growth suppression mechanisms which function within the normal cell. The normal tissue homeostasis is then a balance between growth stimulation and suppression. Malignant transformation is a reflection of an excess in growth factors or failure in the tumour suppression mechanisms with loss of the normal control which keeps tissues in balance. An overview of this process is shown in Fig. 2.1.

There are a large number of identified chemicals which act as growth factors within the cell. One of the more important factors involved in epithelial cell control from which many cancers can arise is epidermal growth factor (EGF). Others include transforming growth factor (TGF), of which there are two forms, alpha, a stimulating factor and beta an inhibiting factor, and fibroblast growth factor (FGF). Other growth factors may be important in stimulating the development of tumour vasculature of which vascular endothelium growth factor (VEGF) and angiopoietin are the best categorized. Each growth factor acts on the cell by binding at a specific receptor on the cell surface.

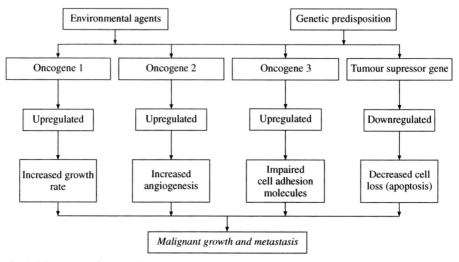

Fig. 2.1 Overview of the malignant process.

Growth factor receptors are protein tyrosine kinases. Abnormalities of growth factor function may arise because of excess production of the growth factor due to upregulation of the gene which controls it or due to changes in the receptor on the cell surface.

Cell loss occurs by necrosis or apoptosis. Necrosis arises because of inadequate nutrition for the cell. This is probably less important in the development of malignancy than apoptosis which is the normal cellular control mechanism by which cells undergo programmed death once they have fulfilled their function within the tissue. There is a complex control mechanism for apoptosis. One of the more important families of proteins which have been identified for this is the Bcl-2 group which are products of the Bcl-2 gene. Mutations in Bcl-2 are found in certain malignant phenotypes. The other important component of apoptosis control is the P53 protein which has been termed the 'molecular policeman' of the cell. This system identifies damaged DNA and enables its repair. Cells which have abnormal P53 function because of mutations in the gene have defective DNA repair and this allows them to accumulate genetic mutations making them more prone to malignant transformation. Aberrant P53 is a well-recognized observation in many malignancies.

It can be seen therefore that changes in growth factor function and the control of apoptosis are fundamental to allowing cellular overgrowth which is the first change towards the malignant characteristics of a cancer or similar type of tumour such as a sarcoma or lymphoma.

The other property of malignancy other than excessive growth is its capacity to invade other tissues and disseminate (metastasize). Invasion is distinct from the changes seen with a benign tumour resulting from local pressure as the mass of cells pushes upon adjacent structures. It implies infiltration of surrounding normal tissue by destruction of the architecture of that tissue and migration of cells within the host cellular framework. Certain products of the malignant cell are important in allowing this to occur, in particular enzymes which break down surrounding connective tissue including collagenases and plasminogen activators. Migration is facilitated by tumour cells being less cohesive than normal cells and this is probably a feature of their deficiency in their cell adhesion molecules (CAMs). These CAMs include the integrins, cadherins and immunoglobin superfamily. Deficiency in CAMs enables the malignant cell to become more mobile, breaking down the connective tissue barriers before it using collagenases to infiltrate the surrounding tissue. They often then follow specific tissue planes for example between muscle bundles or along the connective tissue of nerves resulting in the common observation of perineural invasion.

More sinister than local invasion is the development of metastases which reflects a further step in the infiltration of the tumour cell beyond its site of origin. This results from entry of the cell into the circulation, both lymphatic and vascular, and within the circulation tumour emboli are carried to distance sites where they establish new colonies ultimately presenting clinically as metastatic disease. The process is in fact highly complex requiring the cell to survive a number of hurdles and only a very small proportion of cells entering the circulation are finally established in a distant colony. This is shown in Fig. 2.2.

Key points

- Cancer is essentially a genetic disorder due to a combination of upregulated genes controlling growth rate (oncogenes) and downregulated 'tumour suppressor genes.'
- Upregulation of other genes involved in vasculature growth and reduced cell adhesion properties are also important in enabling the malignant cell to emerge.

Aetiology of cancer

The progressive change from a normal cell to one which is proliferating excessively and thence to a cell which has the properties of invasion and metastases are a result of multiple changes in the cellular DNA with loss of tumour suppression genes and upregulation of growth factor activity, changes in growth factor receptors, upregulation of collagenases and a reduction in cellular adhesion molecules.

Multistage carcinogenesis

The transformation from a normal cell to a malignant cell is not a single event but represents a progressive series of changes; this has been most clearly characterized in

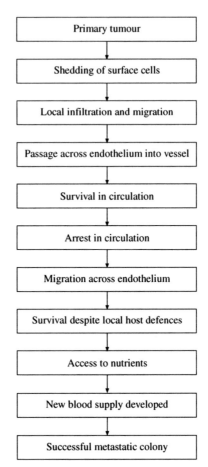

Fig. 2.2 Steps in the process of metastasis.

colorectal cancer where a clear development from normal mucosa to adenoma to dysplasia and ultimately frank malignancy has been elucidated with defined chromosomal events at each stage. This is depicted in Fig. 2.3.

Three distinct stages can be identified in the pathway from benign to malignant: initiation, promotion and progression.

- Initiation occurs when there is damage to DNA which results in mutations in critical genes, enabling the cell to embark on the path towards promotion.
- Promotion occurs as the mutated cells from the initiation process undergo replication with a single cell developing into a potentially malignant clone of cells. This is considered a reversible process if the stimulus to promotion is withdrawn, for example the patient with premalignant dysplastic changes in the epithelium of the aerodigestive tract who stops smoking.
- Progression describes the subsequent irreversible development of an aggressive malignant tumour as additional changes to the genome are accumulated.

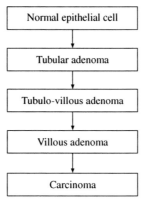

Fig. 2.3 Steps in carcinogenesis in colonic mucosa.

This explains why there is rarely a single cause or event which can be identified to account for malignancy in a given patient, although a wide range of predisposing factors and environmental factors have been identified. These are broadly classified into three main groups: physical, chemical and viral. Environmental factors interact with genetic predisposing features to result ultimately in a malignant phenotype; this may take many years to evolve and indeed the incidence of cancer clearly rises with age, being a relatively rare disease before middle age. Childhood cancer often has a genetic or developmental basis.

Genetic predisposition to cancer

The vast majority of cancer arises as sporadic cases, that is there is no clear pattern of inheritance to account for them. There are however certain rare inherited genes which are recognized to be associated with a high incidence of cancer in patients carrying that abnormality. Examples are shown in Table 2.1.

Environmental factors

Physical factors

Ionizing radiation is an important cause of genetic damage. This is exploited in the use of radiation and for cancer therapy (see Chapter 5). It is however also recognized that genetic damage from ionising radiation results in a higher incidence of malignancy in those individuals who have been exposed. Examples of this include survivors from areas adjacent to the atomic bomb explosions in Japan and individuals exposed to excess diagnostic radiation or inappropriate therapy radiation; examples include the practice of foot radiography to measure shoe size at the beginning of the century and the use of radiation as therapy for scalp ringworm and physiological goitre in the

Table 2.1 Examples of inherited genes and associated familial cancers

Gene	Cancer
BRCA1	Breast, ovary, colon, prostate
BRCA2	Breast, ovary, prostate, pancreas
APC	Familial polyposis coli leading to colorectal cancer
RB1	Retinoblastoma
TP53	LiFraumeni (sarcomas, brain tumours, leukaemia, adrenocortical tumours and breast cancer at young age)
WT1	Wilms tumour
hMLH1 hMLH2	Lynch types 1 & 2 (colon [type 1], other sites also [type 2])
MEN1	Multiple endocrine neoplasia type 1 (parathyroid, pancreas, pituitary)
MEN2	Multiple endocrine neoplasia type 2 (medullary carcinoma of thyroid, phaeochromocytoma)

same era. Other examples are related to occupational exposure, for example, nickel miners exposed to cobalt irradiation and luminous dial painters.

Sun exposure is also important as evidenced by high instance of skin cancers in the skin of those who are exposed to excess hot sun for example white migrants to South Africa and Australia and agricultural workers in particular. There is a clear association between malignant melanoma and sun exposure particularly sunburn in childhood.

Chemical factors

A host of chemicals which can damage the genes predisposing to malignant change have been identified most of which are related to occupational exposure. Historical examples include exposure to cyclic hydrocarbons in soot and oil on the skin of chimney sweeps, mule spinners in the mills of the 19th century. Asbestos inhalation is a further well-recognized carcinogen resulting in malignant mesothelioma. Less common examples include bladder cancer after exposure to aniline dyes and benzpyrene substances found in the cable and rubber industry.

In modern times chemical carcinogenesis from cigarette smoking is undoubtedly the greatest cause of premature death from cancer in both the industrialized and the developing world.

Viral factors

Viral infection is a rare cause of cancer but has been identified in a number of specific examples. These include hepatitis B associated with primary liver cancer, and Epstein Barr virus (EBV) associated with primary hepatocellular cancer and Burkett's lymphoma. Human papilloma virus (HPV) types 16 and 18 have a strong association with carcinoma of the cervix and other primary tumours in the perineal area for example vulval, vaginal and anal cancers.

HIV infection is of increasing importance. There is high instance of malignancy associated with this condition related to the effects on the immune system rather than primary infection by the HIV virus. Herpesvirus has been implicated in HIV patients as the cause of Kaposi's sarcoma amongst other problems. An associated virus and of the same family as HIV, HTLV-I, is a cause of a rare type of lymphoma found in Japan and the Caribbean.

Key points

- Cancer is multifactorial in its causation and in most patients no specific cause or event can be defined.
- Many years of exposure is required to environmental carcinogens, solid tumours typically arising at least 10 years from known exposure.
- Tobacco smoking remains the single biggest cause of cancer world-wide.

Natural history of malignant disease

Malignant cells can vary enormously in their behaviour, some tending to grow and invade locally until a late stage in their life cycle whilst others metastasize at an early stage and can be expected to have micrometastatic disease at the time of presentation with a relatively early primary tumour. Tumours grow at different rates, the clinical volume doubling time reflecting both the rate of cell division and the rate of cell loss. The potential tumour doubling time of a tumour is a measure of its intrinsic rate of cell division and for most common epithelial tumours is only a few days. Clinically however most tumours do not double in size every few days and this is because of a significant cell loss factor for solid tumours; the average clinical tumour volume doubling time is typically between 30 and 90 days being longer for adenocarcinomas and shorter for squamous and undifferentiated cancers.

Exponential growth

Malignant cell colonies grow by exponential growth, that is by a doubling in cell numbers at each division. This can be plotted in an experimental model as shown in Fig. 2.4. This shows that for a single cell to reach the point of being a detectable tumour mass of 1 gm measuring 1 cm^3 around 30 tumour doublings are required; for that tumour to grow to a lethal size beyond this then less than 10 further doubling will be needed. This demonstrates that the clinical phase of a tumour is a relatively small proportion of its natural history, starting with a population of around 10^9 cells and also explains the observation many patients find of concern that as a tumour mass enlarges and doubles

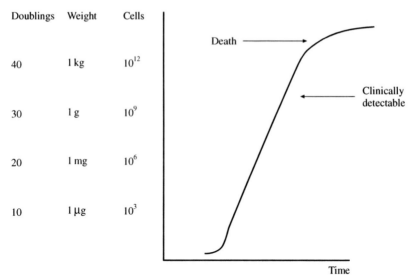

Fig. 2.4 Exponential growth.

in size each time there is an apparent acceleration in growth rate which in fact simply reflects a doubling of a greater number of cells each time rather than an increase in the rate of growth.

Patterns of spread

Traditionally four pathways of tumour spread have been described:

- Local infiltration, with direct migration of malignant cells within adjacent tissues.
- Lymphatic spread occurring in a stepwise fashion to regional draining nodes initially and thence along lymphatic pathways to result in a more widespread lymphadenopathy.
- Vascular spread into venous drainage pathways. Tumours draining into the portal venous system, i.e. those of stomach, bowel and pancreas will spread directly to the liver, others will enter the systemic venous drainage passing to the right side of the heart and thence to the lungs as their first port of call.
  In practice venous spread can involve any organ or tissue in the body, the most common sites being lung, liver, bone and brain. Arterial spread is rarely if ever seen, although direct invasion into an arteriole or artery can result in major haemorrhage.
- Transcoelomic spread, referring to the migration of cells across a body cavity, most commonly seen in transperitoneal seeding from cancers of the stomach and ovary.

Tumours of different sites and histologies are recognized to have a propensity for different patterns of spread often with no apparent mechanism to explain this. Examples include the following:

- Prostate cancer typically spreads via the vertebral venous plexus to bones of the axial skeleton, but rarely involves liver, lung or brain.
- Cervical cancer spreads initially to regional pelvic lymph nodes and only later involves blood-borne sites, typically the lungs.
- Colorectal cancer spreads to regional lymph nodes and the liver.
- Ovary cancer spreads diffusely across the abdominal cavity with multiple peritoneal seedlings, involvement of distant sites occurring rarely and late in the disease.
- Soft tissue sarcomas rarely spread to lymph nodes (with the exception of synovial sarcomas); blood-borne spread to the lungs is the most common pattern seen.

It can be seen then that a knowledge of the natural history of a particular tumour can have important implications for the diagnosis of symptoms and management in the advanced stages of disease. For example a patient with prostate cancer presenting with back pain and confusion is likely to have bone metastases and perhaps associated hypercalcaemia, whilst a patient with cervical cancer presenting with the same symptoms is more likely to have enlarging para-aortic lymph nodes, obstructive hydronephrosis and renal failure.

Key points

- Tumours grow by exponential growth (i.e. doubling) from the initial transformed cell.
- There is a long preclinical phase of growth; the typical tumour will only be detectable as a 1 cm lump after 30 tumour doublings.
- Tumours spread often early in their growth during the preclinical phase.
- Spread is by direct infiltration, lymphatic or blood-borne dissemination or transcoelomic spread.
- Typical patterns of metastases are recognized with different primary sites of origin.

Chapter 3

Epidemiology and cancer trials

The management of any disease is based upon the results of clinical experience in evaluating different interventions and therapies reflected against what is known about the distribution of the disease in a community. The pattern of cancer incidence in the United Kingdom for males and females is shown in Fig. 3.1. There are several different study designs which have varying levels of reliability. This chapter seeks to outline what is known about cancer in a population, the ways in which clinical information is obtained and the levels of certainty with which it can be interpreted. It is important to emphasize that even in palliative medicine where the end-point may not be survival but symptom control it is vital that assessment is based upon sound scientific method which will mean the evaluation of different management options through clinical trials.

Descriptive data

The distribution of cancer within a population can be measured by both its incidence and its prevalence.

Incidence refers to the number of new cases registered in a defined population within a fixed period of time. The usual measure of incidence is cases per 100 000 per year.

Prevalence refers to the number of cases present in a defined population at a single time point. The relation between incidence and prevalence will depend upon the natural history of the cancer; if it has a short rapidly fatal course (e.g. inoperable lung cancer), then prevalence and incidence will be close and prevalence may even be less than the yearly incidence, in contrast for a cancer with a long natural history and low mortality (e.g. low grade lymphoma), then the prevalence may be considerably greater than the incidence.

Human cancer epidemiology

Throughout the developed world large databanks of cancer incidence and distribution are now available through systematic collection of cancer registrations and deaths. There is now an International Classification of Diseases for Oncology so that common codings for the same tumour type and site of origin can be used and data across the world, therefore, compared to review variations in incidence and trends. The situation in an individual country may not reflect world-wide cancer distribution. For example,

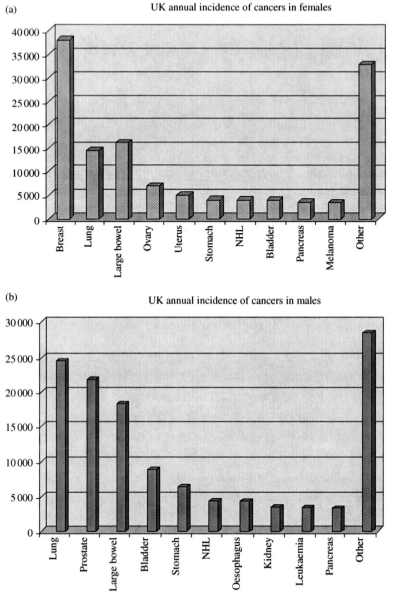

Fig. 3.1 Pattern of cancer incidence in the UK for males and females. (a) UK annual incidence of cancers in females (b) UK annual incidence of cancers in males.

until 1980 stomach cancer was probably the most common cancer world-wide but has always been a relatively rare cancer in the United Kingdom and Western Europe. Stomach cancer incidence is in fact now falling throughout the world and lung cancer is probably the most common cancer world-wide, reflecting the extent of cigarette smoking and other industrial pollution. It is rising particularly in young women born since 1945. It is predicted that because of patterns of smoking habit, this will continue to increase until those born in the 1960s reach middle age as these are the first cohort in which a decline in smoking in developed countries has been observed. In many other parts of the world, however, this is unlikely to occur and a progressive increase in lung cancer for both sexes can be predicted.

Other cancer sites which are increasing in incidence include cancer of the prostate, melanoma of the skin, and non-Hodgkin's lymphoma. Changing patterns of cancer incidence may be related to changes in exposure to aetiological factors, changes in population distribution and migration, and changes in the age and sex distribution within a population. Rarely has medical intervention been shown to influence cancer incidence or mortality with possibly the exception of screening for breast cancer and cervical cancer. The influence of individual factors upon the incidence of various cancers is illustrated in the following.

Age

In general, incidence rates for epithelial cancers increase with age and it is this simple fact which accounts for much of the increasing incidence of cancer seen in the developing world where life expectancy continues to be prolonged. In the European community it is estimated that within the next 20 years the number of cancer registrations will have increased by 15 per cent simply because of the increase in those over the age of 75 years within the population. Because of the major impact which age has upon cancer incidence when comparing cancer mortality for different populations it is important to use age matched or standardized incidence rates.

Sex

With the obvious exception of cancers of the breast, ovary, uterus, testis, and prostate, cancer incidence is generally higher for common epithelial cancers in males than females. No satisfactory explanation for this observation has been forwarded but it is a further important factor when comparing incidence rates.

Exposure to aetiological factors

Mention has already been made of the impact of industrialization and tobacco smoking. Diet is also thought to be important in cancers of the gastrointestinal tract, in particular stomach and colorectal cancer. Very high incidence rates of stomach cancer are seen in Japan and the Far East with a low incidence of colorectal cancer. The opposite is found in Western Europe and the United States. The impact of aetiological factors has been shown by migration studies in which Japanese migrating to the United States are found to lose their risks of their native cancer (e.g. stomach and oesophagus), and acquire those of their country of adoption (e.g. colorectal cancer over two or three generations).

Infective agents may rarely be important and changes in the distribution of infectious diseases may account for changes in incidence. The most striking examples of this are hepatitis B related to hepatocellular carcinoma and HIV related in particular to Kaposi's sarcoma and non-Hodgkin's lymphoma.

Geography and ethnic origin

Whilst in many cases geographical variations can be explained by exposure to aetiological factors it appears that there are clear predilections to certain cancer types in certain racial groups. For example, there is a very much higher incidence of prostatic carcinoma in black Americans than in white Americans. Similarly, malignant melanoma whilst not unknown in coloured races is considerably rarer than in the white races.

The overall trend is for increased levels of cancer incidence throughout the world which reflect a combination of factors including the effects of prolonged survival, the impact of cigarette smoking and other industrial carcinogens, altered lifestyle (e.g. exposure to excess sun), and increasing success at controlling other causes of premature death in particular the infectious diseases. Currently one in three of the population of the developed world can expect to develop a malignant tumour within their lifetime.

Key points: epidemiology

- World-wide lung cancer is the commonest cause of death from cancer.
- There is an increasing incidence in prostate cancer, skin cancers and lymphoma whilst stomach cancer is in decline.
- Cancer incidence is related to age, sex and geographic factors in addition to specific exposure to known carcinogens.

Staging systems

In addition to standardized response criteria it is important that populations can be compared and in particular that the extent of tumour can be compared so that equivalent populations in terms of their tumour burden are evaluated. A common system is vital to avoid misinterpretation of results. For example, if patients in one centre are considered to have stage 2 disease but in another centre this is designated stage 3, then the second centre may claim outstanding results for stage 3 patients which the first centre cannot hope to achieve except in stage 2 patients. For this reason standardized staging systems have evolved the most common of which is the TNM system. This has three parameters as follows.

T stage refers to the extent of the primary tumour. There are usually three or four categories (T1, T2, T3, T4) which follow the format of increasing tumour size from T1 to T3 and extension of the tumour to surrounding local areas for T4.

N stage refers to the regional lymph node status. Typically this extends from N0 to N3 in which N0 refers to the absence of regional lymph nodes, N1 will include mobile first station nodes, and N2 and N3 refer to progressive degrees of both regional involvement, increasing node size and in the N3 category fixation to under-lying structures.

M stage refers to the presence or absence of metastases and is typically denoted by M0 when metastases are absent and M1 when distant metastases are present.

Whilst the TNM staging system is applicable to most epithelial cancer sites there are exceptions. These include the following.

FIGO staging for gynaecological cancer which for each site defines stage 1 through to stage 4. Again this tends to follow a general format with stage 1 reflecting disease local-ized to the organ of origin through to stage 4 where there is involvement of other organs typically bladder and rectum from the cervix or uterus or more distant organs from the ovary.

Ann Arbour staging for lymphoma including Hodgkin's disease which relates disease extent according to distribution of lymphadenopathy. Again, four stages are defined from stage 1 with a single lymph node group involved to stage 2 with multiple groups on one side of the diaphragm involved, stage 3 where nodal disease is present on both sides of the diaphragm, and stage 4 where extranodal organs including bone marrow are involved.

In some sites surgical staging systems are referred to which usually comprise stage 1 and stage 2 reflecting early or more advanced but still operable disease and stage 3 and stage 4 with locally advanced inoperable disease or distant metatases respectively.

Outcome measures

The common end-points in cancer trials are shown in Table 3.1.

Table 3.1 End-points in cancer trials

Survival	Time to death
Overall	Time to death from any cause
Corrected	Excluding deaths from causes other than that being studied, e.g. cancer
Response	Reduction in size of measurable tumour or change in symptom
Complete response	Complete disappearance of tumour or symptom
Partial response	50 per cent reduction in measured parameter
Overall response	Complete + partial responses
Quality of life	Change in objective scores measured by validated quality of life tool, e.g. EORTC QLQC-30 or FACT
Cost effectiveness	Economic consequences of results seen, e.g. cost per year of life gained

Survival data

Survival may be measured in a number of different parameters the common ones being as follows.

Overall survival measures time from enrolment in the period of observation to the time of death. The time at which the observation period starts may vary and should be defined. For example, it may be date of registration, date of diagnosis, date of surgery, or date of randomization. Survival data may be refined measuring only deaths from a specific cause (e.g. lung cancer, when it is termed a *corrected survival*).

Mortality ratios may be used as an alternative way of describing survival. These relate the observed survival in a study group to that of a matched control group. The common measure used is a *standardized mortality ratio (SMR)* which compares the survival in the study group with that of an age and sex matched sample from the general population.

Actual survival measures the period of survival from enrolment to the time of death. It can only be quoted when all the patients within the study group have been observed for the duration at which survival is to be quoted or have died in the meantime. In other words, an actual 5-year survival figure can only be quoted when all patients have either survived for 5 years or died before then.

Actuarial survival is a more accurate measure of survival than actual survival and measures the probability of surviving for each patient within a study group at any time during the period of observation. It is more efficient, in that it allows measures to be made without all the patients having completed the time of assessment, each point on the survival curve being calculated on the basis of all the patients evaluable at that time. This means that data points in the earlier part of the curve are usually based upon more patients being at risk and are therefore statistically more reliable than the tail of the curve where fewer patients may be evaluable. This method gives a better overall picture of survival in a population and is generally that quoted in the results of clinical trials. An example is shown in Fig. 3.2.

Disease-free survival or recurrence-free survival is the time taken from the patient being enrolled in the study to relapse presented as a survival curve. This may be qualified by disease in a specific site so that, for example, in breast cancer where local relapse may be an important end-point this may be recorded as *local disease-free survival*. In general, overall survival will be longer than disease-free survival unless relapse equates with rapid death. Again, this is usually measured by an actuarial survival rate being the most accurate means of analysing the data, as illustrated in Fig. 3.2.

Response data

When the results of treatment are compared with different studies it is important that standardized criteria for response are used. There is now a well-established convention

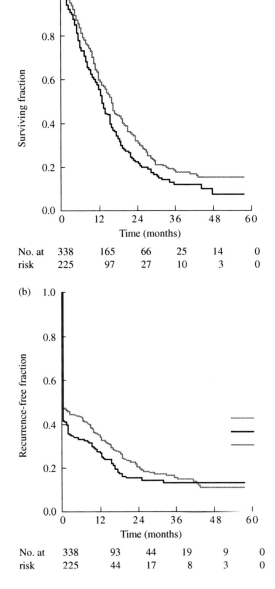

Fig. 3.2 Actuarial survival curves for (a) overall survival and (b) recurrence-free survival for the same cohort of patients with head and neck cancer comparing two forms of radical treatment. Note that each step on the curve represents an event, either death (a) or recurrence (b) and along the bottom of the curve is the number of patients at risk of an event. The greater the number at risk, the greater the reliability of the data at that point on the curve. The y-axis is presented as a probability. This is sometimes better understood as a percentage obtained by multiplying the probability by 100, (e.g. a probability of 0.5 is equivalent to 50 per cent).

to describe the effect of a treatment on a tumour mass. It depends upon a tumour being measurable either clinically or more usually on scan or X-ray.

Complete response is total disappearance of a tumour mass with no new tumour masses developing within a one-month observation period.

Partial response is a reduction in a tumour mass by 50 per cent in at least one dimension, usually the maximum dimension, which is maintained for at least one month after treatment without progression at other sites.

Stable disease is defined when there is no progression of the index tumour mass and when there are no changes at other sites. Within this group, often falls those tumours which have less than 50 per cent regression with treatment, although these are occasionally regrouped into a separate heading of *minimal response.*

Measured response data such as this is essential in the formal evaluation of individual treatment interventions, however there is uncertainty as to how such objective response data can be related to palliation of advanced disease. It is unknown, for example, how much tumour shrinkage is required to improve an individual symptom and how such focussed intervention actually impacts upon the quality of life of patients.

Quality of life assessment

A number of quality of life measures are now available. In many therapeutic trials a simple measure of performance status will be included. Common scales used are either the Karnofsky scale ranging from zero (dead) to 100 (normal) or the simpler 5-point World Health Organization (WHO) performance scale ranging from zero (normal) to 4 (severely disabled), as shown in Table 3.2. More detailed quality of life data can be obtained by formal standardized questionnaires. Perhaps the most widely used of these in Europe is the EORTC QLQ C30 standard questionnaire based on a series of questions relating the effect of the disease or its intervention to everyday activities. This questionnaire has been widely validated in clinical trials including those evaluating palliative treatments. The drawback of such questionnaire-type assessments is the large amount of data collected and the difficulty in succinctly presenting the findings from a large study population.

Key points: assessment of malignant disease

- Amount of disease can be measured by number of cases occurring in a fixed time (incidence) or number of cases at a given time (prevalence).
- Survival data may be presented as a ratio compared to 'standardized' population or a calculated survival rate.
- Extent of a tumour is described by its stage typically combining measurement of primary (T), nodes (N) and metastases (M) to give a TNM stage.
- Performance status describes the activity an individual is capable of in a formal grading system.
- Response to treatment can be measured as formal reduction in measured amount of tumour (compete, partial, minimal, stable) or impact on quality of life.
- Health economic assessments of a new intervention are also important.

Table 3.2 Performance status measures

WHO performance status scale	Karnofsky score equivalent
0 Normal activities	100
1 Restricted but ambulatory; able to carry out light work	70–80
2 Self-caring, ambulatory; up and about >50 per cent of day	60–70
3 Limited self-care; confined to bed or chair >50 per cent of day	40–50
4 Completely disabled; no self-care totally confined to bed or chair	20–30

Sources of data and clinical trials

The above definitions result from the need to document carefully the results of treatment in defined groups of patients. Only if this is carried out with meticulous attention to detail can valid measures of outcome be obtained and reliable predictions of treatment efficacy derived. This is, however, only of use if appropriate comparisons and well-designed studies are carried out. A variety of clinical studies can be performed with a range of reliability in their final results. These are outlined below.

Case reports based on single or small groups of patients often carry undue influence in the minds of practitioners. Their validity however is limited and extends only as far as that individual case. They should be regarded as pointers for more detailed systematic study rather than criteria for change in practice.

Historical series are to be found widely in the medical literature. They usually consist of a single centre's results from a particular treatment over a period of several years. Provided adequate information regarding the make-up of the patient population in terms of age, sex, tumour stage, and any other variables which may influence prognosis are included then they may give a guide to the efficacy of a particular treatment type, but cannot be used to compare that treatment with another from a different series without introducing the possibility of bias. Furthermore many of these series reflect collection of data retrospectively, that is by returning to the patient records long after the treatment has been delivered and attempting to extract the result which may not always be accurately documented. Such studies therefore do have major limitations and undue reliance should not be placed on the results.

Historical comparisons are when the results of treatment A during a particular period are compared with the results of treatment B in a subsequent period. Because the patients do not come from the same group but from a sequential group and because many other factors may have changed over that treatment period direct comparison between the groups is hazardous and should not be performed without careful qualification that any results require further confirmation.

Case control studies attempt to overcome the difficulty of historical comparisons. They allow comparison of treatment A with treatment B in successive cohorts of patients using a control group which is carefully matched to that of the new treatment group for all known parameters that may influence outcome, in particular, age, sex, tumour stage, performance status, and any relevant biochemical factors. They still carry the risk of including other confounding variables in particular changes in supportive care between the two periods.

Randomized control trials represent the gold standard for comparing two different treatments. Bias between different populations is excluded by taking a single group of patients and randomly allocating them to receive either one treatment or the other in a direct comparison. Bias may be eliminated further by the patient being 'blind', in other words not being aware which treatment they are receiving and in some instances both the investigator and patient are blind, a so-called double blind trial. Whilst this is eminently suitable for drug studies in which dummy tablets (placebos) can be given it is more difficult with other interventions or where obvious side effects may distinguish the treatments as is often the case in cancer therapy.

Within a randomized control trial there may be stratification which means that different groups are identified at the outset as potentially those with a different prognosis. This may be related to age or tumour stage. Within each group there is random allocation of the treatments to be compared. This ensures that there is equal randomization within each stratified group and prevents an imbalance of any important prognostic factors appearing by chance.

Randomized controlled trials require a large amount of organization and often depend upon a central trials office which specializes in running such trials. Because for statistical analysis, large numbers extending at least into several hundreds are often required to pick up the relatively small changes seen in therapeutic intervention these trials are typically multi-centre involving many treatment centres both nationally and internationally.

A data-monitoring committee is often incorporated within the trial design. This is a group of independent observers who are allowed to see interim results and if necessary recommend early closure of a trial where either unexpectedly good results from a new intervention are seen or where untoward side effects are being experienced. This takes out the ethical dilemma of patients being disadvantaged when early results are known but the trial continues. At the same it allows the investigators in the trial to remain unbiased without access to such data.

Meta-analysis is a means of incorporating the results from a series of randomized controlled trials which may seek to answer the same question or a similar question. Perhaps the best example of this is in the adjuvant use of tamoxifen or multi-agent chemotherapy in breast cancer. A large number of individual trials have been performed some of which have shown advantage and others a lesser advantage or none.

A meta-analysis involves taking the individual results from each trial, and ideally using the individual data, combining it into a single large analysis which may contain several thousand; for example the breast cancer overview analysed over 15 000 patients in tamoxifen trials and over 5700 patients in poly-chemotherapy trials. It is a general rule that the larger number of individual comparisons that are made the more statistically reliable the results will be. This does not mean that the difference is magnified but simply that any difference seen is a real difference which can be relied upon in clinical practice to reflect the true response when a patient is treated rather than one which has arisen by statistical chance. Thus in the case of the breast cancer overview a highly statistically significant result in favour of chemotherapy in patients under 50 was seen although the actual improvement in survival at 5 years was only 6.4 per cent.

Key points: sources of data in increasing order of reliability

- ◆ Case reports.
- ◆ Historical series and comparisons.
- ◆ Case control studies.
- ◆ Randomized controlled trials.
- ◆ Meta-analysis.

Health economics

The increasing burden placed upon modern health care systems has resulted in greater prominence being given to assessing treatments not only in terms of their clinical efficacy but also their value for money. In terms of cancer treatments this can lead to irreconcilable comparisons in trying to evaluate complex expensive treatments which may benefit only a few percent of a patient population or prolong life by only a few months. Some developments may have no effect on survival but may reduce side effects or inconvenience to the patient although at a greater financial cost.

Health economic assessments have become increasingly sophisticated in attempting to provide objective information on which policy decisions can be based. The simplest form of study is a cost-effectiveness study which measures the cost of different treatments to achieve a single common outcome; this does not however include any assessment of the value of the outcome and is therefore a relatively crude measure of a clinical situation. Cost utility studies in contrast use a measure of the usefullness of the outcome of treatment incorporating a quality scale such as the QALY (quality adjusted life year) so that different interventions can be compared in terms of a consistent end-point.

Clinical research

The basis of sound clinical practice must be the data acquired through clinical research. This applies equally to the management of advanced and incurable malignancy as it does to the evaluation of exciting new cancer cures. The presence of advanced disease and the inevitable limitation of life expectancy this imposes should never be used as an excuse to avoid participation in clinical research and indeed will be welcomed by many patients invited to take part in this exercise. Whilst not to be used as an inducement to patients there is good evidence that patients taking part in clinical trials of cancer treatment have a better outcome than patients receiving the same treatment out of trial. In the palliative setting, trial participation will often include patients in more intensive networks of support and information resulting in recognized 'non-treatment benefits'. Clinical research may take many forms depending to some extent upon the question being evaluated and the availability of subjects and resources.

In the introduction of new clinical interventions there is a well-established convention which defines the steps to be taken in the formal evaluation. This will be applicable not only to new cancer treatments but also to diagnostic agents and supportive agents with recent examples including new bisphosphonates, erythropoietin and fish oils. This follows the following principles:

Phase I trials in which the new treatment is evaluated in patients with advanced disease for whom there is no established treatment remaining. These trials are primarily aimed at establishing the optimal means of administration and, in the case of a drug, the maximum tolerated doses and toxicity profile in a group of patients with the disease to be studied. Clinical efficacy is not a prerequisite for phase I trials. They may also involve pharmacokinetic analyses with blood profiles taken over several hours or many days to determine drug usage under clinical conditions.

Phase II trials evaluate the new treatment under optimal conditions as defined in the phase I trials with a view to determining the efficacy of the new treatment. This will involve patients with advanced disease who have exhausted conventional established treatments. As a result of phase II trials a response rate can be determined and the likelihood of the treatment becoming a useful modality established.

Phase III trials are the natural progression from a phase II trial when the treatment is compared with standard conventional treatment or where there is none available with a control placebo group. This will ideally be a randomized trial and in the case of a drug trial double blind wherever possible. The results of the randomized phase III trials establish the position of the new treatment alongside current treatments.

Phase IV studies continue the acquisition of information regarding efficacy and more particularly toxicity data with the new treatment in widespread clinical use as defined in the phase III trial.

Many patients with advanced disease will be eligible for both phase I and phase II trials. There is sometimes reluctance to offer further treatment to patients who have exhausted conventional options particularly where this may involve chemotherapy with associated toxicity. It is, however, important to allow patients access to such opportunities provided they are clear about the possible impositions in terms of time and toxicity and without unrealistic expectations being placed upon the likelihood of useful benefit. For many patients it is important for them to feel they can still make a contribution to medical research even if there is no personal gain in the last few months of their life.

There may also be the opportunity for patients to be entered into randomized phase III trials particularly those looking at new analgesic or other symptom-orientated treatment methods. There is sometimes concern regarding the randomization of such patients into studies with a placebo arm where they may then receive no active treatment. It is however important to realize that the fundamental principle of any trial design is that it can only be valid in the absence of scientific evidence that one of the treatments being tested in the trial is better than the other, and that entry into a placebo arm does not preclude all standard treatment being given. Well-designed trials will have escape clauses to allow patients adequate treatment if symptoms persist, despite entry into the trial, and all trials allow patients to withdraw at any time should they feel their treatment is unsatisfactory under the conditions of the trial. Further reassurance is included when there is a data-monitoring committee or a sequential analysis design, which allows premature termination of a trial once a robust statistically significant difference is observed even if this is at an early stage of the trial due to the unexpected success or indeed failure of one of the treatment options.

Despite this it is a sad fact that only a tiny proportion of patients eligible for clinical trials are ever entered into them. The reasons for this remain uncertain but undoubtedly a component of this is a reluctance on the part of the health care professionals involved to take part in clinical trial work, and it may be more pronounced in those working in the palliative arena. It should, however, be clear that advances can only be made on the basis of rigid scientific evaluation and indeed there is evidence that patients entered into clinical trials, in general, fare better than those who would otherwise be eligible but are not entered. It is hoped such considerations will encourage greater clinical trial involvement among those dealing with patients having advanced malignancy whether in the field of new cancer treatment or new methods of symptom control.

Key points: clinical trials

- The randomized controlled phase III trial (RCT) remains the gold standard for evaluating a new therapy.
- Phase I and II trials are a prelude to the RCT to confirm safety and efficacy of a new agent.
- Less rigorous information may be obtained from case reports and historical series; these may be the only way to evaluate different approaches in rare instances where very few patients are ever seen.

Chapter 4

The role of surgical and radiological intervention in palliation

Radical surgery is probably the single most effective treatment in cancer management. Cancer surgery however implies complete removal of the tumour with a surrounding margin of normal tissue including any regional lymph nodes which may be involved with an *en bloc* dissection. This will usually entail a major surgical procedure with removal of a total organ such as laryngectomy or cystectomy and the need for reconstructive surgery as seen after many major head and neck cancer resections. Such procedures are rarely appropriate in the palliative setting but nonetheless surgery can have an important role in dealing with some local symptoms and relatively simple procedures can have dramatic results for the patient.

The principle of palliative cancer surgery is to achieve symptom relief without any expectation of complete tumour resection. In some cases surgery will be performed leaving the tumour in situ, for example intubation of obstructing oesophageal carcinoma or internal fixation of a pathological fracture. In these settings consolidation treatment with radiotherapy may be appropriate to delay tumour growth and aid healing after surgery.

Alongside surgery interventional radiology has acquired an increasing role in the management of local tumour related symptoms. One of the major advantages of this approach is the ability to perform procedures percutaneously without the need for deep anaesthesia or skin incisions. Its chief application is in the relief of obstructive symptoms where passage of a stent through an obstructing tumour can give immediate relief of symptoms. Occasionally it may also be used in the control of intractable haemorrhage by embolization.

The indications for palliative surgery in advanced cancer

Pathological fracture is a situation where, when a long bone is involved, surgery is the treatment of choice. Internal fixation enables rapid recovery in terms of weight bearing and mobility and also early pain relief. In most patients therefore who develop a pathological fracture of a humerus or femur immediate orthopaedic referral and internal fixation is the management of choice with the exception of those patients who may have only a very short prognosis who are not expected to regain mobility by virtue of their underlying disease. There may also be a role for prophylactic internal fixation for 'high risk' lytic lesions which would include those >2.5 cm in diameter involving the cortex with associated pain and any metastasis causing >50 per cent erosion of the cortex.

Dysphagia may arise secondary to oesophageal obstruction by an intrinsic primary oesophageal cancer or an extrinsic tumour mass from an underlying bronchial carcinoma or mediastinal lymph nodes. Surgical dilatation of the oesophagus and insertion of a tube will often provide a rapid and satisfactory means of restoring swallowing and is generally associated with little procedure-related morbidity. Various tubes are currently in use, several of which can now be introduced alongside a fibre-optic endoscope an example of which is shown in Fig. 4.1.

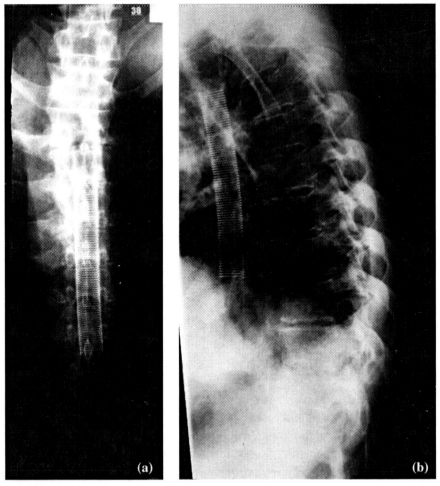

(a) (b)

Fig. 4.1 X-rays demonstrating oesophageal stent *in situ* for an obstructing carcinoma of the oesophagus, passed endoscopically.

There can however be problems associated with the use of such prostheses. They may fail to be retained and pass into the stomach or, if in position for a length of time become invaded by tumour and themselves obstruct. This is sometimes cited as a rationale for post-operative radiotherapy after tube insertion in those patients with a projected survival of several months. Food boluses may also block the tube requiring a further surgical procedure to dislodge them and in general patients rarely return to a normal diet but can manage a semi-solid diet. The management of dysphagia is discussed further in Chapter 11.

Debulking of a proliferative tumour in the oesophagus or at the gastro-oesophageal junction may also be of value using laser or cryosurgery. Laser therapy is also useful in the management of bleeding tumour surfaces.

When normal swallowing is not possible but it is thought appropriate to maintain a high level of nutritional intake a percutaneous gastrostomy (PEG) may be considered. The advantage of a PEG is that it can be inserted relatively simply defining the stomach by the passage of a fibre-optic gastroscope, the light from which can be seen percutaneously, and then inserting through the skin of a self-retaining gastrostomy tube. Initial discomfort and bruising settles within a day or two and feeding through the tube can take place immediately. Complications are few apart from the rare incidence of secondary infection and peritonism when the tube may have to be removed. The major issue surrounding their use lies in selecting appropriate patients; their main role lies in supporting those with advanced head and neck cancer for whom some form of radical treatment may yet be possible. Their place in the management of patients with advanced, progressive and incurable disease is less certain, but in any patient in whom nasogastric hydration or feeding is considered a PEG will often provide a more comfortable and less obtrusive means of reaching the gastrointestinal tract.

Bronchial obstruction may result in distal lung collapse and can be readily treated at bronchoscopy by either cryotherapy or laser therapy to restore the lumen of the bronchus and enable air entry to the distal parts of the lung. Laser therapy can be delivered through a fibre-optic bronchoscope. Cryotherapy may be more widely available being administered through a cryotherapy probe at rigid bronchoscopy. Recurrence after these procedures is not unusual and they may be repeated on several occasions or combined with radiotherapy. When the large airways are involved then tracheal or bronchial stents may be inserted at the time of rigid bronchoscopy which may enable more durable control of airway obstruction in selected patients.

Ureteric obstruction will, if bilateral or in the presence of a non-functioning contralateral kidney, result in renal failure and be ultimately fatal. In some patients this may be part of the natural history of their cancer and intervention inappropriate. In others however restoration of renal drainage will restore kidney function to normal. As a temporary measure percutaneous nephrostomy may be performed and a more permanent solution achieved by the passage of ureteric stents at cystoscopy. Nephrostomies are usually inserted in the radiology department using ultrasound to locate the distended renal pelvis into which a tube is inserted through the skin to drain urine. These may remain in situ for several weeks or even months although they are often prone to being dislodged or falling out during the night whilst the patient moves in their sleep despite elaborate attempts to ensure fixation on the skin surface. Leakage around the entry site is also sometimes a problem and for these reasons a more permanent internal stent is usually chosen with removal of the percutaneous tube at the same time. Ureteric stents should be replaced every six months as they develop encrustation over this time. The management of renal failure and ureteric obstruction is discussed further in Chapter 26.

Haemorrhage may be treated surgically and local cautery, laser or cryotherapy can be of considerable value. Examples include cryotherapy to a carcinoma of the bronchus or transurethral resection of a bleeding bladder or prostatic tumour.

Although used infrequently in the palliative setting, bleeding can also be controlled by embolisation of a bleeding artery. This involves the passage of an intra-arterial catheter, usually introduced percutaneously through the groin, and manipulated to the area of haemorrhage. Particular examples include the renal vessels for bleeding from a renal cell carcinoma or the mesenteric vessels for a bowel tumour. Embolisation is then performed by the injection of a sclerosant or microspheres into the arterial branches responsible. This may also be performed in the liver for primary or metastatic tumours and has been advocated in some instances as a specific means of therapy causing tumour necrosis which may be followed by surgical removal. There are risks in such procedures by affecting the blood flow to normal tissue; a particular concern when it is used for vascular malformations in the nervous system.

Obstructive jaundice may occur due to blockage of the common bile duct by a pancreatic carcinoma or metastatic lymph nodes in this region. Jaundice may be relieved initially by percutaneous drainage directing a catheter into the dilated biliary tree through the skin using ultrasound control. Subsequently more permanent relief of obstruction may be achieved by the passage of an internal stent. For proximal occlusion this may also be percutaneously using ultrasound and X-ray screening to direct the stent to the appropriate area. It is more common in cancer of the head of pancreas or lymphoma for the obstruction to be in the extrahepatic ducts. In these situations a stent is introduced through the ampulla of Vater in the duodenum via a fibre-optic gastroscope; alternatively if there is extensive disease in this region the fashioning of a choledocho-jejunostomy emptying the gall bladder directly into a loop of small bowel will be effective.

Large bowel obstruction may be treated by the fashioning of a colostomy proximal to the obstruction and is usually the only way to overcome this problem when it develops secondary to recurrent colorectal carcinoma.

Small bowel obstruction may present a more difficult surgical problem. If localized then resection may be attempted but in many cases, particularly those secondary to carcinoma of the ovary where it is a common terminal event, there will be multiple levels of obstruction which are not amenable to simple surgical attention. It is often a difficult decision in palliative care to know when it is appropriate to refer a patient with small bowel obstruction for surgery and always an uneasy scenario when a patient with advanced intra-abdominal malignancy is submitted to laparotomy with no benefit ensuing. Equally it is important not to deny those patients with a correctable pathology such as an adhesion or perhaps anastomotic tumour recurrence at a single site appropriate surgical relief of their obstruction. It may be possible radiologically on erect and supine films of the abdomen to diagnose multiple level obstruction and this is the usual case in patients with advanced ovarian cancer. Patients with grossly distended small or large bowel on X-ray, a history of previous abdominal surgery and colorectal primary tumours should be seriously considered for a surgical approach.

Local fungation may be amenable to surgical resection. Perhaps the best example of this is a locally advanced carcinoma of the breast for which a toilet mastectomy may provide the best means of dealing with the chest wall tumour and may be justified even in the presence of metastatic disease if this is causing distress. Extensive reconstructive procedures may be justified where no distant metastases can be demonstrated as the natural history of such tumours may extend for many years. Simple surgical excision can also be the quickest and most satisfactory means of dealing with metastatic skin nodules which become symptomatic unless they are fixed to surrounding structures when radiotherapy may be necessary.

Cerebral metastases are usually multiple and carry a poor prognosis. There is however a small sub-group of patients with solitary cerebral metastases and stable cancer elsewhere who may be best managed with surgical resection of the metastases. Randomized trials have shown that the best survival figures for this group are achieved by craniotomy and surgical removal of the tumour followed by post-operative radiotherapy, although despite this the typical survival in this group of patients will be improved by only a few months with a median of 10–12 months.

Rarely there may be obstructive hydrocephalus due to tumours in the posterior fossa obstructing the fourth ventricle or aqueduct of Sylvius. This may require insertion of a ventriculoperitoneal shunt to drain the dilated lateral ventricles in the cerebrum and relieve headache and associated neurological symptoms. It may be appropriate to consider radiotherapy following this to relieve the obstruction or occasionally an internal shunt may be considered.

Pulmonary metastases are usually associated with advanced disease requiring systemic therapy if treated at all. Again however in a few selected circumstances surgical resection of a limited number of lung metastases may be considered for tumours such as soft tissue and osteosarcoma and renal carcinoma.

Haemoptysis in the setting of multiple pulmonary metastases is always a difficult problem to address unless from a tumour still sensitive to systemic treatment. Local treatment can only be considered if the site of bleeding can be defined which requires a bronchoscopy at which time cryo or laser therapy may be possible. Alternatively if a section of the bronchial tree can be defined then local radiotherapy can be considered.

Pleural effusion causing symptoms of progressive dyspnoea is an indication for pleural aspiration. Frequently however simple aspiration will be followed by recurrent episodes and increasing difficulty in achieving successful drainage. Surgical drainage with thoracoscopy and pleurodesis is a far more effective and permanent solution.

As with any intervention it is important to balance the likely outcome against the potential morbidity of treatment. Inevitably surgery carries greater acute morbidity than many other events in palliative medicine requiring for most procedures a general anaesthetic and each procedure carrying its attendant risk of complications. Despite this, in the examples listed above rapid relief of difficult symptoms may be achieved for the patient who has a prognosis measured in months rather than weeks. In these situations surgery will provide worthwhile symptom-free quality of life.

Key points

- Both surgery and interventional radiology may offer simple but highly effective relief of otherwise troublesome symptoms and should be considered in particular for problems associated with obstruction or haemorrhage.

- Pathological fracture in a long bone should always be considered for surgical fixation.

- Surgical relief of large bowel obstruction will often provide the most satisfactory means of immediate relief; in contrast small bowel obstruction is often not amenable to surgical intervention.

- Surgical resection with post-operative radiotherapy should always be considered for solitary brain metastases.

Chapter 5

Principles of radiotherapy

Radiotherapy refers to treatment with ionizing radiation. Typically this is in the form of X-rays or gamma-rays which on passing through a cell result in ionization and subsequently DNA damage. There are several means of delivering radiation including external X-ray beams and the use of radioisotopes and because radiation is potentially hazardous its use must be carefully controlled within a radiotherapy department able to provide the clinical and physics support for its safe administration. Over 50 per cent of all radiotherapy given in the United Kingdom is with palliative intent. Its major role is in the control of local symptoms in particular pain, haemorrhage, and obstruction.

Types of radiation

Most radiotherapy given in clinical practice today is with high energy X-ray beams produced by a machine called a linear accelerator. Less powerful machines may be used in some circumstances.

Linear accelerators have largely replaced older X-ray and cobalt machines in major centres in Europe and the United States. They are far more sophisticated machines based upon the acceleration of electrons on radio waves to a high energy before focusing them on to a high atomic weight metal target, such as tungsten, as a result of which X-rays are produced; they require intensive maintenance and supervision in their use. Linear accelerators produce X-ray beams ranging from 4 to 25 MV and are highly versatile for the treatment of tumours in most sites of the body, having sufficient penetrating power for the deepest tumours. One characteristic of these high energy beams is that of 'skin sparing' which means that the maximum energy from the radiation beam is deposited not on the skin surface but at a depth below the surface, approximately equivalent to one-quarter of the beam energy in centimetres (e.g. for a 6 MV X-ray beam the maximum will be at 1.5 cm depth). This enables high tumour doses to be delivered without excessive skin reactions developing, in contrast to older techniques using orthovoltage beams.

Despite their technical sophistication it is important to emphasize to the patient that being treated on a linear accelerator differs little from a simple diagnostic X-ray. The patient lies on a treatment couch, is not enclosed, and the machine can rotate around them to achieve the desired angle of beam entry. A modern linear accelerator is shown in Fig. 5.1.

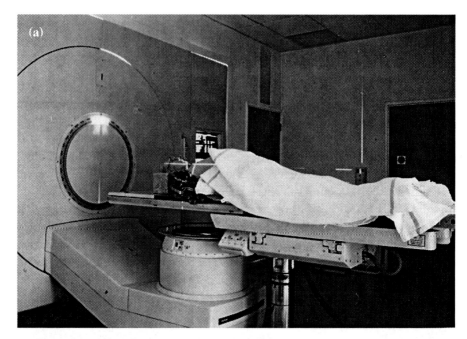

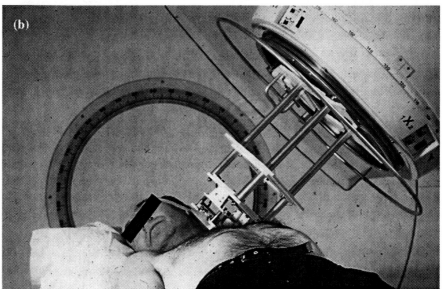

Fig. 5.1 Treatment with a linear accelerator showing (a) patient receiving palliative external beam treatment to the chest and (b) palliative electron treatment to neck nodes.

Electron beams differ from X-rays in having a finite depth of penetration. This depends on the energy of the electron beam and the useful depth of penetration approximates to around one-third of the beam energy. For example a 10 MeV electron beam will penetrate just over 3 cm below the surface of the skin with a very sharp fall in dose beyond this. Electrons are produced in a linear accelerator and many modern linear accelerators can simply switch between producing electrons and X-rays between patients. Low energies of 6–10 MeV are used for treating superficial skin nodules whilst higher energies up to 20 MeV will reach structures 6–7 cm below the surface, which will encompass many lymph node masses as shown in Fig. 5.1. These beams are also of value in treating superficial bones such as the ribs or scapula.

In some departments other sources of external beam therapy may also be available:

Superficial X-rays are produced by X-ray tubes generating energies of up to 150 kilovolts (kV). These X-rays penetrate only 1 cm or so below the surface and are used for treating skin tumours including metastatic skin nodules.

Orthovoltage X-rays are produced by high energy X-ray tubes with energies up to 300 kV. These penetrate 3–4 cm below the surface of the skin and are extremely useful for the treatment of superficial bones such as ribs or the sacrum. One disadvantage of this energy is that the maximum radiation energy is deposited on the skin surface resulting in a marked skin reaction when higher doses are used; this is not a major problem at palliative doses.

Cobalt machines produce gamma-ray beams of 2.5 million volt (megavolt, MV) energy arising from a cobalt source held within the shielded head of the machine. A simple mechanical shutter device opens a collimator in the shielding to allow gamma-rays to escape. These machines have the advantage of mechanical simplicity and require less intensive servicing than the more sophisticated linear accelerators (see below). Their radiation behaves in an identical way to an X-ray beam and penetrates more deeply than superficial or orthovoltage, being able to reach centrally placed tumours in the chest or abdomen. They are, however, less penetrating than the high energy beams produced by a linear accelerator and in order to reach a deep-seated tumour a large surface dose may be necessary to achieve the required central dose.

Key points

- Most patients receiving external beam radiotherapy will be treated on a linear accelerator using 6–15 MV beams.
- Superficial skin and bone lesions may be treated by low energy X-rays or electrons.

Radioisotope therapy

Radioisotopes are naturally occurring substances which decay at a constant rate and release radiation of varying quality. For therapeutic use these may be either:

◆ *gamma rays* such as those produced from the decay of cobalt, caesium, or iridium. These penetrate several centimetres distance from the site of the isotope with the major concentration of dose around the actual source, or

◆ *beta particles* such as those released from phosphorus, iodine, or strontium. These have an effective dose of only a few millimetres from the site of the isotope.

Gamma-emitting isotopes, in particular caesium and iridium, are used for radio-active implants or intracavity treatment whilst beta-emitting radioisotopes such as phosphorus, iodine, or strontium are used for internal radiotherapy in which an isotope is administered systemically and taken up in various sites within the body.

Brachytherapy is a form of radiotherapy in which radioactive sources are placed within or around an area to be treated. This may be achieved in one of three ways:

1 *Intracavitary therapy* refers to the practice of placing a radiation source within a body cavity such as the vagina or uterus when tumours of this area are treated as shown in Chapter 13. Another example relevant to palliative treatment is intra-luminal treatment when a source is placed within the lumen of a hollow organ such as the oesophagus or bronchus (see Chapters 7 and 11).

2 *Interstitial therapy* is when radioactive wires or needles are placed directly within a tumour. This is used for tumours of the floor of mouth, tongue, and anal canal in particular and other sites such as the breast, prostate, and vulva may also be treated in this way.

3 *Surface moulds* are occasionally used to treat locally advanced tumours on the skin and occasionally recurrent chest wall disease in breast cancer. Radioactive sources are typically encased in a plastic moulds shaped to fit accurately the region to be treated.

Internal radiotherapy relies on the property of certain organs and tumour types to concentrate specific isotopes. Examples of this form of radiotherapy include the select-ive uptake of radiodine by both normal thyroid tissue and thyroid cancer cells, and the concentration of bone-seeking isotopes such as strontium and samarium within sites of bone mineralization. Remaining isotope is usually excreted readily through the kidneys and the retained isotope delivers beta particle radiation directly around the site of uptake but not to other parts of the body.

Biological effects of radiation

When ionizing radiation, delivered by any of the above sources, passes through a biological tissue it exerts specific effects upon the cells. These are described as both *direct effects* in which the DNA strands are damaged by the passage of photon energy through them, and *indirect effects* resulting from the ionization of molecules within the cell, in particular water molecules, with the production of toxic chemicals called *free radicals* which themselves damage the DNA. Many cells have the capacity to repair DNA damage but malignant cells are often deficient in DNA repair enzymes and the repair is relatively inefficient. This allows significant damage to accumulate in malignant cells after the passage of ionizing radiation while normal cells may be spared or repair minor degrees of disruption.

The sensitivity of any cell to radiation depends upon a number of factors. Some cells are by their nature more sensitive than others; this is called intrinsic radiation sensitivity. Cells of the central nervous system have very limited capacity to repair damage and are far more sensitive to radiation than those cells with a high repair capacity and cell turnover, such as skin or epithelial linings. The repair process relies not only upon the cell recovering but repopulation of cells within the whole tissue. This explains the clinical observation during radiotherapy that epithelial surfaces within the treatment area become damaged, presenting clinically as skin desquamation or mucositis, but within a few days of completion of treatment they repair themselves by repopulation of the surface and return to normal. The supply of oxygen and nutrients to a cell is also important in determining its radiosensitivity and those cells which have low oxygen supply and poor nutrition are relatively resistant to radiation.

The biological consequences of irradiation express themselves as both early and late reactions in those tissues within the area irradiated.

- *Early events* usually reflect loss of surface epithelial cells resulting in mucositis in the oral cavity and gastrointestinal tract, cystitis in the bladder, pneumonitis in the lungs, and skin erythema followed by desquamation.

- *Late events* reflect progressive tissue damage due to endarteritis resulting in failure of small blood vessels and reduced stem cell activity which may lead to necrosis. Fibrosis is a common end result seen on skin or mucosal surfaces, sometimes with surface telangiectasis. Stricture of tubular structures such as bowel, oesophagus, urethra, or vagina can lead to stenosis or strictures. More serious consequences may arise from damage to the central nervous system causing transverse myelitis or cerebral necrosis, and other sites of tissue breakdown may cause bowel perforation or fistula formation. It is important, however, to emphasize that these events are rare in clinical radiotherapy and only seen after the delivery of radical doses in around 5 per cent of patients.

Late radiation effects are rarely seen before 9 months from treatment and therefore for most patients in the palliative setting are not a major consideration. They are however a major source of concern in radiation therapy generally because they are irreversible and progressive with often catastrophic effects. Examples include the following:

- *Transverse myelitis* when spinal cord tolerance (typically 50 Gy in 25 fractions) is exceeded;

- *Cataract* formation when dose to the lens of the eye exceeds 10–12 Gy;

- *Small bowel* stenosis, haemorrhage or perforation;

- *Large bowel* stenosis, haemorrhage or perforation;

- *Pneumonitis and lung fibrosis* when large volumes of lung receive more than 20 Gy; tolerance of the whole lung is 6 Gy as a single fraction or 12 Gy in 6 fractions.

Management of late effects is usually only by symptomatic means or drastic surgery to remove the damaged areas. Indeed patients cured of their cancer may still require major symptom control support because of intractable post radiation problems, for example severe progressive lymphoedema. For these reasons radiation oncologists are extremely cautious in the use of radiotherapy particularly in certain areas of low tolerance for example the spinal cord and small bowel, and as a result in radical treatment the incidence of symptomatic late effects from radiotherapy is low typically only 2–3 per cent. Other effects are also recognized for example an increased rate of second malignancies is seen 20–30 years after radiation exposure and an increased rate of coronary artery disease after irradiation to the heart. Such events must be kept in the context of treatment for an otherwise fatal illness and their recognition has led to significant changes in modern radiotherapy techniques which are expected to reduce even further their incidence. It is important that palliative treatments are not compromised because of inappropriate considerations regarding late effects in those patients with a short prognosis where it is the acute effects which will have the greatest impact.

Key points

- Acute radiation toxicity occurs during and immediately after treatment and is self limiting.
- Late radiation toxicity may occur at any time after radiotherapy, rarely before 9 months and is a life-long risk.
- Late radiation effects may be progressive, cause major symptoms and rarely contribute to early death.

Fractionation

Large radiation doses delivered as a single exposure are poorly tolerated. Since tumour cure requires high radiation doses this is usually achieved by dividing the total dose into a series of daily treatments allowing the radiation dose to accumulate over a period of 4–6 weeks. The small daily treatments allow normal tissues to recover through repair and repopulation during treatment. This is less efficient in tumour cells and therefore a differential effect accumulates. There may also be some reoxygenation of tumours as they regress, increasing the sensitivity of previously resistant hypoxic cells through a course of treatment lasting several weeks. In general, the greater number of treatments given to provide a given total dose the less damage to normal tissue will result. This is clearly an important consideration when treating patients who may be cured and live for many years.

In contrast, the patient with advanced disease may be able to look ahead only a few weeks or months. It is therefore the radiation effects that occur during this period which are of greatest concern. It is also not usually necessary to achieve high doses of radiation for local symptom control. Because of these considerations palliative fractionation schedules are much shorter and a radiation dose to achieve symptom control may be delivered in a single treatment or a course of 5–10 treatments on a daily basis lasting up to two weeks. In this way the patient is subjected to as few hospital visits as possible and the level of side effects is minimized.

Practical aspects of radiotherapy delivery

Because of the potential hazard of radiation and its effects upon surrounding normal tissue, radiotherapy to a tumour-bearing area must be given in as accurate and precise a way as possible. Whilst in the palliative setting this preparation is minimized as far as possible there are still important principles to apply in order to ensure the best result with the least side effects.

Immobilization of the treated part is important to allow accurate and reproducible treatment. This may simply mean asking the patient to lie still on the treatment couch when treating an area in the spine. However, for more complex mobile structures such as the head and neck area or eye, plastic immobilization shells may be made for the patient to ensure that he/she retains the correct position during treatment.

Localization of the area to be treated is then important to ensure accurate coverage of the affected part. This in its simplest form may mean simply palpating a superficial mass and drawing around it or choosing a radiation cone or applicator to cover it. For deeper soft tissue tumours more complex localization will require computerized tomographic (CT) scanning to define an internal organ such as the bladder, bronchus, or prostate.

Planning of the radiation dose delivery is vital to ensure the appropriate radiation beams are used to focus upon the area requiring treatment. The correct energy of beam, angle of delivery and modifications to the beam must be used to ensure an even coverage of radiation dose to the required treatment volume. The dose to critical structures such as the spinal cord must be accurately calculated and kept within safe limits to minimize or avoid the risk of later damage. This is usually carried out using a computerized reproduction of the shape of the area to be treated and localization of any internal organs. The most accurate way of doing this is by deriving the information from a CT scan, on to which the computer can then overlay radiation beam dose information to permit calculations of dose to tumour volume and other organs to be made. An example of this is shown in Fig. 5.2.

Radiotherapy is becoming increasingly sophisticated in the ways in which it can deliver an accurate radiation dose to an irregular shape avoiding critical normal tissues. This is largely as a result of a series of technical developments over recent years which are now available in routine practice. These include:

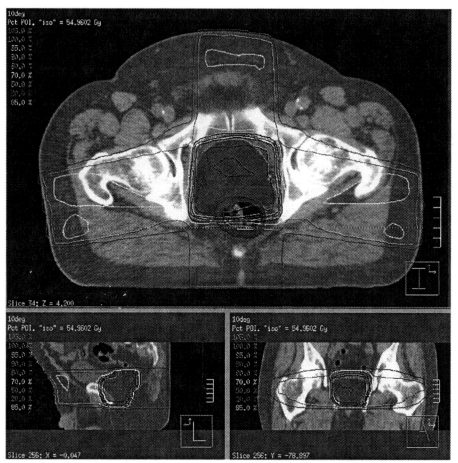

Fig. 5.2 Radiotherapy plans to show distribution of dose from three beams focused on a pelvic volume defined on CT to treat a prostate volume; the large image shows the transverse outline at the centre of the volume, the smaller images the sagittal and coronal distributions through the central plane. Note how in this conformal plan the beams are shaped to give a high dose region covering tumour and avoiding normal tissue as much as possible.

Multileaf collimator (MLC) which is a means of beam shaping built into or fixed onto the head of a linear accelerator. Essentially it comprises between 80 and 120 interleaves which can be moved in and out of the X-ray beam to shape it and also alter the intensity of the beam at any point. Each leaf has an individual electric motor which is co-ordinated through a central computer control. This has replaced the use of large blocks of lead to shape beams being not only more flexible in the possible shapes but also more reliable and reproducable. It is also easier for staff avoiding the need to lift heavy lead trays.

Conformal radiotherapy is treatment in which by using the MLC within the beam irregular and curved shapes to the treatment volume can be accommodated so that high dose volumes can much more accurately 'conform' to the anatomical structures they are attempting to cover, and avoid.

Intensity modulated radiotherapy (IMRT) introduces a variation in dose across the treatment volume. Thus whereas conventional radiotherapy planning seeks to deliver an even dose across the defined volume IMRT allows definition of high dose volume and lower dose areas around this, where for example there may be less bulky or only microscopic disease.

Implementation of the planning and localization brings the patient into the radiation treatment. It is important to check that the above steps have resulted in accurate radiation delivery to the affected area and this will be achieved by either diagnostic X-ray films on a treatment machine simulator or by taking an X-ray film picture using the therapeutic beam during the first treatment. Examples of these are shown in Fig. 5.3.

In palliative treatment where there may be only a single or two treatments to be delivered then these steps are streamlined as far as possible. However, most patients will require a visit to the treatment planning department to have X-ray pictures taken and skin marks made to ensure accurate localization of the treatment. Where internal structures such as the bladder or prostate are being treated which are close to sensitive structures, in this case bowel, more complex planning including CT scanning may still be justified.

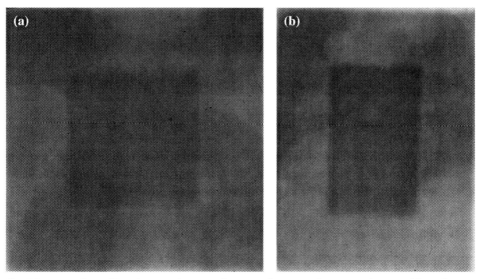

Fig. 5.3 Megavoltage (6 MV) X-ray pictures taken on a linear accelerator to show position of treatment beams for palliative radiotherapy to (a) apical chest mass and (b) spine. Note definition between bone and soft tissue is lost; this is a characteristic of the high energy beam.

> **Key points: radiotherapy delivery**
>
> The key stages in radiotherapy delivery are:
>
> - Immobilization.
> - Localization of area to be treated.
> - Planning of X-ray beams to deliver dose.
> - Implementation of radiotherapy with verification of actual treatment delivered.
> - In palliative radiotherapy simple treatments using clinical or X-ray localization, single or two opposing beams and short treatment times are the ideal.

Palliative and radical radiotherapy

Radiotherapy is a local treatment only. Its effects are limited to the site to which it is directed and indeed as mentioned above, careful steps are taken to ensure its accurate delivery to a limited area. It can therefore offer curative treatment where a tumour is localized to an anatomical region. Examples where this is in common use include areas in the head and neck region such as the larynx, tongue or floor of mouth, localized bladder tumours, prostatic carcinoma, and uterine tumours. It is often combined with surgery to ensure local clearance of an area. In this setting, where the aim of treatment is cure, some disruption to the patient's lifestyle can be justified and inevitable side effects accepted provided these are self-limiting. In contrast, for the patient who has advanced disease and limited survival then the aim of any treatment should be to ensure minimal disruption to lifestyle within the bounds of treatment efficacy. There is therefore a very different philosophy attached to palliative radiotherapy compared to radical radiotherapy.

Clinical indications for palliative radiotherapy

Efficacy

Radiotherapy is appropriate for many local symptoms. It is important to emphasize once more that it has no impact upon systemic disease or survival. Small doses given in one or two treatments, however, can make a major impact upon many of the problems which metastatic disease presents in advanced cancer including:

- bone pain
- pathological fracture
- spinal cord compression
- local haemorrhage including:
  - haemoptysis
  - haematuria

- vaginal or uterine bleeding
- surface bleeding from skin infiltrating tumours
- pain due to tissue infiltration including:
  - hepatomegaly
  - splenomegaly
  - tumour in the pre-sacral space
  - chest wall invasion
- bronchial obstruction causing lung collapse
- dysphagia due to intrinsic obstruction from carcinoma of the oesophagus or extrinsic compression by bronchial tumour or lymph node
- central nervous system symptoms due to cerebral metastases
- choroidal metastases
- advanced fungating lesions on the skin

Availability

The complex nature of radiotherapy as described above means that its delivery has to be concentrated in radiotherapy centres which are not present in all general hospitals and may be some distance from many hospices. The clinical efficacy therefore in some cases has to be balanced against the difficulties and discomfort involved in transporting a patient for radiotherapy. Access to appropriate specialist advice on the possible benefits and side effects of treatment with close liaison between oncologists and palliative care physicians should enable selection of those patients for whom the inconvenience of treatment is outweighed by the possibility of major gains in symptom control.

Patient acceptance

The decision to offer radiotherapy must include the wishes of the patient who in some circumstances may be averse to further active cancer treatment particularly if this does involve transfer and transportation to a cancer centre some miles away. Some patients may also have had radical doses of radiotherapy in the past resulting in significant side effects which deter them from considering this treatment for palliation. It is of course important that patients are given clear and accurate information highlighting the difference between radical and palliative treatment and the attempts to minimize acute side effects in the palliative setting.

Patient management during palliative radiotherapy

Although palliative radiotherapy is given in such a way as to minimize acute reactions these may still occur and require appropriate reassurance and management. These may include the following:

Skin reactions are usually minimal with palliative treatment but some local skin erythema may occur. Generally, this requires no treatment other than reassurance and it will settle spontaneously within two to three weeks after treatment. If there is local itching or dryness aqueous cream may be of value.

Dysphagia may occur from treating the mediastinum or carcinoma of the bronchus or oesophagus. This is due to local oesophagitis. It will resolve itself within two to three weeks of treatment and may be helped by local measures such as the use of soluble aspirin in mucilage, particularly if taken before meals. Rarely, an oesophageal stricture may result in patients surviving for several months if a relatively high dose of radiation has been delivered although very often this development is associated with recurrent tumour. Dysphagia developing more than a few weeks after radiotherapy requires investigation with a barium swallow and oesophagoscopy with dilatation if appropriate.

Oropharyngeal mucositis may arise from treatment to the oral cavity or throat. This also resolves spontaneously and acute symptoms may be helped by local chlorhexidine and benzydamine (Difflam) mouthwashes. It is also important to avoid secondary infection with candida and topical nystatin or clotrimazole may be of value.

Nausea and vomiting may occur where large areas of bowel or liver are included in the radiation field. This may be the case not only when treating an abdominal tumour but also from the beam treating the low dorsal or lumbar spine as it exits beyond the spine. It is best managed with routine anti-emetic treatment such as metoclopramide 10 mg, 4-hourly or, if more severe a 5HT3 antagonist such as ondansetron 8 mg daily. It is invariably self-limiting within a few days of completing treatment. Symptoms persisting beyond this should be further investigated for an alternative cause.

Diarrhoea may occur where the bowel is included in the treatment field, particularly when this includes large bowel and rectum as when the pelvis is treated. Loperamide or codeine phosphate are appropriate treatments. Many patients may already be on a systemic opioid drug (e.g. morphine), and in these patients kaolin mixture may be a more rational treatment for radiation-induced diarrhoea.

Pneumonitis may occur where large areas of lung are treated. This will present with a dry cough and associated dyspnoea with characteristic patchy shadowing conforming to the shape of the radiation field on the chest X-ray. It is best treated with a course of high dose steroids such as prednisolone 40–60 mg, daily over 2–3 weeks with antibiotics as required for secondary infection.

Cystitis may occur when the bladder is included in a radiation field. This is a difficult symptom to treat satisfactorily but is also self-limiting. It is important to exclude coexisting infection and treat this if it develops. Oxybutynin 5 mg, up to four times daily may help with frequency and bladder spasm as may other drugs with anticholinergic activity such as tricyclic antidepressants or phenothiazines.

Virtually all *acute* side effects from radiation are a result of transient damage to epithelial surface which will invariably repair itself after the low doses of radiation delivered for palliative purposes. These events are therefore self-limiting and within the life cycle of the basal epithelial cells will resolve themselves. It is important therefore to reassure the patient regarding this effect and provide suitable symptomatic treatment during the acute phase.

Key points: management of acute toxicity

- Most acute toxicity is self-limiting and simply requires supportive treatment for a short period.
- Where appropriate anti-emetics and anti-diarrhoeal agents should be used in the usual way.
- Local irritation of mucous membranes is best treated with topical analgesics and anti-inflammatory agents.
- Skin reactions are best left alone as far as possible; aqueous cream or weak hydrocortisone cream may reduce irritation; other skin preparations should be avoided but gentle washing is not harmful and should be encouraged.

Chapter 6

Systemic therapy: chemotherapy, hormone therapy, biological therapy

Systemic therapy may take the form of chemotherapy, hormone therapy or biological agents such as interferon or interleukin. The major advantage of systemic therapy over local treatment such as surgery or radiotherapy is the ability to deliver tumouricidal therapy throughout the body so that all sites are exposed to therapy. Inevitably the consequence is that there is increased exposure to normal tissues with concomitant increases in the extent of toxicity. For this reason systemic therapy is often regarded warily in palliative medicine but it is important to realize that there are a number of drug schedules which have limited toxicity and considerable efficacy, for example oral melphalan in myeloma, CMF (cyclophosphamide, methotrexate and 5-fluorouracil) chemotherapy in breast cancer, oral etoposide in small cell lung cancer and hormonal therapies such as tamoxifen or megestrol in breast cancer and goserelin in prostatic cancer. These will be considered in more detail below.

Key points

- Systemic therapy includes chemotherapy, hormone therapy and biological agents.
- Wider exposure to tumour cells is balanced by greater toxicity.

Chemotherapy

Chemotherapy is a wide ranging term encompassing the administration of cytotoxic chemicals to the patient. These may at one extreme be intensive regimes requiring continuous infusion chemotherapy and bone marrow support with a high incidence of major toxicities and even mortality, or in contrast simple oral chemotherapy with few if any side effects. There are various classifications for chemotherapy drugs. The common chemotherapy agents are shown in Table 6.1 classified according to their mode of action.

The wide range of drugs perhaps reflects as much as anything the limited efficacy of individual agents for the common solid tumours. Examples of the spectrum of chemosensitivity are shown in Table 6.2.

Table 6.1 Classification of chemotherapy drugs by mode of action

Antimetabolites: interfering with nucleic acid synthesis
Methotrexate
5-Fluorouracil
Capecitabine
Irinotecan
Gemcitabine
Cytosine arabinoside
Fludarabine
Alkylating agents
Cyclophosphamide
Chlorambucil
Melphalan
Nitrosoureas (BCNU, CCNU)
Intercalating agents: binding to helical structure of DNA
Antracyclines (doxorubicin [adriamycin], epirubicin, mitozantrone)
Etoposide
Cisplatin
Carboplatin
Oxaliplatin
Drugs acting on spindle microtubules: preventing passage through mitosis
Vinca alkaloids (vincristine, vinblastine, vindesine, vinorelbine)
Taxanes (paclitaxel, docetaxel)
Others
Bleomycin
Procarbazine
Mitomycin C

Chemotherapy agents may be used alone or in combination. Single agent use has obvious advantages in the palliative setting being simpler, and usually associated with fewer side effects. Examples of this include oral melphalan or cyclophosphamide for myeloma, etoposide in small cell lung cancer, gemcitabine or vinorelbine in non small cell lung cancer and cisplatin or carboplatin in ovarian carcinoma.

Combination chemotherapy consisting of three, four or more drugs given together is more usual in practice and enables drugs of modest efficacy to be combined improving the overall efficacy. The further principle of combination chemotherapy is that drugs with differing toxicities are chosen so that where possible, the spectrum of toxicity can also be spread and minimized.

Table 6.2 Chemosensitivity of common tumours

Highly sensitive (>70% response rates)	Moderately sensitive (30–60% response rates)	Poorly sensitive (10–30% response rates)
Lymphoma	Breast cancer	Prostate cancer
Germ cell tumours	Colorectal cancer	Pancreatic cancer
Small cell lung cancer	Bladder cancer	Gliomas
Myeloma	Cervix cancer	Endometrial cancer
Leukaemias	Ovary cancer	Melanoma
	Non small cell lung cancer	Renal cancer

In general, combining drugs results in simple addition of their effects rather than a superadditive effect. There are however, examples of drug combinations where the efficacy of one drug can be enhanced by the addition of a modulator. The most common of these is the use of folinic acid which is a non-chemotherapy agent and a precursor in the methyl folate synthesis pathway important in nucleic acid synthesis. The use of folinic acid with 5-FU can approximately double the efficacy of 5-FU by increasing its incorporation into the nucleic acid chain. As a result of this, mistakes in replication are made and the cell becomes non viable. This is now the standard chemotherapy for both adjuvant and metastatic colorectal cancer although there remains a debate as to the optimal schedules to achieve the maximum response with least toxicity with some favouring weekly injections of 5-FU/folinic acid and others advocating two day infusions.

There are also examples of specific antagonists to chemotherapy the most common of which is again the use of folinic acid to 'switch off' the effects of methotrexate. This is because methotrexate works by inhibition of dihydrofolate reductase which again interrupts the methyl folate synthesis pathway. This is important in nucleic acid replication and by replenishing folate stocks with folinic acid the block caused by methotrexate can be overcome. This can be useful in minimising side effects of methotrexate and often a short course of folinic acid is given orally in a dose of 15 mg 6 hourly for 24 h starting 24 h after administration of methotrexate.

Because chemotherapy is a systemic treatment to which every tissue in the body is potentially exposed it can be associated with a wide range of side effects. Chemotherapy will affect to varying degrees the bone marrow with a reduction in red cell, white cell and platelet production after administration. The typical pattern is for a gradual fall in counts to reach a nadir at 10–14 days after treatment returning to normal levels between days 21 and 28. This pattern is principally responsible for the timing of chemotherapy at 3–4 week intervals. Important exceptions to this pattern are mitomycin C and the nitrosoureas (BCNU and CCNU) which cause a much later nadir in white cells at 4–5 weeks after administration as a result of which they must be given at no less than 6 week intervals.

Key points

◆ Chemotherapy drugs may be classified by mode of action including: antimetabolites; alkylating agents; intercalating agents; spindle microtubule poisons.

◆ Chemotherapy may act on specific phases of the cell cycle (phase specific) or throughout the cycle (cycle specific).

◆ Chemotherapy drugs may be used alone or in combination when drugs from different classes may be synergistic.

◆ With few exceptions (e.g. bleomycin and vincristine) chemotherapy will cause bone marrow depression.

Chemotherapy administration

Most common chemotherapy drugs are toxic agents. In their simplest form they can be administered on a outpatient basis as an oral formulation, but even in this setting careful monitoring of blood count is required since the bone marrow is generally the most sensitive organ to chemotherapy in the body and falls in blood count must be monitored and treatment withheld unless there are adequate levels of circulating cells.

The majority of chemotherapy drugs require intravenous administration. This should only be carried out in an experienced unit dedicated to chemotherapy administration preferably by a nurse specialist trained in chemotherapy administration and its side effects. It is important to have secure venous access, and administration into a fast flowing drip can reduce local venous irritation and the chances of extravasation which can have catastrophic effects within soft tissues. This is particularly severe with certain drugs including the anthracyclines (adriamycin, epirubicin) and vinca alkaloids (vincristine and vinblastine).

Where venous access is difficult because of poor veins in patients who are needle phobic and in those requiring repeated or continuous infusional treatment, an indwelling central venous catheter may be preferable such as a Hickman line. Continuous infusion chemotherapy is given using a small battery-powered pump or an infuser system using a vacuum bottle and rubber reservoir. Hickman lines can be inserted under radiographic control with local anaesthetic or at open operation under general anesthetic and having multiple channels provide a permanent means of both blood sampling and venous access. A Hickman line *in situ* is shown in Fig. 6.1 together with a schematic representation of its anatomical positioning.

Patients who have a Hickman line *in situ* need to be seen weekly for the line to be flushed with heparinized saline to maintain patency and administration of warfarin 1 mg daily is also recommended to reduce the rate of thrombotic complications. Central venous catheters are a potential route for infection and, particularly in patients at risk of infection due to neutropenia or immunosuppression, should be carefully inspected

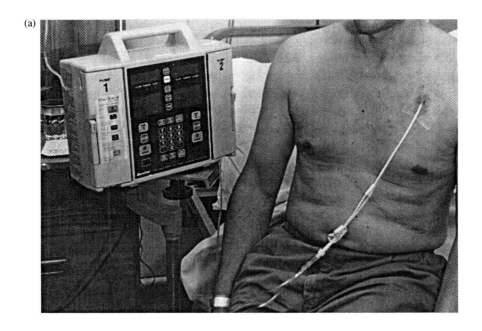

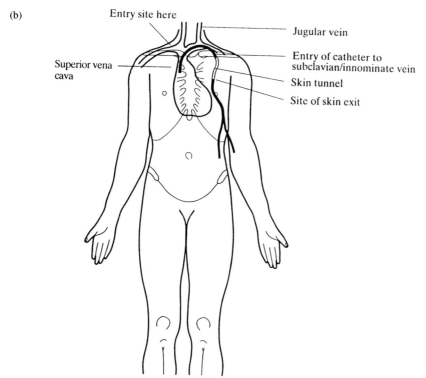

Fig. 6.1 Hickman line *in situ* connected to infusion pump (a) and diagram (b) to show route of line.

for signs of sepsis around their entry site. Early infection may be cleared by the use of flucloxacillin in the immune competent and teicoplanin in the immunosuppressed but once infection is established along their track lines it must be removed with continued antibiotic cover. Plastic clamps will be found on the line which must always be closed when the line is opened to prevent air entering the vein or if the patient is supine, blood pouring out. Once connected to a syringe or infusion system the clamps are then opened. When blood sampling, the initial few millilitres should be discarded as these will be contaminated with heparin from the flush; after sampling the line should always be flushed to ensure patency is maintained.

Removal of a line is a simple process which can be performed in the ward or a clinic room. With reference to the figure it can be seen that there is a fibrous cuff mid-way along the tunnelled portion of the line which is the sole means of retention. Whilst there are advocates for simply tugging on the line to free the consolidated cuff frequently, it will not free itself readily and it is usually less traumatic to free the cuff first.

Key points

- Chemotherapy may be given orally or intravenously.
- Certain drugs if injected outside a vein will cause severe soft tissue damage (vesicants) and these include anthracyclines and vinca alkaloids.
- Continuous infusions through a central Hickman line may be given.

Palliative versus radical chemotherapy

As with any intervention in patients with advanced disease and limited survival the probability of benefit must be carefully balanced against the inevitable intrusion and toxicity of treatment. In addition, the wishes of the patient must be considered and many patients are anxious to receive all possible treatments despite advice to the contrary where the probability of response is low. These issues are particularly pertinent in the use of chemotherapy where major responses in advanced disease are unusual outside those highly sensitive tumours shown in Table 6.2. There is some evidence that objective response defined by a 50 per cent or greater reduction in tumour mass is not always necessary for the patient to have improved quality of life, and symptom control may result from a lesser response albeit often relatively short-lived. Toxicity from chemotherapy can be significant and multiple hospital attendances, if not inpatient admissions, will usually be required. For this reason it is essential that response is closely monitored and that if no significant response, whether objective or subjective, is seen after two or three courses, ineffective treatment is discontinued.

Against this background it is possible to define indications for palliative chemotherapy as outlined in Table 6.3.

Table 6.3 Indications for palliative chemotherapy

Symptoms attributable to locally advanced primary or metastatic tumour.

Local radiotherapy inappropriate (either scattered sites or previous radiation failure).

Significant (>30%) response rate anticipated for symptoms (rather than tumour shrinkage).

Toxicity acceptable to patient.

General medical condition adequate to tolerate procedure and toxicity.

Patient wishes to proceed.

New agents are also often available for evaluation and it is those patients with advanced disease, particularly who have failed previous treatments, who will be considered for Phase I and early Phase II studies (i.e. those looking at the pharmacology of the drug and seeking to determine its efficacy in certain tumours). This again raises the dilemma of offering treatment that may be ineffective and associated with known toxicity to a patient with advanced disease and limited survival. There is however an important role for the patient who wishes to have all possible treatment and more generally in furthering knowledge and developing new treatments which may be applicable in a more radical format, once properly evaluated. It is important to establish an honest rapport with the patient to reach the best decisions for each individual. Whilst relatives and many health carers may wish to protect the patient from 'experimentation', for some individuals it is an important contribution for them to be allowed to make.

Management of patients during chemotherapy

Aside from the administration of chemotherapy, patients receiving such treatment require careful monitoring as specific complications may arise requiring active intervention.

Neutropenic sepsis is the most serious potentially fatal complication of chemotherapy which occurs in a significant number of patients particularly those receiving combination chemotherapy. The reported incidence of neutropenic sepsis from common chemotherapy schedules is shown in Table 6.4.

Because the bone marrow is one of the most active sites of cell division in the body, most chemotherapy drugs cause bone marrow suppression. The extent of this varies considerably between individual patients and is also influenced by existing bone marrow reserve as a result of previous treatment and tumour infiltration. Patients in whom the total neutrophil count falls below $1.0 \times 10^9/L$ are at considerable risk of sepsis often from their own bowel or skin organisms rather than extrinsic organisms. This may initially present with minor symptoms or simply an asymptomatic fever. It is vital that these early signs of neutropenic sepsis are not ignored and any patient feeling unwell or presenting with a fever having had recent chemotherapy requires an urgent full blood count. If neutropenic, usually defined by an absolute neutrophil count below

Table 6.4 Incidence of neutropenic sepsis with different chemotherapies

CHOP (cyclophosphamide, adriamycin, vincristine, prednisolone)	lymphoma	35%
LOPP/EVAP (chlorambucil, vinblastine, procarbazine, prednisolone etoposide, vincristine, adriamycin, prednisolone)	Hodgkins disease	31%
CMF (cyclophosphamide, methotrexate, 5-FU)	breast	5%
MMM (mitozantrone, methotrexate, mitomycin C)	breast	22%
CAV (cyclophosphamide, adriamycin, etoposide)	small cell lung cancer	12%
5-FU/Folinic acid	colorectal	5%

1.0×10^9 then admission to a unit experienced in the management of such complications is mandatory and high dose intravenous broad spectrum antibiotics are required without delay using combinations such as gentamicin and ticarcillin or a broad spectrum cephalosporin such as ceftazidime. Cultures should be taken prior to the treatment but antibiotics should not be delayed awaiting results. Within only a few hours a previously well patient may deteriorate rapidly and become moribund with neutropenic sepsis and it is therefore essential to have a high index of suspicion for this condition in any patient receiving chemotherapy.

This applies equally to patients within the palliative care service and any non-specific symptoms in a patient within two to three weeks of chemotherapy requires investigation with an urgent full blood count.

Failure to treat this situation aggressively will result in septicaemic shock and death. The usual pattern of white count fall after chemotherapy is for it to reach a trough 10–14 days after administration, recovering in the subsequent week; during this period, in particular, vigilance is required to detect early signs of sepsis. Patients with a low neutrophil count ($<0.5 \times 10^9$/L) should be kept under close observation with monitoring of their temperature at least twice daily; if a single reading $>38.5°$ or two reading of $38°$ are seen then antibiotics should be started without delay. Whilst there is no good evidence to support the practice many of these patients will be started prophylactically on broad spectrum oral antibiotics such as ciprofloxacillin. This should be considered if there have been previous episodes of sepsis or there is a potential infective focus such as a catheter in situ; it is however no substitute for continued close surveillance.

Patients at particular risk of myelosuppression due to their disease, the chemotherapy agents being used or previous episodes of neutropenic sepsis may be treated with granulocyte colony stimulating factor (GCSF) (see page 64); again it is important to be aware that this does not prevent neutropenia but may shorten the period of a very low count. Close surveillance is still required however.

Key points

- Patients who have recently received chemotherapy will be at risk of neutropenia and neutropenic sepsis.
- Procedures which cause bacteraemia, e.g. rectal examination, dental treatment may provoke septicaemia in a neutropenic patient.
- Any patient in this category who presents with a fever of >38° requires an urgent blood count.
- Fever in a patient with an absolute neutrophil count <1.0×10^9 is an indication for immediate hospital admission and high dose broad spectrum intravenous antibiotics.

The profile of other common side effects seen with different agents is shown in Table 6.5. Typical problems and their management are outlined below:

- Nausea and vomiting for which routine anti-emetics will usually be successful using either metoclopramide, cyclizine, prochlorperazine or ondansetron.
- Mouth dryness and oral ulceration which will usually heal spontaneously and is eased with oral chlorhexidene and benzydamine (Difflam). This is seen particularly with methotrexate or 5-FU.
- Diarrhoea will be controlled with loperamide or codeine phosphate. This is seen particularly with methotrexate, 5-FU, irinotecan and cisplatin.
- Peripheral neuropathy may cause tingling and numbness of the fingers and toes. This is seen particularly with vincristine and cisplatin. It is important that such symptoms are made known and if they persist the offending drug substituted by another less neurotoxic agent. In the early stages spontaneous recovery is usual. Typically it is a sensory neuropathy and may result in neuropathic pain, often during the recovery phase. This should be treated pharmacologically in the same way as other cases of neuropathic pain.
- Tinnitus may occur with cisplatin and again its identification is important so that further exposure is avoided to prevent worsening of the symptoms.
- Bleomycin can cause characteristic skin changes with increased pigmentation and peeling of the skin over the palms and soles of the feet. Occasionally discolouration of the nail bed is seen and in some patients total nail loss occurs.
- Alopecia occurs with many chemotherapy agents. Scalp cooling by the use of an ice cap during administration can reduce the probability particularly when anthracyclines (adriamycin, epiribucin or idarubicin) are used. It is important to

Table 6.5 Non haematological toxicity with common chemotherapy agents (score 0 to 3 refers to arbitrary designation of none (0), mild (1), moderate (2) and severe (3))

	Nausea vomiting	Diarrhoea	Mucositis	Cardiotoxicity	Pneumonitis	Peripheral neuropathy	Alopecia
Methotrexate (standard iv dose)	1	2	3	0	0	0	1
5-Fluorouracil	0	2	2	2	0	0	0
Capecitabine	0	1	1	0	0	0	0
Irinotecan	1	3	2	0	0	0	0
Gemcitabine	0	0	1	0	0	0	0
Cytosine arabinoside	1	0	1	0	0	0	2
Fludarabine	0	0	0	0	0	1	0
Cyclophosphamide	2	0	0	0	0	0	3
Ifosphamide	2	0	1	0	1	0	3
Chlorambucil (oral)	0	0	0	0	0	0	0
Melphalan (oral)	0	0	0	0	0	0	0
Nitrosoureas (BCNU, CCNU)	2	0	0	0	0	0	3
[1]Antracyclines	2	0	0	[4]3	0	0	[5]3

Etoposide	2	0	0	0	0	3
Cisplatin	3	2	0	0	2	0
Carboplatin	3	1	0	0	1	0
Oxaliplatin	2	1	0	0	0	0
²Vinca alkaloids	0	0	0	0	3	0
³Taxanes	2	2	1[6]	0	2	3
Bleomycin	0	0	0	3	0	0
Procarbazine	1	0	0	0	0	0
Mitomycin C	1	1	1	0	0	1

[1] doxorubicin [adriamycin], epirubicin, mitozantrone
[2] vincristine, vinblastine, vindesine, vinorelbine
[3] paclitaxel, docetaxel
[4] dose related, least with mitozantrone, greatest with adriamycin
[5] may be reduced by scalp cooling (not mitozantrone)
[6] paclitaxel only

pre-empt alopecia and provide appropriate alternatives either in the form of a wig or, in men, a suitable hat is often the preferred choice. It is equally important to reassure patients receiving chemotherapy which does not usually cause alopecia, that such measures will not be required. Examples where alopecia is rare include CMF and MMM chemotherapy for breast cancer, carboplatin or cisplatin as single agents in ovary cancer, 5-FU or capecitabine as single agent in colorectal cancer, gemcitabine or vinorelbine for lung cancer and oral alkylating agents such as melphalan, cyclophosphamide and chlorambucil in haematological malignancies.

Hormone therapy

Certain malignancies are dependent upon their hormonal environment for growth and development. The most common examples of these are breast and prostate. Endometrial carcinoma is also dependent upon oestrogen and occasionally renal carcinoma may respond to hormone treatment also.

Hormone therapy may take several forms

1 Positive hormone stimulation to alter the hormonal environment as in the use of progestogen or oestrogen for breast cancer.

2 Hormone antagonists to block the action of hormones as in the use of anti-oestrogens such as tamoxifen in breast cancer or anti-androgens in prostate cancer.

3 Modification of hormone release or activation as in the use of gonadotrophin releasing hormone analogues in prostate cancer or the use of aromatase inhibitors which prevent the peripheral conversion of precursors to oestradiol in breast cancer.

Most hormone therapies can be given orally and unlike chemotherapy they are often relatively free from major side effects. Because of this they may have an important role in palliative medicine but in many cases would have already been used by the time patients reach the final stages of their disease. Often patients will be inadvertently left on hormonal therapy without good evidence of efficacy and there may even be a tendency to use them in a placebo fashion because of their low toxicity. This should in general be avoided and where there is no good evidence of response their use discontinued. The role of continued anti-androgen therapy in prostate cancer is controversial and there may be justification for continuing treatment on the basis of a residual hormone sensitive population despite the emergence of hormone resistant cells; this is an area currently under evaluation in clinical trials.

Other tumours

Renal carcinoma is sometimes considered hormonally responsive but in practice significant responses are rare and may be no more common than spontaneous remissions. Because the behaviour of renal carcinoma is unpredictable it is difficult to document the true incidence of hormone sensitivity. It has been claimed that up to

Table 6.6 Indications for hormone therapy in malignant disease

	Breast cancer	Prostate cancer	Endometrial cancer
Tamoxifen	Yes	No	No
LHRH angonist/antagonists, e.g. Goserelin	Yes	Yes	Yes
Progestogens	Yes	No*	Yes
Aromatase inhibitors, e.g. anastrozole	Yes	No*	No
Antiandrogens, e.g. cyproterone, flutamide, bicalutamide	No	Yes	No

* responses to both progestogens and aromatase inhibitors may be seen, but not used routinely

20 per cent of patients will respond to progestogen treatment and this will often be tried in patients with advanced disease for whom there is no other active treatment option.

Differentiated thyroid cancer is stimulated by the thyroid stimulating hormone released from the pituitary. For this reason patients with differentiated thyroid cancer are treated with thyroxine to suppress the feedback mechanism at the pituitary and prevent release of TSH.

Key points

- Many breast cancers are hormone sensitive and will respond to oestrogen antagonists.

- Commonly used effective drugs in breast cancer include tamoxifen, toremifene, anastrazole, letrozole, megestrol and medroxyprogesterone.

- Second or third line hormone treatment may be worthwhile after relapse on initial treatment.

- Most prostate cancers are dependent on androgens and respond to anti-androgen treatment.

- Androgen blockade can be achieved by oral peripheral antagonists, e.g. cyproterone, flutamide or bicalutamide, LHRH agonist-antagonists such as goserelin or orchidectomy.

- Progestogens may be useful on metastatic endometrial cancer.

Biological agents

In recent years there has been increasing interest in the development and use of biological agents based on naturally occurring substances within the body. There are two major groups of biological agents currently in use.

- *Lymphokines* such as interleukin 2 (IL2) and interferon. These are part of the normal inflammatory response and increase the immune reaction in the body which may be important in removing the malignant cells. The efficacy of these agents in advanced disease is poor and there are very few incidences where they are of great value outside experimental schedules.

  Interferon has a role in the primary treatment of hairy cell leukaemia which is a rare form of leukaemia characterized by circulating leukaemic cells with hair like projections on their surface. It may also have a role in selected patients with metastatic melanoma and carcinoid syndrome and is used as an adjuvant treatment after initial response to chemotherapy in chronic myelocytic leukaemia and myeloma. Administration is thrice weekly by subcutaneous injections often self-administered; side effects are variable but a disabling chronic flu-like illness may be encountered. There is a relative contraindication to the use of steroids with interferon.

- *Growth factors*, in particular granulocyte colony stimulating factor (GCSF) will increase white blood cell production from the bone marrow and are used as an adjunct to myelosuppressive chemotherapy to enable more frequent treatment or higher doses than would otherwise be possible or to prevent the complications of severe neutropenia. They are also valuable in mobilizing peripheral blood progenitor cells which can be collected from the circulation and stored. This technique allows very high dose chemotherapy to be given resulting in ablation of the normal bone marrow which can then be re-seeded by infusion of the stored peripheral blood progenitor cells collected prior to exposure to the chemotherapy. Other uses for GCSF are under investigation for example in the treatment of severe mucositis. Keratinocyte stimulating factor has also been used for this problem.

- *Erythropoetin* is now available in a synthetic form. Given by subcutaneous injection thrice weekly it will increase and maintain haemoglobin levels provided there are sufficient iron stores and bone marrow activity. It is effective in reducing chemotherapy-associated anaemia and in advanced disease, particularly where there is extensive bone marrow involvement, for example low grade lymphoma, myeloma and prostatic cancer it will reduce transfusion requirements and the syndrome of 'transfusion dependence' which can develop. Even where there is only modest anaemia reduced symptoms of fatigue with improved quality of life scores are reported.

There is considerable expense associated with these agents. The use of GCSF is therefore limited to selected circumstances where neutropenia is a major hazard. Their role is limited in the palliative setting. The use of erythropoetin is more controversial since, whilst there are clear gains for the patient in improved quality of life, the cost of its widespread adoption in advanced cancer patients would be prohibitive for many health care systems. One important practical application is in the management of the patient with symptomatic anaemia who refuses blood transfusion on religious grounds for whom erythropoeitin is an alternative.

Monoclonal antibody therapy uses antibodies to surface receptors specific to the malignant clone of cells to target deliver of a toxic molecule to the malignant cells. In recent years two examples of this form of treatment have become established in clinical practice. The first uses antibodies to the CD20 cell surface marker for B lymphocytes expressed by malignant lymphoma. This agent is called Rituximab and is given as an intravenous infusion in predominantly low grade but also some high grade lymphomas resistant to conventional chemotherapy. Response rates of around 50 per cent are reported albeit relatively short-lived. There may be reactions to the foreign protein but in general the treatment is well tolerated and of particular importance in this group of patients it does not cause bone marrow depression. Herceptin is an antibody to the c-erbB2 receptor found on some breast cancer cells. Its presence is associated with a relatively worse prognosis but such patients can respond to antibody therapy using this agent. Whilst currently predominantly used in the palliative setting both these monoclonal antibodies are being evaluated in their role as primary treatment.

Key points

- Immune augmentation using interferon or interleukin may be of value in hairy cell leukaemia, renal cancer and melanoma. Neutropenia ($<1.0 \times 10^9$/L) must be excluded in any unexplained fever or infective episode.
- Colony stimulating factors enable bone marrow stem cell harvesting for high dose chemotherapy and will reduce periods of neutropenia in susceptible patients struggling with conventional chemotherapy.
- New approaches with monoclonal antibodies offer additional low toxicity treatment in lymphoma and breast cancer.

Chapter 7

Lung cancer and mesothelioma

Lung cancer

Incidence

The incidence of lung cancer in the United Kingdom is over 40 000 new cases per year, and the number of deaths from this disease is very similar in number to the incidence, reflecting its poor prognosis. It is invariably associated with a history of tobacco smoking and clear correlations between number of cigarettes, tar content and filter use, and lung cancer have been demonstrated.

Pathology and natural history

Lung cancer generally refers to primary carcinomas of the bronchial tree, of which there are two main types, non-small cell lung cancer (NSCLC) and small cell lung cancer (SCLC). NSCLC includes squamous cell cancer, adenocarcinoma and anaplastic cancers.

SCLC is characterised by widespread metastases which develop by blood-borne spread at an early stage of its development. This means that almost all patients presenting with SCLC have metastases even if not clinically apparent and their management is based primarily on systemic treatment. NSCLC also has a high rate of metastatic spread but may present with a localised disease and in a few patients it may be possible to offer radical treatment with a chance of cure.

Local growth of carcinoma of the bronchus may cause obstruction to the bronchus and collapse or infection of the distal lung. There may also be local haemorrhage causing haemoptysis. Infiltration of the lungs and surrounding mediastinal structures may involve the oesophagus and pericardium resulting in pain and dysphagia.

Lymph node involvement occurs at an early stage, spreading to hilar and mediastinal nodes in 60–70 per cent of cases with NSCLC. The development of mediastinal node masses may cause oesophageal obstruction. Pressure on the recurrent laryngeal causes vocal cord palsy with associated hoarseness and on the phrenic nerve affects diaphragmatic movement.

Blood-borne metastases can occur to all sites, in particular the bone, liver and central nervous system. These are seen at an early stage in SCLC, but also develop in many patients with NSCLC. (Fig. 7.1)

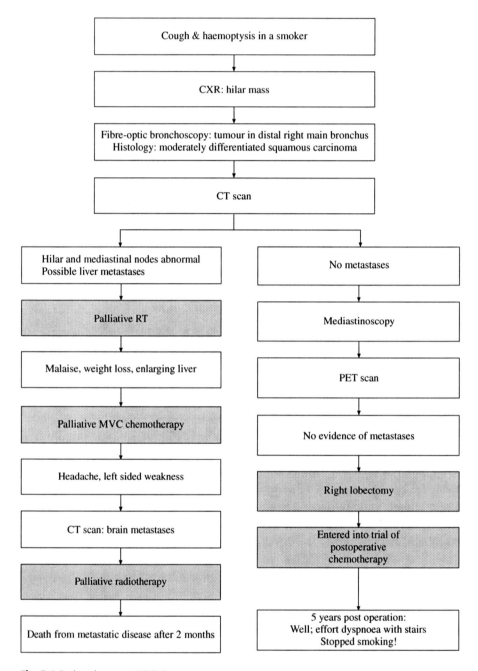

Fig. 7.1 Patient journey: NSCLC.

Prognosis

The overall prognosis of patients presenting with lung cancer is poor, with median survivals of less than one year. Approximately 20 per cent of patients with NSCLC may have disease limited to the lung, in which case radical surgery is appropriate. If these patients do not have involvement of lymph nodes up to 50 per cent may be cured, but involvement of nodes reduces this probability significantly; patients with only hilar nodes which are resected have a 30 per cent five year survival falling to only 15 per cent when mediastinal nodes are involved. For the remainder of patients with more advanced disease, the chances of surviving one year from diagnosis are less than 20 per cent.

In SCLC patients disease limited to the hemithorax may be treated with intensive chemotherapy, thoracic irradiation and cranial irradiation; 5-year survival in this group is however only around 10 per cent and this may be associated with significant alterations to their life style and performance status. The remainder of patients often have rapidly growing disseminated disease which, although sensitive to chemotherapy, progresses over a period of only a few months.

Key points

- Small cell lung cancer is typically widely disseminated at presentation.
- Non-small cell lung cancer may present with localised disease when surgery can be curative, but the majority of patients also have more widespread disease at presentation for which only palliative treatment is appropriate.
- Survival is poor for both types of lung cancer, worse for SCLC than NSCLC; even with the earliest stages only 10–20 per cent of patients are cured.

Common symptoms

Pain

There are well recognised pain syndromes in lung cancer associated with apical tumours infiltrating the brachial plexus, and peripheral tumours invading and eroding the ribs and chest wall. There may also be chest pain associated with the development of a more central bronchial carcinoma, though this is a relatively rare symptom and is often poorly localized with no specific features.

Metastatic disease most commonly causes pain from bone metastases. Headache may accompany brain metastases and rapid expansion of the liver may cause hepatic pain.

Pressure

Local growth of the tumour in the bronchus may result in distal collapse of the lung, or retention of secretions and accompanying infection. Irritation of the bronchial lining results in cough, and there is usually associated dyspnoea.

Oesophageal compression will result in dysphagia, either due to infiltration of the primary tumour, or involvement of surrounding mediastinal lymph nodes.

Extensive mediastinal disease may present with the syndrome of superior vena cava obstruction (SVCO) due to obstruction of veins returning blood from the upper part of the body to the heart. There is extensive venous dilatation and oedema above the nipple line, including the upper limbs, neck and face, and this presentation demands active treatment (see Chapter 24).

Metastases may cause spinal cord compression from extradural deposits, and pressure symptoms may arise from the growth of liver metastases or brain metastases.

Haemorrhage

Local haemorrhage will present as haemoptysis, which is rarely severe, although may be extremely distressing for the patient. Less frequently haematemesis may arise from oesophageal infiltration, and intrahepatic and intracerebral haemorrhage is a recognized complication of metastases in these sites.

Other symptoms

Symptoms commonly associated with lung cancer include hypercalcaemia, often as a result of a parathyroid hormone like peptide production and inappropriate ADH secretion (SIADH) causing drowsiness and confusion.

Pleural effusions are common resulting in progressive dyspnoea. Other paraneoplastic syndromes are recognised with lung cancer. These include myositis, myopathy, peripheral neuropathy and skin rashes of which the most striking is erythema gyratum characterised by erythematous whorls arising over the trunk. More generalized skin rashes may arise and erythroderma may be seen.

Hypertrophic pulmonary osteoarthropathy (HPOA) is particularly associated with NSCLC. The most common manifestation of this is finger clubbing but other bones may also be involved with a periosteal reaction seen as periosteal elevation on X-ray which may be painful.

Eaton-Lambert syndrome is also associated with lung cancer which presents with muscle fatigue similar to that seen in myasthenia gravis.

Key points

- Cough, haemoptysis, shortness of breath and chest pain are the common symptoms.
- Systemic symptoms of malaise and weight loss are common.
- Bone, liver and brain metastases are common.
- Metabolic and para-neoplastic symptoms are also well recognized.

Symptom management

Radiotherapy

Radical (high dose) radiotherapy may be given for localised NSCLC which is inoperable either because of local infiltration or the general condition of the patient but which is nonetheless confined to the thorax without extensive lymph node involvement. Typically, doses of 55–60 Gy in 4 to 6 weeks will be given. Recent trials have shown that better results can be obtained using shorter more intensive schedules such as CHART. This comprises radiotherapy treatment given thrice daily at 8-h intervals delivering a total dose of 54 Gy in 12 days. A randomized trial has shown a three year survival of 20 per cent with CHART compared to 12 per cent with conventional treatment delivering 60 Gy in 6 weeks, and a median survival of 16 months compared to 12 months. These represent the best results currently available with radical radiotherapy and are similar to other intensive combined radio-chemotherapy schedules.

For patients who have more advanced inoperable NSCLC, there is no advantage in giving radiotherapy to the asymptomatic patient and 30 per cent will die from progressive metastatic disease without developing chest symptoms. This 'watch policy' approach may however be difficult to accept for some patients who know that they have an advanced lung cancer and these will often receive 'prophylactic' radiotherapy which may prevent symptoms in many cases. Specific indications for treatment include lung collapse, haemoptysis, dysphagia and local pain.

There is good evidence from randomized studies performed by the MRC in the United Kingdom that one or two treatments is as effective as a more prolonged course in patients with advanced disease, and a single dose of 10 Gy, or a total dose of 17 Gy in two fractions one week apart are adequate and effective in controlling symptoms. Between 70 and 80 per cent of patients will report an improvement in local symptoms after such treatment.

The major acute toxicity of chest irradiation in such doses is transient dysphagia, usually lasting for no more than 7–10 days with spontaneous resolution. This can be managed with local agents such as mucaine or soluble aspirin if particularly troublesome. The technique of endobronchial irradiation is increasingly being evaluated in this setting. This involves the passage of a plastic catheter via a bronchoscope into the affected bronchus so that it passes alongside the tumour. This catheter is then used to direct a radiation source along the segment of bronchus affected by tumour, and in this way delivers a localized high dose of radiation. This is demonstrated in Fig. 7.2.

Treatment is a relatively simple single step procedure. However, one randomized trial has shown that it is less effective than external beam in the management of cough and chest pain, and its main role is retreatment after previous palliative or radical external beam therapy. The highly localized nature of the radiation means that further treatment may be delivered to the bronchial wall without added risk from damage to lung, oesophagus or spinal cord.

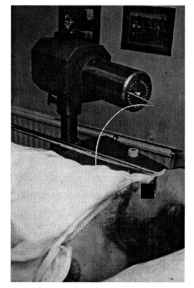

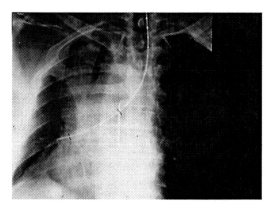

Fig. 7.2 Patient undergoing endobronchial radiotherapy (a) with endobronchial catheter passing from afterloading radiation machine to patient and (b) showing route of endobronchial catheter on chest X-ray.

Case History 7.1

A 74-year-old man has complained of an itchy purplish rash on his head and backs of hands for some months. This seemed to improve with topical steroid creams. The following year he coughs blood and lung cancer is diagnosed. He is given palliative radiotherapy to his chest for a locally advanced squamous carcinoma. The field encompassed his mediastinum and a mass at the right hilum. Seven months later his general practitioner requests admission to the hospice for symptom control. He is distressed by noisy breathing and has been coughing up blood on several occasions. Until the past week, he had been active in his allotment and maintaining his weight. Now he has stridor but no palpable nodes in his neck and no evidence of superior vena caval obstruction.

The symptoms suggest progressive tumour within the bronchial tree with narrowing of the main airway. He is sent across to the hospital. While his chest X-ray shows little change, bronchoscopy confirms endobronchial tumour growing from the right main bronchus into the trachea. It is possible to pass a catheter to deliver endobronchial radiotherapy and he has this in a single session under local anaesthetic.

He had been commenced on high dose steroids at the hospice and these are quickly reduced.

Case History 7.1 (continued)

There is noticeable symptom improvement within the next 2 weeks and he returns home. This is maintained for the following 10 weeks but he dies suddenly one day from a massive haemoptysis.

Practice points

- Dermatositis is a recognized paraneoplastic condition, characterized by a violaceous rash worst on sun-exposed areas. It may resolve with treatment of the cancer.

- Intraluminal radiotherapy is a useful technique where symptoms are directly caused by tumour in the airway. It is not effective for airway narrowing caused by external tumour compression.

- It can be used when external beam radiotherapy has been give previously but a reduced dose is used.

- Massive haemoptysis is caused by erosion of a major vessel into the bronchial tree. Endobronchial radiotherapy may increase the risk of haemorrhage but it is a well-recognized development in advanced disease.

Radiotherapy is also indicated for metastatic disease in the brain and bone which is symptomatic (see Chapters 20 and 23).

Radiotherapy also has a role in SCLC. Radical treatment will involve intensive chemotherapy but those patients responding well to this may be offered consolidation chest irradiation. There is little doubt that this reduces the rate of relapse in the chest and a recent overview suggests that there may be an improvement in 3-year survival of around 5 per cent. Prophylactic cranial irradiation may also be given to those patients responding well to chemotherapy. This will reduce the incidence of intracranial relapse from 23 per cent to 7 per cent with a smaller improvement in survival from 21 per cent to 16 per cent. (Fig. 7.3)

Palliative radiotherapy in SCLC will offer useful palliation of chest symptoms and problems from bone and brain metastases. Although not subject to the same systematic study as NSCLC, this is generally a very radioresponsive tumour often with rapid regression seen and similar low, hypofractionated regimes are used.

Key points

- Patients with localized tumour may achieve long-term survival with radical radiotherapy; accelerated treatment, e.g. CHART or chemoradiation is more effective than standard radiotherapy.

- Asymptomatic NSCLC unsuitable for radical treatment does not benefit from immediate radiotherapy.

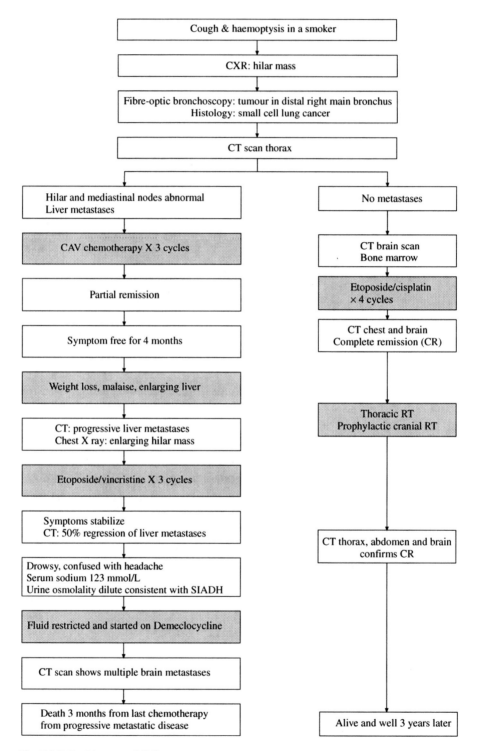

Fig. 7.3 Patient journey: SCLC.

- Radiotherapy given in one or two treatments will provide effective palliation for most patients with local symptoms, but for those with bronchial obstruction initial bronchoscopy with cryotherapy or laser therapy may provide more rapid relief of symptoms.
- Endobronchial brachytherapy may be considered for recurrent local symptoms after previous external beam radiotherapy.

Chemotherapy

Chemotherapy is the primary treatment for SCLC. A number of different drug combinations are in use, none of which has emerged as markedly superior. They commonly contain three or four drugs including cyclophosphamide, etoposide, adriamycin, cisplatin, vincristine or methotrexate. The common schedules are CAV (cyclophosphamide, adriamycin and vincristine or EP (etoposide and cisplatin)). Most patients will receive four to six cycles at three to four weekly intervals, and those achieving complete remission will proceed to thoracic and prophylactic cranial irradiation.

In recurrent and advanced disease there is good evidence to suggest that the quality of life for the patient is improved by giving chemotherapy, compared with simple symptomatic measures alone. A small advantage for combination chemotherapy using etoposide with vincristine or CAV (cyclophosphamide, adriamycin, vincristine) over oral etoposide alone has been shown in a large MRC trial with a median survival of 183 days compared to 130 days although the palliation of symptoms was equivalent and one year survival was 13 per cent and 11 per cent. For many patients therefore who present with advanced or relapsed disease simple treatment with oral etoposide may be entirely appropriate.

Whilst relatively non-toxic, even these simple chemotherapy schedules can result in bone marrow depression, with the risk of neutropenia and sepsis. It does, therefore, require careful monitoring by a unit experienced in the complications of chemotherapy.

Chemotherapy also has a role in NSCLC. Meta-analysis suggests a small but definite improvement in survival of around 5 per cent when chemotherapy is given after radical surgery or radiotherapy and current trials are addressing the role of cisplatin based schedules in this setting. There is also an increasing evidence that concomitant chemotherapy enhances the results of radiotherapy compared to using radical radiotherapy alone and increasingly chemoradiation is being used in this setting using cisplatin based chemotherapy during a course of radiotherapy.

In the palliative setting, chemotherapy should also be considered. A combination of mitomycin C, vinblastine and cisplatin (MVC) has been shown to improve tumour related symptoms in 69 per cent of patients when given three weekly for up to six cycles; 19 per cent of patients reported moderate or severe nausea and vomiting secondary to the chemotherapy. Small improvements in median survivals have also been demonstrated when chemotherapy is compared to 'best supportive care'. Many of the newer chemotherapy agents have been tested in NSCLC and have activity; common schedules now in use include gemcitabine, paclitaxel and vinorelbine in combination with either cisplatin or carboplatin. A direct comparison between chemotherapy such as this and radiotherapy has not been carried out; for most patients with local symptoms radiotherapy will offer high response rates and will usually be associated with less systemic toxicity when delivered as one or two fractions, for multiple systemic symptoms chemotherapy should be considered and may offer a small survival benefit also.

Key points

- SCLC is invariably disseminated at presentation. Patients with limited disease localized to one hemithorax may benefit from intensive chemotherapy followed by thoracic and prophylactic cranial irradiation, but cure rates are low around 10 per cent.
- Patients with SCLC may have better quality of life with chemotherapy at relapse than supportive treatment alone.
- Chemotherapy also has an increasing role in the palliative treatment of NSCLC.

Surgery

Surgery is the only curative treatment for early NSCLC and should be considered for all patients presenting with disease localised to the bronchus or with only hilar node involvement. Chest wall involvement and presentation with superior vena cava obstruction are not absolute contraindications to radical treatment. Careful staging including CT scanning and mediastinoscopy is essential to prevent patients with incurable disease, being submitted to thoracic surgery which depending upon the extent of the tumour will involve either lobectomy or pneumonectomy. Positron emission tomography has recently been shown to improve the accuracy of staging further over CT and MR alone and is increasingly being used to select patients for radical surgery. In addition, patients must be medically fit for surgery and have adequate lung function to cope with the loss of lung tissue which will result.

The major role of surgery in advanced disease is in the management of local symptoms due to progressive endobronchial tumour. Bronchoscopy with cryotherapy or laser therapy of the endobronchial growth can be highly successful in re-establishing a patent bronchus where this is obstructed, thereby allowing re-expansion of a collapsed lung or drainage of an area of infection. It may also be valuable in controlling persistent haemoptysis. Endobronchial stents may be used to maintain the lumen of a recurrently blocked bronchus and stenting of the superior vena cava is the best means of re-establishing venous drainage when mediastinal tumour has caused obstruction (SVCO) (see Chapter 22).

Other indications for surgery in advanced lung cancer may include intubation for dysphagia secondary to oesophageal involvement, and for metastatic disease fixation of pathological fracture or resection of solitary brain metastasis.

> ## Key points
>
> ◆ Radical surgery is the best curative option for localized NSCLC.
> ◆ Good palliation of local endobronchial symptoms can be achieved by laser, cryotherapy, intubation and stenting.

Hormone and other treatment

There is no role for hormone therapy in lung cancer which is universally hormone-resistant. Biological therapy has not been shown to be of value in this situation either.

Mesothelioma

Although rare mesothelioma can result in major problems for symptom control. This is a malignant tumour arising from the pleural or peritoneal surfaces. Intrathoracic mesothelioma is by far the most common form encountered and there is a very clear association between the development of this tumour and exposure to blue asbestos (crocidolite). A careful occupational history is therefore important when encountering patients with mesothelioma, not least because they are entitled to industrial compensation if the diagnosis can be confirmed. Despite this, however in up to a third of patients no history of asbestos exposure is ever demonstrated.

There are around 6000 cases of mesothelioma in the United Kingdom each year, the vast majority occurring in men who have had industrial exposure to asbestos. There has been a gradual rise during the century mirroring the utilisation of asbestos. This may be anticipated to fall in the forthcoming decades as awareness and careful regulation of asbestos use have developed.

Natural history

Mesothelioma develops as flat plaques growing on the surface of the pleura or less frequently on the peritoneum. It is often multi-focal with adjacent plaques eventually coming together to form a sheet of tumour encasing the pleural surface. Direct invasion of chest wall, mediastinum and diaphragm is common but distant metastases are rarely a major feature. There may also be involvement of the pericardium and primary mesothelioma of the pericardium is also recognised. In the abdomen, involvement of mesentery and bowel will result in obstruction and secondary ascites.

Clinical features

Pain

Pain is often a prominent feature of intrathoracic mesothelioma often pleuritic in nature and with more advanced cases becoming continuous and intractable.

Dyspnoea

Dyspnoea is also an inevitable feature as the lung is restricted by the encasing tumour. There may also be secondary pleural effusion further compromising lung function. Ascites from intra-abdominal mesothelioma or in reaction to a pleural effusion may add to the difficulties with respiration. Pericardial involvement with an associated pericardial effusion or constrictive pericarditis will create further problems with cardiac function and impaired exercise tolerance.

Other symptoms

Cough may be associated with the intrathoracic complications of mesothelioma. Invasion of the mediastinum can result in dysphagia and, if the recurrent laryngeal nerve is involved, vocal cord palsy with associated hoarseness and bovine cough. Involvement of mediastinal sympathetics may cause Horner's syndrome.

Key points

- Mesothelioma usually affects the pleural surfaces, but may also occur in the pericardium or peritoneum.
- Pain and shortness of breath are usually the most prominent symptoms.

Symptom management

Unless in its early stages, mesothelioma is rarely curable. Small intrathoracic plaques may be removed by pleurectomy but the disease is rarely localised with multiple plaques over the pleural surface being the usual case. There are advocates for extensive *en bloc* removal of lung, pleura and even associated chest wall and diaphragm in the hope of achieving local control. Despite this long term survivors are rare and most patients will present with more advanced disease.

Surgical intervention

Surgical intervention may still be appropriate to obtain control of progressive symptoms in the chest. Bronchoscopy and pleurectomy or surgical pleurodesis to seal the pleural cavity and prevent progression of secondary pleural effusion may be of value. There have been advocates for installation of various agents including mechanical irritants such as talc, chemical irritants such as tetracyline or bleomycin and intrapleural radioisotopes such as colloidal gold in the hope of achieving better control of intrapleural disease. The use of intrapleural chemotherapy and radioisotopes has not been shown to have advantages over mechanical pleurodesis which is usually more complete and effective.

Radiotherapy

Radiotherapy has only limited value in the management of pleural mesothelioma and is not used for intra-abdominal mesothelioma. Painful plaques of tumour may respond to palliative radiotherapy although there is limited data on its true efficacy. Doses of 20–40 Gy in 1 to 4 weeks have been advocated but there seems no advantage to high dose treatment over more pragmatic palliative schedules for palliation. There have been advocates for high dose radical radiotherapy to localised disease and combination chemoradiation has also been tried, but the results from this remain poor. Irradiation of the drain site after pleurodesis has been recommended and there is some evidence that this reduces the likelihood of seeding and tumour growth through the track.

Chemotherapy

Few chemotherapy agents have any impact upon mesothelioma. Occasional responses are seen with anthracycline drugs such as adriamycin and other combinations have included cyclophosphamide, cisplatin and mitomycin-C. Attempts have been made to use chemotherapy with radiotherapy or surgery to improve the poor results obtained with either modality alone but no evidence has yet emerged to support the routine use of either chemotherapy alone or combined modality treatment.

Other treatments

Pleural and pericardial effusions and ascites may require repeated drainage. This can be a difficult procedure as the chest wall is often encased with tumour so that drainage has to occur through tumour. Seeding with chest wall nodules growing through the drain sites can develop. Local radiotherapy to such sites should be considered if tumour growth is found to develop. Repeated procedures become increasingly difficult as scarring and loculation develops and appropriate pharmacological support in the management of the ensuing severe and often frightening dyspnoea with associated chest pain is essential.

Dysphagia due to mediastinal invasion may require intubation but this is rarely a problem featured in the absence of progressive respiratory symptoms.

Small bowel obstruction may be a feature of intra-abdominal mesothelioma. This is usually multiple level obstruction for which surgery can offer little and conservative management alone is indicated.

Key points

• Early disease may benefit from radical surgery with pleurectomy but typically disease is multifocal and cannot be completely cleared.

• In advanced disease local radiotherapy may be of value for pain relief and to prevent seeding along pleurodesis tracks.

• There is no proven role for chemotherapy in mesothelioma.

Case History 7.2

A 63-year-old electrician developed left sided chest pain and some shortness of breath. His general practitioner sent him for a chest X-ray which showed pleural thickening and a basal effusion. There were also calcified plaques and he had a history of exposure to asbestos nearly 40 years earlier. He was referred to the thoracic unit with a probable diagnosis of mesothelioma. This was confirmed by biopsy and a pleurodesis was performed after drainage of the effusion.

Although this improved his breathlessness, chest wall pain was an ongoing problem. Initially this was helped by weak opioids and anti-inflammatory drugs, but gradually worsened. Unfortunately he proved to be very intolerant of stronger analgesics. A repeat chest X-ray showed evidence of tumour destruction of several ribs. Palliative radiotherapy was given, covering the area of rib involvement, which coincided with the site of worst discomfort.

There was some improvement in pain for a few weeks after this but he gradually developed unpleasant hypersensitivity around his chest wall and a burning sensation. It was recognized that he now had a clearly neuropathic pain. Although the introduction of amitriptyline helped, he subsequently gained more relief with the addition of oral ketamine. It was possible to keep his pain under reasonable control until his death 12 weeks later.

Practice points

• Pain is often a difficult problem in mesothelioma and often has combined nociceptive and neuropathic components.

• Radiotherapy can be useful if there is localized, painful disease to target such as the site of chest wall invasion or tumour growing along biopsy tracks.

• Intrathecal alcohol injections can also be useful when pain is confined to a section of the chest.

• Deaths associated with mesothelioma must be notified to the coroner.

Chapter 8

Colorectal cancer

Colorectal cancer is the second most common malignancy in the United Kingdom, with an incidence of 30 000 cases each year and is responsible for over 20 000 deaths annually. The risk of developing this cancer rises sharply with age, doubling each decade from the age of 50 onwards.

Aetiology

It is believed that all bowel cancer develops by a sequence of events from dysplasia through to malignant transformation within an adenomatous polyp. This process is linked to predisposing genetic factors and exposure to environmental carcinogens. Asymptomatic polyps are probably present in 10 per cent of adults in middle age and beyond. The risk of carcinomatous change is greater in larger lesions (20 per cent in adenomas of 2 cm and more) and is 40 per cent in villous adenomas.

Cancer is a well-recognized development in people with familial polyposis coli; affected family members are identified as young as possible and are protected by surveillance and elective colectomy. However, 25 per cent of cases of polyposis appear to arise as a result of spontaneous genetic mutation and have no family history. The other important familial link is described as hereditary non-polyposis colon cancer (HNCC) and this probably accounts for 5 per cent of all cases. These individuals have a family history of frequent bowel, breast, and ovarian cancer. Among the population as a whole, bowel cancer in a first degree relative is associated with a threefold increase in risk. Inflammatory bowel disease is also associated with cancer, particularly in long-standing ulcerative colitis where the entire colon is affected.

Dietary causes have long been implicated to explain the high incidence in affluent Western nations. These include alcohol and a high saturated fat intake, which may lead to the production of certain carcinogenic bile acids by bacterial degradation. A low fibre diet reduces transit time and so lengthens the duration of exposure to carcinogens.

Efforts to reduce mortality from this common cancer by earlier diagnosis are hampered by the low specificity of screening tests such as faecal occult blood, and by the presenting symptoms which are often indeterminate and may be caused by other common bowel disorders. As yet there is no national screening programme for colorectal cancer within the general population, 75 per cent of whom have no obvious predisposing risk factors. Table 8.1 identifies the groups for whom counselling and possible active surveillance is indicated.

Table 8.1 Risk indicators for colorectal cancer within families

High risk (counselling and regular surveillance)		
Family with known genetic disorder		
◆ Familial adenomatous polyposis		
◆ Gardner's syndrome		
◆ Peutz–Jegher's syndrome		
◆ Hereditary non-polyposis colon cancer		
Family cluster of 3 or more cases of colon/endometrial cancer		
Ulcerative colitis (risk increasing with extent of disease and duration)		
Medium risk (require further assessment)		
Family history of bowel cancer		
◆ two or more relatives who presented with their cancers under 45 years of age		
◆ consider regular screening follow-up for first degree relatives of a patient who themselves are aged 50 or more.		
Low risk (no intervention)		
Only 1 case within a family, presenting in elderly relative		

Pathology

Adenocarcinoma of the bowel arises in the sigmoid colon and rectum in 70 per cent of patients. Of these, 15–20 per cent are mucin-secreting and may cause problems with discharge if arising in the distal bowel and rectum. The tumour may be polypoid, an ulcer or a stenosing lesion that has involved much of the circumference of the bowel. Spread is through the submucosal layers into and through the muscle layers of the wall; these features are used in the staging classification (see Table 8.2). The depth of invasion correlates with prognosis and the risk of lymph node involvement which is present in 60 per cent of cases where the tumour has extended through the entire wall. At this point, seeding can occur within the peritoneal cavity. The gut is drained by the portal venous system and this explains why the liver is the commonest site for distant spread. This is followed by systemic dissemination to the lungs and then other sites such as brain and bone. Rectal cancers can also invade the axial skeleton through the vertebral venous plexus, but for the majority of patients, the clinical course of the illness is dominated by the progression of intra-abdominal or pelvic disease.

Staging correlates well with survival following treatment. Only 10 per cent of patients have stage 1 disease at diagnosis and 20 per cent present with advanced cancer.

Carcinoembryonic antigen (CEA) is a serum marker of low specificity but is elevated in bowel cancer and this can be used in monitoring of patients after the primary treatment; levels of 20 μg/ml or more are significant. A rise in CEA predicts tumour recurrence in 75 per cent of relapses, sometimes months before clinically apparent.

Table 8.2 The staging of bowel cancer (TNM categories and Dukes' classification)

TNM (tumour, nodes, metastases)			Dukes
Stage 1	T1N0M0	Confined to mucosa	Stage A
	T2N0M0	Invades muscle layer	Stage B
Stage 2	T3N0M0	Invades beyond mucosa	Stage B
	T4N0M0	Invades other viscera	
Stage 3	T1–4, N1M0	Nodes involved	Stage C
	T1–4, N2–3, M0		
Stage 4	Any T,N + M1	Distant metastases	Stage D

Presentation

This depends upon the site:

- *Rectal tumours* produce symptoms of bleeding and mucoid discharge. As they enlarge, there is tenesmoid discomfort and a sensation of incomplete evacuation.
- Cancers of the *left side of the colon* may lead to altered bowel habits with episodes of constipation and diarrhoea as stool passes through a narrowed lumen. There may be abdominal distension and obvious blood in the stool. Up to a third of cases present with large bowel obstruction.
- *Right-sided* tumours present with small bowel obstruction and sometimes as 'appendicitis' with a palpable mass in the right iliac fossa. Others may develop iron deficiency anaemia and weight loss and the colonic cancer is found to be the underlying cause.

Management

Surgery is the mainstay of curative treatment and is often the best means of palliation. Whenever possible there is resection of the tumour with margin and re-anastamosis of the bowel to avoid a stoma. Depending on the site, a hemicolectomy or sigmoid colectomy is performed. Eighty per cent of patients undergo surgery with curative intent but half will subsequently relapse, hence the use of adjuvant treatment to reduce the risk of this. At least a quarter of cases are initially dealt with as an emergency procedure; these are associated with a higher complication rate, particularly in the elderly. In cases with obstructed bowel, there is a risk that the anastomosis may breakdown and therefore a temporary loop colostomy may be formed to bypass the obstruction which and can be reversed at a later date.

The surgery for rectal cancer depends upon the level of the tumour above the anal margin. If possible an anterior resection is carried out with anastomosis of the sigmoid to the rectal stump; tumours that arise 6 cm or less from the anal margin require an abdominoperineal resection and end colostomy. The mesorectum is also cleared to remove adjacent lymph nodes. Autonomic fibres may be damaged as a consequence of surgery and lead to subsequent impotence. The management of inoperable rectal cancer is discussed later in the chapter.

Adjuvant treatment

Radiotherapy

This has an important role in reducing pelvic recurrences in Dukes' stage B and C tumours of the rectum; in one series the recurrence rate was reduced from 35 to 15 per cent compared with a control group although the incidence of distant metastases remained the same. There is now evidence that it improves both disease-free survival and overall survival. Radiotherapy is given by either a low dose treatment immediately before surgery, or a longer post-operative course when the full extent of disease is known. It is not used as adjuvant treatment to sites elsewhere in the colon, as dose is greatly restricted by the tolerance of surrounding tissues in the abdominal cavity and the localization of the high risk area is more difficult.

Some cytotoxic drugs, including 5-flurouracil and capecitabine are radiosensitisers when given concurrently with radiotherapy. This may improve control of the local tumour but with increased side-effects.

Chemotherapy

Any attempts to improve outcome in colorectal cancer have focused on the use of systemic therapies, particularly for patients with evidence of lymphatic invasion. 5-Fluorouracil is a well-tolerated drug with a response rate of around 20 per cent in bowel cancer. This is increased if given by continuous infusion or in combination with folinic acid (leucovorin). Some studies have shown benefit from 5-fluorouracil and levamisole, an immunomodulator. Another approach is to insert a catheter into the portal vein at the time of surgery and infuse 5-fluorouracil over a 7-day period post-operatively. In patients with rectal cancer, this is also combined with radio-therapy.

It is now established practice for all patients with Dukes' C carcinomas (a third of all cases) to be offered 6 months of adjuvant chemotherapy with 5-fluorouracil and folinic acid. Large studies indicate that this may increase the survival for this group at 5 years from diagnosis from by a further 5–6%. It is generally well toler-ated but the side effects include stomatitis, diarrhoea, and neutropenia. Adjuvant treatment may be given to those with Dukes' B disease but is not used for Dukes stage A disease.

It is probable that the developments with new cytotoxic agents such as capecitabine and oxaliplatin for advanced disease will before long influence adjuvant therapy in colorectal cancer.

Results of treatment for operable disease

The outlook depends upon operability and stage at the time of surgery. Early cancer is certainly curable; over 80 per cent of patients with Dukes' stage A tumours are alive 5 years post-operatively. This falls to 60 per cent for stage B and around 35 per cent for stage C. Unfortunately, over half of all cases are in the latter category. The overall cure rate for all colorectal cancer is 30 per cent.

Most recurrences develop within 3 years and are seen in 40–60 per cent of those with positive lymph nodes. They may be heralded by a rising CEA level and in the absence of obvious tumour on CT scanning, a second laparotomy is sometimes performed. This might offer a further chance of surgical salvage for those with a recurrence at the site of the bowel anastamosis, or if there is a solitary metastasis, but probably does not help the outcome for many patients.

An individual with one colorectal malignancy is at greater risk of another. These can be multiple at diagnosis: 3–4 per cent of patients will develop a secondary bowel primary by 10 years after their initial surgery. While a colonoscopy should be performed at the time of, or following initial diagnosis, there is no recommendation for routine repeat examinations unless the individual has bowel polyps.

Problems associated with recurrent and late disease

These may be due to:

+ advanced or locally recurrent rectal cancer
+ recurrence at the site of the anastamosis
+ intraperitoneal disease
+ distant metastases

Around 10 per cent of patients with cancer of the rectum or sigmoid colon have advanced and unresectable tumour at diagnosis. The bowel lumen is narrowed by circumferential infiltration of the wall or by bulky tumour within it. Bleeding is common and mucin-secreting tumours may produce considerable discharge and often this is associated with an offensive smell and local pain; fistulae can develop between bowel, vagina, and bladder.

Locally advanced disease or recurrence in rectal cancer produces pain which may be in the perineum, localized to the sacral area, or radiating to one or both feet. This may be followed by foot-drop. Others develop urinary hesitancy and dribbling. A CT scan of the pelvis confirms the recurrence, typically in the pre-sacral area and often shows a distended bladder. Small bowel loops may become adherent to the pelvic mass with subsequent obstructive symptoms (see Fig. 8.1). In other patients, cutaneous infiltration of the perineum is sometimes apparent.

Many patients also have problems due to tumour deposits outside the bowel but within the peritoneal cavity. Those with tumour extension beyond the serosa or

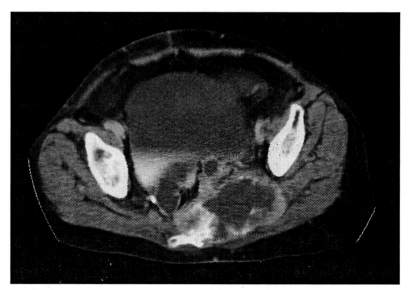

Fig. 8.1 CT scan of the pelvis showing recurrent rectal cancer which is invading the sacrum and causing obstruction of adherent loops of small bowel.

node involvement on the resected specimen are at particular risk. These may be associated with widespread intraperitoneal disease, ascites, and tumour invasion of the abdominal wall itself. Direct infiltration of the mesentery or secondary thrombosis can be a cause of pain. Confluent masses affect bowel motility can lead to obstruction. A second laparotomy is sometimes performed in these cases to establish the cause of symptoms as there is also a possibility that these could be due to post-operative adhesions or local recurrence at the anastamotic site. In some cases a colostomy provides good palliation but in others the tumour is too extensive for this to offer any benefit.

In advanced disease fistulae may develop adding to the distress of the individual patient. These can arise between adjacent bowel loops or from bowel to exterior abdominal wall, occasionally with a relief from obstruction. Communication between the transverse colon and stomach can cause faeculent vomiting.

The liver is the commonest site of distant spread following resection of bowel cancer and is the only detectable site in 40 per cent with recurrent disease. Other sites of metastases are lung, bone, and brain.

Most patients who die from colorectal cancer will do so about 3 years from diagnosis; the median survival from presentation of distant metastases is 8–9 months. However, some individuals do live longer with their disease and there are modest gains from systemic treatments such as chemotherapy.

Case History 8.1

A 45-year-old man develops recurrent abdominal pains, weight loss and anaemia. For some months his symptoms are managed as Crohn's disease but when he develops a right-sided inflammatory mass he undergoes a laparotomy. At operation he is found to have a carcinoma of the caecum which is invading to the outer surface of the bowel, although surrounding lymph nodes are found to be free of tumour. The primary is resected.

Twelve months later he again develops right iliac fossa pain. A CT scan shows recurrent tumour and also liver metastases. He commences chemotherapy with 5-fluorouracil but develops painful mucositis and diarrhoea. His pain proves difficult to control despite NSAIDS and high doses of opioids. His wife is extremely angry about the sequence of events and is fearful of any adjustment to his medication because he has been sleepy. She refuses professionals entry to the house and on one occasion disconnected a diamorphine subcutaneous infusion. This precipitated an emergency admission to hospital because of uncontrolled pain. It is clear that the patient himself is profoundly depressed.

The oncology and hospital palliative care team work closely together to help the patient and support his wife. An intrathecal injection of alcohol proves to be the best way of reducing pain and opioid requirements but has to be repeated at intervals of a few weeks. The depression also responds to treatment and he continues with chemotherapy. Although there is only a partial response on CT scan appearances, he copes well with treatment. Over a year later, there are lung metastases on his scan. Although not well enough to return to work, he has had a good quality of life and the couple have a better relationship with community and hospital staff. He continues treatment with oral capecitabine.

Practice points

- Tumours arising from the proximal bowel are less likely to obstruct the passage of stool and so may be diagnosed comparatively late.

- Intrathecal alcohol injection at T12 level blocks somatic pain arising from tumour invading the lower abdominal wall.

- Some patients with advanced bowel cancer may live several years alongside their slowly progressing disease.

Management of late disease

Surgery

Even if resection of the primary bowel tumour is not feasible, surgical palliation is often possible (Table 7.3). While survival is likely to be longer in those for whom resection has been possible, a diverting colostomy may be used and will dramatically improve the quality of life for patients with obstruction or fistulae. Median survival figures for palliative resective and non-resective surgery are 7 and 15 months respectively, although there are a small number of patients who survive several years with slow growing tumours.

Patients who present with extensive and fixed rectal tumours may obstruct, as the proximal bowel contents cannot pass through the narrowed canal. A palliative end colostomy may be necessary to prevent obstruction. This leaves the rectal cancer *in situ* and the distal bowel is closed and returned to the abdominal cavity as in a Hartmann's procedure. Palliative radiotherapy is usually given subsequently. The median survival for this group is 14–16 months and falls to 8 months for those with coexistent liver metastases. Fungating tumour involving the perineum, when radiotherapy has failed, is very difficult to palliate. Surgical resection and tissue coverage using myocutaneous flaps have been performed but this is a major procedure and would be suitable in only a very small number of patients.

A minority of patients who relapse with metastases apparently confined to one site such as lung or liver may have prolonged survival, and possibly cure, if all the disease is resected. This applies to those with a solitary metastasis or up to 4 deposits within one lobe; 5-year survival rates of 20 per cent have been described. This is discussed in more detail in Chapter 22.

Palliation by laser

Laser treatment has a place in palliation of rectal cancer, particularly when the patient is frail or declines to have surgery. It is of most benefit in dealing with small lesions, which are sometimes completely ablated. It can effectively control mucoid discharge and bleeding as might occur with progression of unresected disease in the rectal stump. This has also been used de-bulk tumour to increase the bowel lumen in rectal cancer and more proximal tumours of the sigmoid colon. Treatment can be performed under light sedation but complications include perforation of the bowel and haemorrhage; it is not suitable for disease close to the anal sphincter. Most patients undergo a number of treatment sessions especially if the aim is to maintain patency of the lumen. Larger, circumferential tumours are probably better palliated by a colostomy. Cryotherapy may also offer similar benefits.

Use of stents

Some elderly patients present with tumour obstructing the bowel. In those individuals who are too frail to undergo operation – or who would not be able to cope with a stoma – it may be possible to insert an expandable metal stent through narrowed segments from sigmoid colon up to the splenic flexure. In some this may enable a planned resection after relief of the obstruction. As with laser palliation, this is limited to the accessible left colon.

Case History 8.2

A frail 92-year-old lady presents with anaemia and altered bowel habit. She has mild dementia and lives in a nursing home, but co-operates well with examination and subsequent investigations. A barium enema reveals a carcinoma of the colon at the splenic flexure.

  She is successfully managed by laser treatment to the primary tumour under light sedation; this is repeated at three monthly intervals. This prevents development of bowel obstruction and reduces her occult blood loss.

Radiotherapy

Inoperable rectal cancer may be treated with pelvic radiotherapy. In the absence of documented metastases, a radical course of treatment is given over several weeks. The main side effect from this is the inevitable radiation proctitis which causes diarrhoea and tenesmoid discomfort. Radiotherapy is unlikely to cure inoperable patients, but in some, subsequent surgery becomes possible and will give the best chance of local tumour control. Radiotherapy can give good palliation of pain, bleeding, and discharge associated with a recurrent rectal cancer. Unlike a surgical bypass operation or laser therapy, it shrinks the bulk of tumour both within the bowel wall and in the adjacent pelvic tissues. The majority of patients will have improvement in pain, tenesmoid discomfort, and bleeding or discharge. This is likely to be maintained for several months.

  Fractionated treatment over several weeks is justified for patients whose general condition is good, in order to achieve a good and sustained result, especially as it may take several weeks to obtain the full benefit. Patients with a colostomy are spared troublesome proctitis. Radiotherapy is sometimes combined with chemotherapy, especially where there is both local and distant recurrence.

  In patients with extensive disease, single treatments with radiotherapy are sometimes given for pain and bleeding. Radiotherapy treatment which encompasses the pelvis cannot be repeated, but it may be possible to give a further palliative treatment to a localized perineal nodule or to bone destruction of the sacrum using a single field technique. Endoluminal brachytherapy can also be used to deliver single doses of 10 Gy to the mucosa to control bleeding; this is feasible even after prior pelvic radiotherapy.

  Radiotherapy may be used in other situations such as palliation of bone or brain metastases. Localized treatment can be used to treat symptomatic tumour masses involving the abdominal wall or recurrent disease around a stoma.

Chemotherapy

5-Fluorouracil with folinic acid has been the most widely-used regimen in palliative therapy. In many patients this is delivered by continuous infusion via a central venous catheter. The response rate is 20 per cent and people tend to continue treatment for at least 6 months or until there is evidence of progressive disease. Capecitabine is another pyrimidine analogue with the advantage of oral administration.

New drugs offer improved results, including those with disease resistant to fluorouracil. Irenotecan achieves responses in up to 15 per cent of the latter group and in one study comparing this with no active treatment there were twice as many patients alive at a year; for some this was a survival increase of 6 months. Oxaliplatin is another alternative option and now patients with progressive colorectal cancer are undergoing second and third line chemotherapy, not unlike those with advanced breast cancer. Significantly increased responses of 40 per cent, although with increased toxicity, come from combination of 5-fluorouracil with irinotecan or oxaliplatin as the initial treatment for those with recurrent disease.

The role of chemotherapy as palliative treatment in patients with inoperable recurrences or advanced disease at diagnosis is now well established with the potential benefits (to responders) of reduction and control of active symptoms due to the tumour burden, and improved survival. This must be set against the burden of toxicity although for many people there is an important psychological benefit of continuing with some form of treatment. Unfortunately some trials have omitted to evaluate quality of life parameters while others have included few elderly patients (75 or over) who make up a significant proportion of the population with colorectal cancers. It does appear that if chemotherapy is to be offered, it should be given early rather than waiting for major symptoms to develop but this may only be achieving an overall increase in life expectancy of 3–6 months.

Chapter 9

Breast cancer

The diagnosis of breast cancer is made in over 34 500 women in the United Kingdom each year and over 6000 of these are detected through screening programmes. It is responsible for the deaths of almost 15 000 women annually. Clearly breast cancer is one of the major malignancies seen by oncologists and palliative care professionals; its importance lies not just in the numbers, but also in the range of therapeutic opportunities for control of disease and relief of symptoms even in incurable patients.

Over 90 per cent of tumours arise from the epithelium of the terminal duct and lobule. Carcinoma *in situ* describes cells with malignant features that have not breached the basement membrane; those that have are invasive carcinomas. Paget's disease of the nipple is an eczematous condition which can cause bleeding and ulceration and is nearly always associated with an underlying duct carcinoma.

Several histological subtypes are described which may influence prognosis. Lobular carcinoma appears to be associated with multi-focal malignancy and more frequent metastatic involvement of the meninges and peritoneum compared with other types. Inflammatory carcinomas, as the name suggests, present with a red, swollen breast and can be misdiagnosed as infection. They behave in an aggressive fashion and have a poor outlook. Malignant tumours other than adenocarcinomas are rare but include lymphoma and soft tissue sarcoma. Cystosarcoma phylloides is an unusual tumour which comprises benign epithelial elements with sarcomatous change in a fibrous stroma and a third of these show malignant behaviour. This chapter discusses the identifiable causes of invasive carcinoma of breast and provides an outline review of treatment approaches in early and late disease.

Aetiology

Patients often search for an answer as to why they have developed cancer; in this particular malignancy a number of risk factors are known but even so it is rarely possible to determine the cause in one individual.

Although breast cancer is the commonest cause of death among women aged between 40 and 50, most cases develop in post-menopausal women and 40 per cent occur in patients aged over 70. While the incidence increases with age, the rate of increase actually slows with the onset of menopause. A small but increased risk is linked with obesity (in post-menopausal women), use of high oestrogen oral contraceptive pills and prolonged hormone replacement, and also to alcohol intake. Exposure to ionizing radiation has a well-documented carcinogenic effect but is rarely an identifiable factor in the cause of the disease.

It has been observed that post-menopausal women who are prescribed adjuvant treatment with tamoxifen develop fewer new primary tumours in the contralateral breast than might be expected. This apparent protective effect has lead to prospective administration of tamoxifen and newer anti-oestrogens to healthy women in an attempt to reduce the incidence of breast cancers. Results of on-going trials are awaited.

Genetic risks

As this is a common cancer there are always anxieties concerning other female family members and in some cases, genetic screening and surveillance is justified.

Many people worry about their family history but it should be remembered that breast cancer is a relatively common disease and in Britain only 5 per cent is linked with genetic susceptibility. This should be suspected if the family history includes the following:

- breast cancer in a first degree relative (doubles the risk),
- breast cancer in more than one generation,
- bilateral breast cancer in one or more individuals,
- diagnosis in second and third decades,
- familial clustering of cancers of the ovary, bowel, and prostate.

Transmission appears to be through either sex by an autosomal dominant gene but incomplete penetrance, so that affected individuals do not always develop cancer but can pass on the gene. Several genetic markers have been identified (e.g. the BRCA 1 on chromosome 17 and BRCA 2 on chromosome 13). Mutations involving the p53 gene occur in the Li–Fraumeni syndrome; members of affected families develop bone and soft tissue sarcomas, adrenal tumours and leukaemia, as well as breast cancers. It is worth referring individuals who appear to be at increased risk for assessment and advice from a medical geneticist.

Case History 9.1

Helen, age 37, has just completed a course of radiotherapy following lumpectomy for an early breast cancer. Although well-adjusted to her own situation, she confides to the breast nurse specialist that she is worried about her 9-year-old daughter – as she put it, 'It's struck our family again'. Further questioning revealed that Helen had previously lost an elder sister and their mother from breast cancer. Both women had been diagnosed under 40 years of age. The family history also recorded the death of a maternal aunt from ovarian cancer. Helen's sister (44) and brother were apparently well. Was her daughter at risk?

Practice points

- This family history, with a cluster of affected close relatives who developed cancer when comparatively young raises suspicions that there is an inherited gene responsible. Further research into the family history may uncover additional records of breast and ovarian cancer on the maternal side. With at least four affected individuals, a blood sample from Helen may establish that a BRCA1 mutation is responsible. If so, there are significant implications for this family.

♦ Helen herself is at increased risk of another cancer in the other breast and also of the ovary.

♦ Helen's daughter, remaining sister and brother each have a 50 per cent chance of having inherited the gene: if genetic testing is confirmatory with Helen, this can be offered to other family members with appropriate counselling. Those who are found to carry the gene have a greater than 50 per cent risk of developing breast or ovarian cancer in their lifetimes. They may be offered increased screening and some may wish to pursue prophylactic surgery (such as oophorectomy).

Principles of management

The aim of treatment in any patient with cancer is to strive for the best chance of cure. In breast cancer, a secondary and important objective is to achieve control of disease at the primary site and regional lymph nodes. The appropriate management will depend on the extent or stage of disease and the widely used classification is summarized in Table 9.1. In early breast cancer the incidence of detectable distant metastases at the time of diagnosis is very small and so investigations beyond blood profiles and a chest X-ray are not performed routinely. For patients without obvious dissemination,

Table 9.1 Staging of breast cancer (UICC and TNM)

UICC	TNM
Stage I	T1, N0, M0
Stage II	T1, N1, M0; T2, N0–1, M0
Stage III	T1–4, N2–3, M0; T3, N0–3, M0
Stage IV	Any T, any N, M1

where,

T1 = <2 cm

T2 = >2–5 cm

T3 = >5 cm

T4 = involvement of chest wall/skin or inflammatory carcinoma

N1 = ipsilateral axillary nodes

N2 = fixed ipsilateral axillary nodes

N3 = ipsilateral internal mammary nodes

M1 = ipsilateral supraclavicular nodes or distant metastases a further practical distinction is between those with operable disease (80 per cent) and locally advanced, inoperable disease. The surgical oncologist is best placed to define operability in an individual case, but characteristics of inoperable disease include:

- disease fixed to chest wall,
- satellite skin nodules,
- fixed axillary nodes or arm oedema,
- supraclavicular or parasternal node involvement,
- inflammatory carcinoma.

However, operable disease comprises stages I, II and a number of stage III patients with considerable differences in prognosis, as shown in Fig. 9.1.

Management of early (operable) breast cancer

The main options in early breast cancer are simple mastectomy or wide local excision of the tumour followed by radiotherapy to the whole breast. Without radiotherapy, 30–50 per cent would recur within the breast and irradiation reduces this to less than 10 per cent. Breast conservation is combined with surgical clearance of axillary nodes if these are involved; alternatively the axilla and supraclavicular area are treated with radiotherapy if sampled nodes are positive but an axillary dissection has not been performed. The histological status of the axillary nodes is important in order to define the stage and the need for additional systemic treatment.

The importance of informed patient choice is now recognized and respected, but considerations such as breast size, size, and position of the tumour and evidence of multi-focal disease will also determine whether breast conservation can be an option for that individual. For example, it may not be suitable for women with small breasts especially with large primary tumours. Some will in any case choose to have mastectomy, when possible breast reconstruction should also be discussed with the patient.

It is now accepted that local excision plus radiotherapy or simple mastectomy achieve similar results for local control and long-term survival. Radiotherapy may be given after mastectomy if the tumour was large, close to margins of excision, high grade, or involving lymph nodes. There is some evidence that post-operative radiotherapy to regional nodes may increase survival.

Prognostic factors

Over 50 per cent of patients with operable breast cancer will develop distant metastases and the extent of treatment to the primary disease does not appear to influence this. Even the more extensive surgical procedures – the so-called 'radical mastectomy' of the past did not achieve more long-term survivors than current conservative techniques. Overall, 55 per cent of women will survive 5 years and 35 per cent reach 10 years from

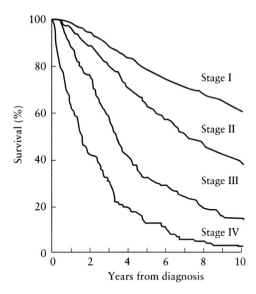

Fig. 9.1 Survival of breast cancer patients from diagnosis: effect of stage.

diagnosis, but late relapses continue. Important prognostic factors are stage and in particular, the status of the axillary lymph nodes. Other factors are differentiation of the tumour, age, and menopausal status. The effect of stage upon survival is shown in Fig. 9.1: 45 per cent of women with stage I disease are alive at 15 years but the results continue to decline with increasing stage. Those developing breast cancer when under 35 do less well and pathological features such as poor differentiation, vascular invasion, lack of oestrogen receptors and expression of epidermal growth factors all have an adverse effect on outlook.

Adjuvant therapies

The belief that we fail to cure breast cancer because of early dissemination of undetectable malignant cells has led to use of additional systemic treatments in the hope of improving results. Adjuvant treatment as either hormone therapy or chemotherapy is now a standard practice following the initial surgery and radiotherapy. This is given to all stage II and III patients and also those in stage I with poor prognostic indicators.

Post-menopausal women are given adjuvant hormone therapy with tamoxifen 20 mg, daily for 5 years. There is concern that this may be associated with a small risk of developing endometrial cancer but this has to be balanced against reduction in the chances of dying from breast cancer compared with untreated groups. For those with positive nodes, this approaches a 9 per cent reduction in the probability of dying from breast cancer at 10 years. The rates of local recurrence are also significantly less. Women who are still menstruating in their late 40s and early 50s might be offered ovarian irradiation as an alternative to tamoxifen; this will induce the menopause and periods usually cease within 3 months.

Pre-menopausal women who have positive axillary nodes are given adjuvant chemotherapy, usually over a 6-month period. A typical combination treatment is the CMF (cyclophosphamide, methotrexate, and 5-fluorouracil) or FEC (fluorouracil, epirubicin and cyclophosphamide) regimens administered on a monthly basis. The absolute survival benefit from chemotherapy appears to be around 6 per cent at 10 years from diagnosis. If adjuvant chemotherapy is administered to patients with stage 1 disease or to post-menopausal women, there is still discernible benefit, although less. However, for a chance to improve her outlook, an asymptomatic patient has to undergo the morbidity of frequent blood tests, hospital attendance, and side effects which include nausea, occasionally vomiting, hair loss, and increased infections among others. Some may also develop menopausal symptoms and cessation of periods. High dose chemotherapy is under evaluation in current trials, for women with more than 10 positive axillary nodes who are at very high risk of recurrence and distant spread. Another area of interest is whether endocrine manipulation combined with chemotherapy will prove superior to endocrine therapy alone.

Chemotherapy as primary treatment

The use of chemotherapy as the initial treatment of breast cancer is well established for patients with inflammatory carcinomas and younger women with locally advanced and potentially inoperable disease. For other women with operable tumours, there is an argument for administration of systemic therapy as early as possible, since more succomb to distant metastases than as a result of local recurrence. This also offers an opportunity to document the chemosensitivity of the individual tumour *in situ*; for some patients with larger tumours, this approach may improve surgical results by prior shrinkage of the tumour mass. There is a counter-argument that those individuals who do not respond are disadvantaged by the delay in surgery, which could result in loss of local control. However the response rates to primary chemotherapy appear to be as high as 70 per cent. This approach is not established for the majority of women who have early stage disease at diagnosis.

Problems associated with treatment for early disease

Surgical complications In the majority of patients, there are few complications following simple mastectomy once the wound has healed although, for some, the psychological morbidity may be considerable. However, this also applies to conservative treatments, as a similar proportion of women have difficulties in psychological adjustment. Damage to peripheral cutaneous nerves (e.g. section of the intercostobrachial nerve in the axilla), produces areas of numbness and neuropathic pain may follow in a few cases. A full surgical clearance of nodes entails dissection up to the axillary vein and lymphoedema of the arm is seen in 5–10 per cent of patients after surgery alone. The range of shoulder movement may be reduced and some will require intensive physiotherapy. Full dissection of the axilla may be superceded by sampling of the lowest, or sentinel, nodes. If negative, involvement of higher lymph nodes is less likely and this approach may spare patients from more extensive procedures.

Post-radiation problems Radiotherapy treatment is generally well tolerated but a skin reaction is to be expected during the latter part of the course and may take a further 4 weeks to settle. This is because the treatment must encompass the skin and superficial soft tissues. Techniques are used to keep the dose to the underlying lung to a minimum. The final cosmetic result, particularly for women opting for breast conservation, is usually very good.

The late effects of radiation produce increased fibrosis and vascular changes. These may range from telangectasia of skin capillaries to a shrunken or oedematous and painful breast in a very small number of women. Radiotherapy can also lead to a frozen shoulder and to lymphoedema of the arm after treatment to the axilla, especially if given after surgical dissection, which is discussed later in this chapter. For this reason the combination is avoided unless it is necessary to deal with residual or recurrent disease.

Late effects are insidious and progressive, often developing some years after the treatment, and women have been indignant about failure to discuss potential problems when treatment is proposed. Serious late damage includes rib necrosis and brachial plexopathy leading to a painful and functionless arm. Such major complications develop in less than 3 per cent and improvements in technique, and more restricted selection of patients for axillary irradiation, will reduce this further.

Case History 9.2

Peggy developed a lump in her breast 2 years ago, just after her marriage to her second husband. She has large breasts and so wished to have breast conservation. Axillary sampling was negative so she underwent a 5-week course of radiotherapy to the breast alone.

She developed a brisk, sore skin reaction during and after treatment which took some weeks to heal. Despite reassurance, her breast continued to be tender and painful. Peggy could not tolerate wearing a bra and was constantly fearful of someone knocking against her. Nearly 18 months later, the situation was even worse: she avoided any use of her arm on the affected side and had developed shoulder problems with limitation of movement. There were marital tensions and she was tearful and desperate, constantly searching for relief of her problems. A number of analgesics had been prescribed, from weak opioids to morphine, NSAIDS and steroids, all with lack of success.

On examination, Peggy had a tender breast, slightly reduced in size in comparison with the other, but no redness. The skin on her upper breast, around the lumpectomy scar was exquisitely sensitive and even light touch felt unpleasant.

> **Case History 9.2 (continued)**
>
> ### Practice points
>
> - Exploration of Peggy's anxieties: first to exclude recurrence of her cancer, which may require MR imaging as she could not tolerate mammography.
> - Review of the radiotherapy records with Peggy to answer questions about her treatment. This would confirm that there had been no errors leading to over-dosage of radiation. Unfortunately a very small proportion of patients do experience such problems following radiotherapy and this may be related to the larger volume of breast tissue that was treated in her case.
> - Such problems may gradually improve with time, but the immediate task is to focus on ways to help her live with the situation. Peggy had asked about mastectomy but agreed to try other approaches first.
> - Formal pain assessment looked at the impact on her sleep, psychological state and daily activities. She scored high on both anxiety and depression and agreed to an antidepressant.
> - Opioid analgesia was slowly withdrawn. Instead she responded well to a trial of topical capsaicin cream, targeting areas of hypersensitivity.
> - She underwent a programme of physiotherapy to improve the range of shoulder movements and to reduce musculoskeletal discomfort. She also responded well to complementary therapies.

Late effects of chemotherapy Adjuvant chemotherapy given to the pre-menopausal woman will cause temporary or permanent amenorrhoea, depending upon age. Permanent effects are likely in women over 40 years although the younger women may develop a premature menopause. Rare long-term effects are a small risk of congestive heart failure and also of myelodysplasias and acute myeloid leukaemia. This develops in less than 1 per cent of patients and is more likely if high dose therapy has been given.

Detection of recurrent disease Many recurrences occur within 2 years of the initial treatment but in breast cancer there is continued relapse, sometimes 10 years or more from diagnosis. The routine follow-up in an oncology clinic consists of a general enquiry followed by clinical examination of the breasts or chest wall and nodal areas; general practitioners are encouraged to share in the process to cut the number of hospital visits. Surveillance includes mammography; breast cancer patients have an increased risk of developing breast cancer in the contralateral breast and this occurs in 6 per cent within 10 years from the initial diagnosis.

Recurrence rates within the breast itself are low but affect 1–2 per cent of women annually after breast conservation. This may be manifest as a discrete mass, a cutaneous nodule, or increase in breast size and an inflamed appearance. Sometimes there is difficulty in distinguishing relapse from late effects of radiotherapy especially if there is oedema and induration of breast tissue. Clinical suspicions should be pursued by mammography and fine needle aspiration for cytology or biopsy; a number of patients can still be offered a chance of cure by further surgery. The appearance of chest wall recurrence may vary from one or more tiny nodules, perhaps in the line of the scar, or a small erythematous patch. Again biopsy is needed to confirm the relapse.

Other patients will relapse with an enlarged node in the ipsilateral axilla or supra-clavicular fossa. Some medially placed tumours may lead to subsequent involvement of the internal mammary nodes and present with parasternal swelling. A solitary mobile node would be excised to confirm the diagnosis, or alternatively a needle biopsy of a fixed mass is performed. Nodal involvement is an ominous finding as these patients often have more widespread dissemination, particularly once the supraclavicular nodes are enlarged.

Problems affecting the ipsilateral arm A difficult situation to deal with, is the patient who develops lymphoedema, pain, or a combination of both in the ipsilateral arm without any obvious clinical disease in the neck or axilla. Is this due to recurrent dis-ease high in the axillary nodes, or is it a late effect of treatment? Swelling of the arm in itself may be a sign of relapse, but can be due to fibrosis after surgery or radiotherapy given to nodal areas. It does not, however, result from radiotherapy to breast or chest wall alone. When surgical clearance and radiotherapy are combined, lymphoedema develops in at least one-third of patients.

Radiation-induced brachial neuropathy is fortunately a rare problem but has been seen as a result of a localized high dose at the junction between fields. In these cases the upper trunk of the brachial plexus is usually damaged, producing shoulder pain and symptoms affecting the C5 and C6 dermatomes. Thus, patients may develop paraes-thesiae and sensory change affecting thumb and forefinger, together with wasting of the muscles of the hand. Up to two-thirds of women with brachial plexus damage have subsequently lost function in the limb and hand.

In most patients, pain in combination with lymphoedema is due to recurrent cancer in association with spread to upper axillary and supraclavicular nodes. This is most frequently found in close proximity to the lower brachial plexus so that the distribu-tion of pain or any neurological signs is therefore more likely to affect C7–T1 der-matomes and will progressively worsen.

When there is no obvious palpable disease, a magnetic resonance imaging (MRI) scan is the investigation of choice in order to distinguish between active disease in the apex of the axilla and post-treatment fibrosis (Fig. 9.2) although it may still be difficult to make a diagnosis, particularly when there is diffuse infiltration. A CT-guided biopsy of abnormal areas may sometimes be necessary. Involvement of the upper thoracic and cervical spine is another cause of pain in the shoulder and arm, often accompanied by neurological signs. Metastatic disease in the spine can of course coexist with local

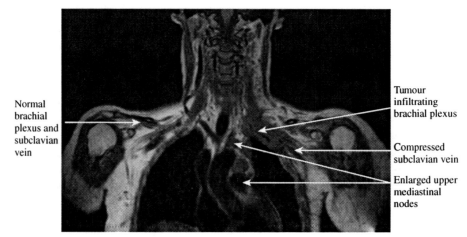

Normal brachial plexus and subclavian vein

Tumour infiltrating brachial plexus

Compressed subclavian vein

Enlarged upper mediastinal nodes

Fig. 9.2 MRI scan showing invasion of the left brachial plexus by recurrent breast cancer.

recurrence. Investigations should include plain X-rays followed by an isotope bone scan if the films show no obvious abnormality.

Failure of initial treatment Patients attending follow-up clinics often ask anxiously if they should be 'having a scan' and there may also be anger when distant spread has been discovered as a result of a symptom such as pain – 'I was seen 4 months ago . . . why wasn't this picked up sooner?' This is not surprising in times of increasing public awareness and also widespread community fund-raising for CT scanners. The reality, which perhaps clinicians are reluctant to discuss with patients, is that the incidence of distant spread detectable by present methods is too low in early stage disease to justify routine use, and in any case metastatic disease in breast cancer is incurable. For example, the incidence of abnormal findings on an isotope bone scan is less than 5 per cent in early stage disease. In contrast, the majority of patients with stage III disease will develop a positive bone scan within 2 years. However, it is difficult to justify treating an asymptomatic patient who would also be burdened with knowledge of her prognosis earlier than would otherwise be the case, especially as there is no evidence that earlier treatment would prolong survival. On the more positive side, patients with symptoms from metastatic disease can at least be offered effective treatment that may enable them to have several years of relatively symptom-free life.

Management of locally advanced breast cancer

Locally advanced disease at presentation

Patients with stage III disease at initial diagnosis are a heterogeneous group and more than 50 per cent will quickly develop evidence of metastases. The management of locally advanced breast cancer should be tailored to the individual situation and may involve several treatment modalities. Every effort is made to achieve control of the local disease and a toilet mastectomy provides immediate palliation of fungating tumour. As there is a substantial likelihood of recurrence, surgery is followed by radiotherapy and adjuvant treatment as previously described. Primary radiotherapy may also palliate symptoms, but two-thirds will have progression of the disease and so surgery is a better option where possible unless refused. Elderly patients should also be considered for appropriate surgery if the absence of other serious medical problems. To give these women tamoxifen alone is sub-optimal treatment for many.

Thirty per cent of surgically treatable patients survive 10 years but less than 15 per cent of patients with inoperable breast cancer are alive at 5 years. Fortunately, only a small proportion of women have inoperable disease at presentation although this may still be the result of ignorance, embarrassment or fear of treatment, particularly mastectomy. Tumour which deeply invades and is fixed to, the underlying chest wall is usually inoperable although in some cases extensive resection followed by flap reconstruction may be possible. In other cases, surgery may not be an option because of extensive satellite nodules beyond the breast or axillary nodes which may be fixed. Uncontrolled breast cancer is extremely distressing. Treatment in these situations is palliative but contributes greatly to the quality of life of the individual and so should be considered even in the presence of metastatic disease.

Radiotherapy can achieve good palliation of bleeding and ulcerated tumour, and sometimes subsequent mastectomy is possible following a good response to irradiation of the breast. This can, of course, be combined with hormone treatment or chemotherapy. Since patients may live a year or more with progressing local disease, the course of radiotherapy will be carefully planned and delivered over several weeks. Radiotherapy can produce regression of nodal disease that would otherwise cause lymphatic and venous obstruction and of course, pain.

Regional perfusion of cytotoxic drugs through the internal mammary artery has been used in selected patients to temporarily control disease. Younger patients with advanced disease and a poor prognosis are given systemic chemotherapy, sometimes as part of an intensive initial approach and then have surgery or radiotherapy to residual tumour in the breast. Chemotherapy is also given as the initial treatment to women who present with inflammatory breast cancer.

Some patients are found to have distant metastases at the same time as the diagnosis of advanced regional disease. They require a systemic approach and the primary disease may respond to this without any additional local measures; in the presence of serious problems such as brain metastases, local treatment of the asymptomatic primary breast tumour becomes pointless.

Locally advanced recurrent disease

Management will depend upon the previous treatment. Radiotherapy is not repeated to previously irradiated areas although some overlap might be acceptable with careful judgement (e.g. to deal with a parasternal mass). Occasionally low dose treatments to achieve growth restraint may give good palliation. A common finding is that the cutaneous disease is extensive over the trunk and there is little point in treating isolated small areas unless discrete lesions are painful or bleeding. Usually better palliation is achieved by hormone therapy or chemotherapy. Occasionally major surgical excision and reconstruction using flaps are possible for chest wall recurrence. Unfortunately, a number of women have to live with persistent disease, having exhausted these options, and local radiotherapy to symptomatic nodules is all that can be offered.

Metastatic breast cancer

Sites of disease

Ten per cent of women have overt metastatic disease at presentation. In others, evidence of dissemination precedes or coincides with local recurrence at the primary site in 45 per cent of patients. Local recurrence is the first site of relapse in one-third of patients. The most common first sites of distant relapse are bone, followed by lung. Metastatic breast cancer can involve a number of different tissues in the body although bone involvement is the most common site and often dominates the illness. Marrow failure due to infiltration is comparatively unusual, but may cause anaemia and thrombocytopaenia and this may limit the scope for chemotherapy.

In over 60 per cent of patients at post-mortem examination there is evidence of liver, lung, and pleural infiltration. There are adrenal metastases in half the cases although these are not so often detected before death. Up to 30 per cent of patients develop central nervous system involvement, which includes leptomeningeal as well as cerebral metastases. Visual field loss may be due to choroidal deposits which are found to be bilateral in 10 per cent of affected patients.

Patients with abdominal distension may have ascites. Although this is commonly associated with liver metastases, peritoneal deposits and secondary (Krukenburg) tumours in the ovaries are well described. Lobular carcinoma is a category of breast cancer which is well recognized in producing intraperitoneal disease. Sometimes there may be infiltration of the stomach and bowel itself although this is uncommon. Other organs that can be the site of metastatic deposits include the skin, heart and pericardium, thyroid, and even the uterine cervix.

Lymph node involvement is present in 70 per cent of patients with advanced breast cancer. As well as axillary node disease, regional nodes include supraclavicular, cervical and internal mammary groups. Involvement of mediastinal lymph nodes can cause hoarseness, dysphagia, and a picture of superior vena caval (SVCO) obstruction. Sometimes upper abdominal nodes are enlarged and can cause extrahepatic biliary obstruction.

Prognosis

The prognosis in women with metastatic disease is worsened by:

◆ short duration from initial treatment to relapse (disease-free interval)

◆ visceral metastases rather than bone

◆ multiple sites of disease

Examples of reported median survival times are given in Table 9.2.

Treatment options

Decisions about the best plan of treatment for an individual patient will be based on the following considerations:

◆ localized or multiple symptomatic sites of disease

◆ the general condition and performance status of the patient

◆ age and menopausal status, which will influence the use of hormone manipulation

◆ previous treatment (e.g. radiotherapy, or adjuvant chemotherapy)

◆ the presence of progressive visceral disease and other indications for urgent intervention (e.g. hypercalcaemia, fracture, cord compression)

Metastatic breast cancer is incurable but there is considerable useful treatment to be offered. This will consist of direct local intervention (e.g. by surgery or radiotherapy), together with systemic treatment by hormone manipulation or chemotherapy.

Hormone manipulation

Breast cancer is one of the few malignancies that responds to changes in the hormonal environment. This is due to the presence of hormone receptors on the surface of the nuclear membrane of breast cancer cells. The mechanism of response is complex and many different hormone manoeuvres may be effective in the management of breast cancer. This is explained by the altered sensitivity of oestrogen receptors, loss of oestrogen receptors, or varying expression of other hormone receptors that are as yet unidentified.

Table 9.2 Median survival times from relapse in breast cancer patients

Site	Median survival (months)
Local recurrence only	34
Bone (no other site)	20
Lung	10–12
Liver	2–6
Brain	3–6

Hormone therapy is used to improve survival as adjuvant therapy for early cancer, while in later stages it can bring about control of widespread disease and palliation of symptoms. It is also fortunate that, in general, hormone therapies are well tolerated and can be given with benefit to ill patients of poor general condition and in the very elderly. However, they are not without side effects; the gain is in useful regression of disease rather than cure and the time to obtain a useful response may be 2–3 months – too long if there are distressing or life-threatening problems. They are therefore most valuable in treatment of slowly progressing cutaneous and nodal disease or bone metastases.

The earliest hormone treatments were achieved surgically, by removal of the ovaries in pre-menopausal women with metastatic breast cancer. Subsequently, it was found that bilateral adrenalectomy produced a response in post-menopausal patients and also that hypophysectomy was effective. An easier and more acceptable alternative to oophorectomy was the 'radiation menopause' produced by irradiation of the ovaries and still in use today. In most patients, pharmacological treatments are used to alter the hormonal environment and these are reversible on discontinuation of therapy. All hormone treatments, when used initially, achieve an overall response rate of 30–40 per cent; this is lower in pre-menopausal women and may reach 70–80 per cent in the elderly.

Benefit is predicted by the presence of oestrogen receptors in the tumour; this is determined using immunohistochemical staining of the receptors on tissue sections from the primary tumour. Those tumours which exhibit high levels of the receptor are in general most sensitive. However, this information is not always available and around 10 per cent of receptor-negative patients also do respond, so that a trial of hormone treatment is often given without knowledge of the receptor status. There should be evidence of a useful clinical response within 2–3 months (e.g. bone pain may lessen or there is visible regression of skin nodules). After this has been achieved, treatment is continued until there is evidence of disease progression. These patients are then likely to have a beneficial response to subsequent hormonal manoeuvres, which are used in sequence when there is evidence of further relapse. However, the proportion of good responders is less with second- and third-line therapies and the alternative is then a trial of chemotherapy.

The order in which endocrine therapies are used is usually to start with those with least side effects and easiest administration. Options are as follows:

Tamoxifen This is probably the most common hormonal therapy in use and major advantage is its relative lack of side effects. Taken orally in a dose of 20 mg daily, the major problems are occasional nausea, hot flushes, and weight gain. Endometrial hyperplasia may occur with long-term use resulting in vaginal discharge or bleeding and, rarely, endometrial carcinoma has been reported. Another rare complication is retinopathy and, visual disturbances whilst taking tamoxifen should always be formally evaluated by slit lamp examination. Occasionally patients notice a flare of their symptoms when tamoxifen is first started and this reflects the fact that tamoxifen has both stimulatory as well as oestrogen-blocking effects. This results in some advantageous side effects including the fact it maintains bone mineral density and provides cardiovascular protection in a similar way to the naturally occurring oestrogen in the pre-menopausal woman. Few women find tamoxifen difficult to tolerate although occasionally hot flushes become unacceptable.

Newer drugs, which are non-steroidal analogues of tamoxifen, have been developed in the hope of reducing the agonist effect while maintaining the anti-oestogen action. Of these, *toremifene* is now licenced for use in post-menopausal patients but the clinical advantage is uncertain. More promise is shown by another group of compounds, steroidal anti-oestrogens, which may be more effective than tamoxifen. *Faslodex* has a high affinity for the oestrogen receptor, has no stimulatory action and also leads to 'down regulation' and reduction of receptors. Women with advanced disease whose tumours have become resistant to tamoxifen are shown to respond to this drug, with lasting remissions of up to 2 years.

Progestogens An alternative to tamoxifen therapy in breast cancer is the use of a progestogen such as *megestrol* or *medroxyprogesterone acetate*. They may be used as primary treatment in breast cancer but more commonly are given to patients who relapse whilst on tamoxifen. Patients who have previously responded to tamoxifen will respond to a change to progestogen in up to 50 per cent of cases. Either megestrol 80 mg b.d. or medroxy-progesterone 200 mg t.d.s. are commonly given. Side effects may include water retention, weight gain, and depression and some women develop a cushingoid appearance with prolonged use. However, a beneficial effect of progestogens can be an improvement in well-being and appetite.

Aromatase inhibitors These drugs inhibit the action of peripheral aromatase enzymes which are important in the production of oestradiol from its precursors synthesized in the adrenals. They therefore block oestrogen production in tissues other than the ovary and are used in post-menopausal patients. *Aminoglutethimide* was an early example of an unselective inhibitor which also blocked corticosteroid production so that hydocortisone replacement was necessary. It also tended to produce more side effects than tamoxifen or progestogens, including nausea, a flu-like illness, liver dysfunction, and a characteristic skin rash (usually of short duration). Newer aromatase inhibitors are more selective and steroid replacement is not required, but their use remains confined to post-menopausal patients. Steroidal compounds include *formestane* and *exemestane*. Formestane has the disadvantage of requiring a 2-weekly injection but is often associated with fewer side effects than aminoglutethimide. Exemestane is given orally.

The non-steroidal aromatase inhibitors such as *letrozole* and *anastrazole* show effective anti-oestrogen activity with low toxicity; they do not cause the weight gain seen with progesterones and have better results than megestrole acetate as second-line therapies. Anastrazole (Arimidex) may even displace tamoxifen from its place as first-line endocrine therapy for both advanced disease and as an adjuvant treatment in early breast cancer.

Androgen therapy Occasionally, androgen therapy is used as a further means of altering the hormone environment in breast cancer and achieving additional hormone responses. *Deca-Durabolin* is a depot preparation administered by intramuscular injection every 3 weeks. It is generally well tolerated but some women do notice changes from the androgen stimulation with increased hair growth, deepening of the voice, and increased libido.

LHRH agonists These are being used in pre-menopausal patients as a means of completely suppressing ovarian oestrogen production, comparable with castration. Any means of ovarian ablation in younger women can produce distressing menopausal symptoms; this approach has the advantage of being reversible if a response is not achieved. *Goserelin* 3.6 mg is given by a subcutaneous depot injection every 4 weeks. Superior response rates have been claimed for LHRH agonists in combination with tamoxifen.

Corticosteroids Before other effective endocrine therapies became available, it was recognized that there was a response to cortisone and prednisolone in low doses. This can still be given as a useful adjunct to other treatments for metastatic disease.

Case History 9.3

Sequential therapies in progressive breast cancer

A 51-year-old woman has a lumpectomy followed by radiotherapy to the breast for a 2.5 cm carcinoma. The tumour tissue has oestrogen and progesterone receptors present.

Within a few months she has developed an enlarged node in the ipsilateral supraclavicular area. Further radiotherapy is given to this site. Further relapse is likely and so options for systemic treatment are considered. As the tumour is likely to be hormone responsive, this is chosen as likely to be better-tolerated than chemotherapy. She is still menstruating although cycles are becoming erratic. She is offered a single radiotherapy treatment to the pelvis to induce a complete menopause. This is acceptable to her. Within 3 months menstruation has ceased and she has frequent sweats and hot flushes. HRT is not recommended in this situation but fortunately low dose clonidine is helpful.

10 months later she develops persistent backache. Plain X-rays show wedge collapse of T12 vertebral body. There are several areas of increased uptake on an isotope bone scan consistent with metastases.

Local radiotherapy is given to the lower thoracic spine and she commences anastrazole 1 mg daily. She remains well for some time after this, but multifocal sites of bone pain flare up 18 months later and her bone scan indicates progressing disease, although there are no other sites of metastases. This time the hormone therapy is switched to tamoxifen 20 mg daily and the plan is to give monthly bisphosphonate infusions (pamidronate 90 mg). Her symptoms at this stage respond to a weak opioid – NSAID combination.

However within a further 6 months there is evidence of skin nodules on her scalp and abdominal wall, and asymptomatic lung metastases on her chest X-ray. A further switch in treatment is made to exemestane 25 mg daily but on this occasion the response is poor. Within weeks she is becoming breathless as her pulmonary disease progresses. It is evident that her tumour is now resistant to endocrine manipulation and at this point she commences chemotherapy.

Systemic chemotherapy in advanced breast cancer

Chemotherapy can improve and control symptoms associated with metastatic spread and uncontrolled local breast cancer, with useful responses seen within a few weeks. While there seems to be a correlation between response and median survival in some series, the benefit is small and the aim of chemotherapy in advanced breast cancer is to improve quality of life rather than to prolong it.

Chemotherapy is used in younger women who are less likely to obtain a useful response to hormone manipulation or in situations such as symptomatic lung metastases in which a response is needed as quickly as possible. Systemic chemotherapy is more effective than local instillation of drugs in cases with effusions or ascites. It is also used for recurrent disease in previously irradiated areas when further radiotherapy or surgical salvage is not feasible. Older patients with progressing disease who have failed to respond to hormone therapy may also benefit from chemotherapy; general health and performance status are more important than absolute age when considering treatment options.

A number of cytotoxic drugs are active against breast tumours, of which the most effective single agents are anthracyclines (e.g. adriamycin or epirubicin), which produce a response in 30–40 per cent of women. Taxoids (docetaxol, paclitaxel) are a newer group of compounds that have produced responses even in heavily pre-treated women; this argues for their use as first line but this is undergoing careful scrutiny because of their expense. Combinations of drugs are given to improve the response rate further. Examples of commonly used regimens are:

CMF: cyclophosphamide, methotrexate, and 5-fluorouracil (5-FU)
AC, FAC or FEC: 5-fluorouracil, adriamycin/epirubicin, and cyclophosphamide
MMM: methotrexate, mitoxantrone, and mitomycin

Such treatments can produce good responses in over 50 per cent of patients who have not previously been treated with chemotherapy, although complete regression of disease is uncommon. Evidence of a beneficial effect should be apparent by the second or third course and treatment is usually continued for about six courses in total to maintain the benefit. The median duration of response is 6–8 months and these patients have a median survival of 18 months. As with endocrine therapy, second-line chemotherapy may be given but the chances of a useful response are smaller but are possible; some patients may continue with third- or fourth-line treatments. Other drugs with activity in breast cancer include vinorelbine, gemcytabine and capecitabine. These alternative drugs may offer useful responses in women who have become resistant to anthracyclines.

Specific toxicity depends on the drugs and doses given. Hair loss is not a problem for patients treated with MMM but is a disadvantage of using adriamycin, although this can be countered by scalp-cooling during administration. Nausea and myelosuppression are frequent problems and as much as possible is done to support the patient through this. This includes the use of effective anti-emetics, particularly the 5HT3 antagonists, and the use of central venous lines for easier venous access.

The use of higher doses of cytotoxic drugs is often limited by marrow toxicity and fatal infection as a result of severe myelosuppression. This can be circumvented by the use of haemopoietic colony stimulating factors or harvested peripheral blood progenitor cell support in autologous bone marrow transplants. Early data on high dose chemotherapy in patients with advanced cancer suggests that this can achieve a higher response rate, more complete responses and prolonged duration of benefit. Unfortunately, the benefit in terms of longer survival is at present doubtful and such procedures have significant associated morbidity.

In general, chemotherapy is useful as a palliative treatment in advanced breast cancer and there is evidence that improvements in symptoms and quality of life do correlate with tumour response. Treatment may also prolong survival, for example in patients with liver metastases. While elderly patients with advanced breast cancer may benefit from chemotherapy after failure of hormone manipulation, it is important that regimens of low toxicity are used.

Sometimes a trial of different regimens is given one after the other even though at best these might only offer a chance of slowing inexorable disease progression with no prolongation of life. In such situations there should be honest discussion about the aims of treatment and the drawbacks; even so a number of patients decide that active treatment is worthwhile and will continue with it as long as it is offered.

Herceptin Between 20–30 per cent of breast cancers over-express a protein, HER2, which is an epidermal growth factor. This is associated with increased cell proliferation and metastatic spread. Such tumours are less likely to respond to endocrine treatments, and tend to be associated with a worse prognosis.

Herceptin (trastzumab) is the product of monoclonal antibodies directed against the HER2 protein. It is given as an intravenous infusion to patients whose tumours show such activity, based upon immunohistochemical staining of the cell membrane. This may achieve responses even in women who have been through considerable prior treatment and may prove to be even more useful in combination with chemotherapy by increasing response rates with little or no increase in toxicity.

Bisphosphonates These drugs, initially introduced for the treatment of hypercalcaemia, appear to offer a significant improvement to the quality of life for women with incurable breast cancer. Both oral clodronate and intravenous clodronate or pamidronate, administered over a 12–24 months, appear to reduce skeletal morbidity in terms of a 30–40 per cent reduction in vertebral collapse, other pathological fractures, hypercalcaemic episodes and a reduction in requirement for radiotherapy for symptomatic sites. The expense of the drugs may be offset by fewer hospital admissions and less need for orthopaedic surgery in particular. It would be desirable to institute such treatment in all patients with progressing bone disease before significant structural damage has occurred, and presumably to continue indefinitely; this would be in addition to other systemic anti-tumour therapy. Not surprisingly, bisphosphonates are not in routine long-term use but an attempt has been made to identify those patients who might benefit most. The Guidelines of the British Association of Surgical Oncology (BASO) for management of bone metastases in breast cancer include recommendations from the Yorkshire Cancer Group (YCRC). The latter offer a practical approach in selection of patients for 'pre-emptive' use of bisphosphonates (Table 9.3). These prioritise those patients who have symptomatic metastases which are not responding to endocrine therapy, but in whom disease is mainly confined to bone. In contrast, a patient who also has lung or liver metastases is unlikely to survive long enough to benefit from long term bisphosphonates. However in all patients with multifocal bone pain, clodronate or bisphosphonate infusions have been tried for short term symptom relief and improved pain has been noted within 2–4 weeks.

Newer agents such as ibandronate and zoledronate are becoming available and are more potent than the previous drugs. The possible benefits of combining bisphosphonates with chemotherapy remain to be seen.

Treatment decisions in metastatic breast cancer

Once widespread cancer has been diagnosed, the management plan for the individual patient will be a combination of therapeutic manoeuvres:

- Systemic therapy, i.e. endocrine or chemotherapy in an attempt to control the overall pace of disease: this in turn is influenced by the likelihood of response to hormone manipulation, previous treatments and the clinical urgency
- Localized treatment, i.e. radiotherapy, directed at specific sites of disease which are causing actual or potential problems (Table 9.4)
- Other palliative interventions, which are not directed at tumour control but enhance quality of life.

Table 9.3 Use of bisphosphonates in breast cancer with bone metastases: a scoring system to select those who might benefit from long-term use
Local guidelines of the YCRC in The Management of Metastatic Bone Disease in the United Kingdom by the Breast Specialty Group, British Association of Surgical Oncology. [European Journal of Surgical Oncology 1999; 25:3–23]

	Score
Disease Extent	
Bone (marrow) only	3
Bone and soft tissue	2
Bone and visceral disease	1
Bone Morbidity	
Previous skeletal event +/− bone pain	3
Bone pain	2
Asymptomatic	1
ECOG Performance Status	
1, 2	3
0, 3	2
4	1
Underlying Treatment	
Chemotherapy/endocrine resistant	2
Potentially endocrine sensitive	1
Good Prognostic Factors	
Disease-free interval >3 years	1
Pre-menopausal	1
Ductal grade 1 or 2 or lobular carcinoma	1
Bone metastases at initial presentation	1

Total score and interpretation:
>11 Highest priority for long-term bisphosphonate treatment
7–11 Moderate priority
<7 Low priority

It is important that from the time of recognition of incurable disease, the potential for useful life prolonging and life-enhancing approaches are emphasised but also that treatment of the tumour is but part of a spectrum of help and support to patient and family. This becomes increasingly important as the oncological options become exhausted.

Table 9.4 Role of palliative radiotherapy in advanced breast cancer

Control of locoregional disease: *Usually fractionated treatment to breast and/or regional lymph nodes*

◆ Massive tumour within breast

◆ Tumour fungation

◆ Enlarged SCF, axillary or internal mammary nodes

◆ Brachial plexus involvement

◆ Mediastinal tumour

◆ Chest wall recurrence after surgery

Symptom-directed palliation of distant metastases: *Single treatments often used for bone pain*

◆ Bone metastases

◆ Spinal cord compression

◆ Bleeding/painful skin nodules

◆ Choroidal metastases

◆ Cerebral metastases

Radiotherapy rarely used or unhelpful: *Consider systemic treatment, i.e. hormone manipulation or chemotherapy if appropriate*

◆ Previously irradiated site

◆ Liver metastases/ascites

◆ Lung metastases/effusions

◆ Bone marrow infiltration

◆ Short prognosis, e.g. less than 4 weeks

Chapter 10

Urological cancer

Bladder cancer

This is a relatively common cancer with over 10 000 cases in the United Kingdom each year, affecting twice as many men as women. It encompasses a wide spectrum of disease from the very good prognosis, superficial well-differentiated bladder tumours to very aggressive muscle invasive tumour with a poor prognosis.

Pathology and natural history

The majority of bladder cancers are transitional cell carcinomas arising from the epithelial lining of the bladder. Rarer forms are squamous carcinomas seen particularly in relation to chronic inflammatory conditions, such as schistosomiasis, and even rarer are adenocarcinomas.

The common transitional cell carcinoma is related to a number of aetiological factors suggesting that in many cases it is a response to exposure of the urothelium to certain chemicals in particular products of the cable and rubber industry, aniline dyes, smoking, and drugs such as cyclophosphamide. Most tumours probably arise as a dysplastic change which progresses to an in situ carcinoma and subsequently invasive carcinoma. Whilst many bladder cancers present with an established invasive carcinoma, a significant number of patients have a superficial tumour on presentation which is limited to the mucosa. In around one-third of these there will be progression to a more sinister muscle-invading tumour but the remainder will be cured by local resection at cystoscopy and surveillance.

It is the muscle invasive bladder cancer and the high grade superficial bladder cancer which is likely to lead to metastatic disease and ultimately be fatal. These tumours disseminate through pelvic lymph nodes and blood-borne metastases particularly involving lung, liver, and bone. Progressive local disease within the bladder and involving the ureteric orifices may result in hydronephrosis and ultimately renal failure.

A small number of patients have a generalized change in the urological epithelium and multiple tumours develop throughout the tract from the renal pelvis through the ureters and bladder to the urethra.

The prognosis from bladder cancer depends upon the degree of invasion and histological grade. Well-differentiated superficial bladder cancers are invariably cured unless they progress to more sinister types. The overall outlook for muscle invasive bladder cancer or high grade superficial bladder cancer, whether treated by radical radiotherapy or surgery, is for a 5-year survival of around 40 per cent. Death may be from widespread metastatic disease or renal failure secondary to bilateral ureteric obstruction.

Key points: bladder cancer pathology and primary management

- Common bladder cancers are transitional cell cancers; may be low or high grade. Divided into superficial or deep, having invaded muscle wall.

- Superficial bladder cancer can be managed by cystoscopic resection and observation unless progression to a high grade tumour or muscle invasion is seen. This develops in around 30 per cent initially presenting with superficial disease.

- High grade superficial bladder cancer (T1G3) and muscle invasive tumours (T2 or T3) may be managed with either radical radiotherapy reserving cystectomy for salvage if this is unsuccessful or primary radical cystectomy.

- Renal failure is not necessarily a contraindication to radical treatment which can be given following the insertion of a percutaneous nephrostomy or intra-ureteric stent. In advanced disease, however, intervention may be inappropriate.

Common symptoms

Haemorrhage

The most common presenting symptom of bladder cancer is haematuria. Any patient presenting with this symptom requires urgent investigations to exclude bladder cancer or indeed neoplasia elsewhere in the urogenital tract. The bleeding itself is usually self-limiting or will be readily controlled following cystoscopy and trans-urethral resection of the tumour. In advanced tumours, or the later stages of recurrent disease, however, it can be persistent and troublesome, causing bladder spasm and clot retention.

Pain

Bladder cancer may cause local pain due to bladder spasm and occasionally in more advanced cases infiltration into the extravesical tissues and even the pelvic bones. Involvement of pelvic and para-aortic nodes may cause deep pelvic or back pain as they enlarge. Dysuria may be a feature and is often associated with frequency and nocturia due to bladder irritation from the tumour mass. Ureteric obstruction may result in painful distension of the proximal tract and hydronephrosis with loin pain. Bone metastases are a feature of the natural history of bladder cancer and local bone pain may occur.

Pressure symptoms

The main problem which may arise is due to ureteric obstruction causing obstruction to renal outflow and ultimate hydronephrosis and renal failure. Pelvic lymphadenopathy may result in lower limb oedema and must be distinguished from deep venous thrombosis as a cause of leg swelling; this may be obvious clinically or require venography to determine the patency of the leg veins.

Other symptoms

The development of renal failure may be associated with a wide range of symptoms including nausea, diarrhoea, confusion, drowsiness, and itching. In patients receiving a wide range of medication problems may arise from impaired drug clearance. In the palliative setting it is particularly important to remember the increased sensitivity to morphine which develops due to accumulation of the active metabolite, morphine-6-glucuronide, as a result of which doses will need to be reduced and the dosing interval may have to be prolonged.

Symptom management

Radiotherapy

This is of value both for radical and palliative treatment. For muscle invasive bladder cancer and high grade superficial bladder cancer, radiotherapy may be chosen as the primary treatment of choice. Radical doses to the bladder are given which may in themselves result in local radiation cystitis causing frequency and dysuria and some associated proctitis with bowel frequency. The side effects will usually settle spontaneously. With radiotherapy alone up to 40 per cent of patients will achieve cure remaining disease-free for at least 5 years. Following radiotherapy regular surveillance by cystoscopy is recommended to detect early relapse since salvage cystectomy can be successful in many cases. The major advantage of radiotherapy as primary treatment is in allowing the patient to retain their bladder and normal urinary function. Post-radiation changes, however, may result in bladder fibrosis with reduced bladder volume, haematuria from telangiectasis and occasionally urethral strictures. These are usually self-limiting and amenable to simple local treatment, but in severe cases of bladder fibrosis and shrinkage a permanent indwelling catheter or even cystectomy may be required.

In the palliative setting, radiotherapy has a role in locally advanced bladder cancer in the control of symptomatic local diseases despite widespread metastases.

Haematuria responds to relatively low doses of radiation. A large randomised trial has shown that a dose of 21 Gy in 3 fractions given on alternate days over one week is as effective as 35 Gy in 10 fractions over two weeks with an overall rate of symptom improvement of 68 per cent. Single doses of 10 Gy are also used particularly for troublesome haematuria with good palliation of bleeding. Such doses have little associated morbidity although transient bowel upset may occur. Pelvic pain due to extravesical extension of bladder tumour or lymph node involvement may also be usefully treated with radiotherapy using similar dose schedules to those described above. Local radiotherapy is less successful in achieving control of cystitis-like symptoms or urethral obstruction, and these problems alone would not generally be considered indications for palliative radiotherapy.

Pain from enlarged pelvic or para-aortic nodes will respond to a short course of radiotherapy delivering doses of 20–30 Gy in 1–2 weeks, however since this is often a feature of more widespread disease, chemotherapy may be preferred in this setting as initial treatment. Transient nausea and diarrhoea may be a side effect of larger field radiotherapy to the pelvis and abdomen due to inclusion of overlying small bowel in the treatment volume. Palliation of painful bone metastases with local radiotherapy is always of value.

Chemotherapy

Bladder cancer is sensitive to certain chemotherapy agents and combination schedules are now established which have response rates of over 50 per cent with up to 30 per cent of patients achieving complete tumour regression. The common effective schedule for bladder carcinoma is based on cisplatinum, methotrexate, and vinblastine (CMV) to which other drugs such as adriamycin are sometimes added. Short hospital admissions for hydration are usually required with cisplatinum, and common side-effects include nausea, stomatitis, and some degree of alopecia. Less often, peripheral neuropathy, tinnitus, and bone marrow depression may be troublesome. An alternative schedule with equivalent response rates is cisplatin and gemcitabine which may be better tolerated particularly in the older patients and those with renal impairment, and does not cause alopecia. The role of chemotherapy in the palliative treatment of bladder remains uncertain. It may offer useful palliation for extensive symptomatic metastatic disease in selected patients.

There is no evidence that chemotherapy as adjuvant treatment for either surgery or radiotherapy improves survival and it is now not generally recommended in the primary treatment of bladder cancer, although it may enhance the effects of radical radiotherapy and its role in this setting remains under investigation.

An alternative means of giving chemotherapy to bladder cancer is to deliver the drug directly into the bladder – intravesical chemotherapy. Whilst attractive, however, this is only of value for superficial bladder tumours and patients are selected for this treatment if they have multiple areas of disease or several recurrences after transurethral resection. In these patients control of the local disease can be achieved in 70–80 per cent of patients using intravesical mitomycin C, adriamycin, or BCG, although later relapse is quite frequent. It is, however, a simple treatment with little associated morbidity other than mild cystitis following treatment. It has no role for advanced local disease in the palliative setting.

Surgery

Surgical intervention plays an important role in the diagnosis and treatment of bladder cancer. The diagnosis depends upon cystoscopy and biopsy. Transurethral resection of the bladder tumour (TURBT) at cystoscopy may in itself be curative for superficial disease.

For muscle invasive disease, cystectomy is the surgical treatment of choice. Control rates are at least as good as with radical radiotherapy but this is a major surgery involving resection of the bladder, perivesical tissues, and either the prostate in men or the uterus, ovaries, and upper vagina in women. In many circumstances the entire urethra will be removed in men although externally the penis is preserved. Urine drainage thereafter is through an ileal conduit, a reservoir made from a small loop of ileum, opening onto the abdominal wall into a collecting bag. More elegant valve-type reconstructions are now possible but still require urine drainage through the abdominal wall. It may, however, be possible with this approach to avoid the need for continued wearing of a bag, using intermittent catheterization through the abdominal valve to drain the reservoir. Primary cystectomy may be required for very bulky tumours in young patients and those causing ureteric obstruction and hydronephrosis. There is some evidence that the combination of pre-operative radiotherapy and cystectomy improves local control rates, and the two treatments may therefore be combined in these circumstances.

Occasionally, partial cystectomy may be considered. This may be the case for a tumour developing in a diverticulum of the bladder when it is possible to achieve radical resection while preserving a useful amount of bladder.

In the palliative setting, TURBT can be a very useful means of stopping haematuria from advanced tumours. This is a relatively minor procedure performed under general anaesthetic but even in the patient with advanced metastatic disease it can be of great value in preventing local symptoms. Through the cystoscope the tumour is shaved off the bladder wall and the surface cauterized by the hot wire used for resection.

Surgery may also be required following radiotherapy for complications such as bleeding from telangiectasia, which can be cauterized at cystoscopy, and the dilatation of urethral strictures.

Tumours encroaching upon and invading the ureter may require a stent to be passed at cystoscopy through the area to maintain urine drainage prior to definitive treatment.

Key points: treatment interventions for advanced bladder cancer

- Radiotherapy for bleeding, pelvic pain or lymphadenopathy: 21 Gy in 3 fractions.
- Chemotherapy for symptomatic metastatic disease: cisplatin with methotrexate and vinblastine (CMV) or with gemcitabine (CG).
- Surgery for persistent bleeding from tumour or telangiectasis and ureteric or urethral obstruction.

Other treatment

Persistent haematuria can present a very difficult problem. Local radiotherapy and TURBT may be effective as may chemotherapy. Occasionally, however, haematuria persists despite these interventions. Bladder irrigation with normal saline through a two-way catheter may reduce the bleeding and allow a brief respite but it will frequently recur when the irrigation is discontinued. Sometimes success may be achieved with the use of oral haemostatic drugs of which ethamsylate is preferred over antifibrinolytic drugs, such as tranexamic acid, which carry a greater risk of thrombosis both within the bladder and elsewhere; a particular concern in debilitated immobile patients. Other measures which have been described include irrigation of the bladder with 1 per cent precipitated alum, irrigation of the bladder with formalin, and the use of local pressure from a hydrostatic balloon introduced into the bladder. None of these methods are supported by a significant body of evidence but may be worth a trial in intractable cases.

Progressive renal failure from ureteric obstruction may present a dilemma. In principle, urinary diversion either through a percutaneous nephrostomy or by the use of internal stents introduced from the bladder into the ureters will provide relief of obstruction, and is discussed in Chapter 26. In practice technical difficulties can arise when percutaneous tubes fail to be retained and stents are impossible because of occlusion of the ureteric orifice by tumour within the bladder. In addition attempted correction of the biochemical disturbance may be considered inappropriate in the setting of incurable advanced malignancy. As a general rule, attempts should be made to restore renal drainage in medically fit patients for whom radical treatment of their bladder cancer has yet to be attempted and where there is no metastatic disease. In patients with recurrent or metastatic disease conservative management of renal failure, maintaining fluid balance and controlling other symptoms with medication as necessary, may be more appropriate.

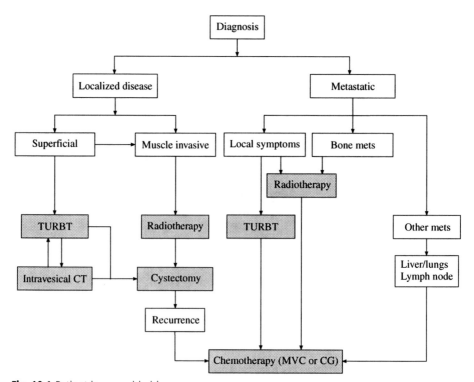

Fig. 10.1 Patient journey: bladder cancer.

Case History 10.1

A 58-year-old man was investigated because of haematuria and multiple bladder papillomas were discovered. Initially these were controlled by diathermy and he has been on regular cystoscopic follow-up. He was never too worried about his 'warts' as the surgeon called them. A further check after an interval of six months finds a solid tumour which is invading into the bladder wall. The pathology confirms a high grade transitional cell carcinoma.

He has a course of radical radiotherapy over four weeks; during this and for several weeks afterwards he is bothered by dysuria, urinary frequency, and also loose stools. These problems gradually resolve apart from his frequency which increases by day and night. At follow-up cystoscopy, four months after his radiotherapy there is residual tumour and quite small bladder capacity. A cystectomy is planned but a CT scan demonstrates pelvic and retroperitoneal nodes. Instead a palliative urinary diversion is performed, as his bladder symptoms are likely to worsen.

Within weeks, he has increasing backache and swelling of his legs.

He understands that the situation is now incurable but is keen to pursue further treatment with chemotherapy. There is some tumour regression after three courses, but not much improvement in his lymphoedema and his mobility is becoming worse. He decides, together with his oncology team, not to carry on with treatment.

It is only at this point that a referral is made to a community nurse specialist in palliative care and she persuades him to be admitted a hospice for management of his lymphoedema. By this time he has low grade cellulitis and is leaking fluid through the skin. The infection responds to penicillin V and after this, a period of bandaging achieves enough reduction in volume to fit compression stockings.

His back pain had been well-controlled by controlled-release oxycodone but he starts to complain of pain at a higher level than previously. He is sent for an X-ray and this shows metastatic involvement of a lower dorsal vertebral body. He is referred for a single palliative radiotherapy treatment which leads to improved pain control. Not long after this episode, he is admitted to the hospice because of nausea and vomiting. The cause of this is hypercalcaemia and on this occasion it is felt to be appropriate to treat with intravenous fluids and bisphosphonates. Although there is short term improvement, he is never well enough to return home. He and his family agree that he would not want further intervention should the hypercalcaemia recur and he dies 15 days later.

Practice points

- Invasive bladder cancer behaves very differently from papillomas and can be aggressive in behaviour with metastatic spread.
- Urinary diversions can offer useful palliation of severe dysuria and frequency.

Case History 10.1 (continued)

◆ Lymphoedema treatment should be commenced as early as possible together with prompt antibiotics for even low grade infection.

◆ Problems such as bone metastases and hypercalcaemia are not uncommon in bladder cancer.

Prostate cancer

Cancer of the prostate gland is the second most common malignancy in men and is increasing in incidence each year. It is a disease of predominately elderly men and may be a universal finding in those over 80 years. Currently, there are over 12 000 cases in the United Kingdom each year, of which 30–40 per cent present with locally advanced disease and 50 per cent present with metastatic disease; only 10 per cent have early localized disease at diagnosis.

Pathology and natural history

Virtually all prostatic carcinomas are adenocarcinomas although rarely transitional cell carcinoma of the prostatic ducts is seen. Adenocarcinoma of the prostate grows locally extending ultimately through the capsule of the gland into surrounding pelvic tissues. Distant spread is lymphatic draining to the pelvic lymph nodes and venous blood-borne dissemination characteristically through the vertebral plexus resulting in a pattern of bone metastases being established in the pelvic and vertebral bones before disseminating to the rest of the skeleton. Bone metastases from prostatic carcinoma are characteristically sclerotic with an exaggerated osteoblastic response. Complications such as pathological fracture, spinal cord compression, and hypercalcaemia are common. Soft tissue and lymph node metastases are less common in prostate cancer but occasionally pelvic and para-aortic nodes and lung and liver metastases are seen.

The prognosis from early prostatic carcinoma is good with many patients cured or having sufficiently long survival for it not to limit their life expectancy. Fifteen-year survival rates from early prostatic carcinoma (T1, T2) are of the order of 70–80 per cent with local treatment alone. Metastatic carcinoma of the prostate has an overall median survival of 18 months to 2 years although occasional long-term survivors 8–10 years after original diagnosis of metastatic disease are well-recognized.

Key points: prostate cancer

◆ Prostate cancer is the second commonest cancer in men and in Europe 50 per cent present with advanced disease.

◆ There is as yet no evidence that screening and early detection reduce death rates.

- Localized disease has a good prognosis with either radical radiotherapy or radical surgery.
- In patients with asymptomatic, early, well-differentiated disease who have an estimated life expectancy of less than 10 years there is a case for deferring treatment until symptoms arise.

Diagnosis and the asymptomatic patient

An increasing number of patients are diagnosed with asymptomatic disease having had the level of their prostate specific antigen (PSA) measured either during investigations for another condition or, as a 'screening' test. The optimal management of such patients is unknown. Undoubtedly, given the prevalence of prostate cancer, a significant number of these would otherwise remain asymptomatic with death from another cause and there is concern that as a result many men diagnosed in this way receive unnecessary intervention often with associated treatment-induced toxicity. Large trials into the utility of prostate cancer screening are currently underway but due to the long natural history of the disease critical answers as to the effect on prostate cancer survival are many years away.

Common symptoms

Pressure symptoms

The most common symptom of prostatic carcinoma is that of urinary outflow obstruction causing frequency, hesitancy, poor urinary stream, nocturia, and in more severe cases urinary retention. These are all features of 'benign' prostatic hypertrophy also and many cases are diagnosed during the investigation of benign prostatic symptoms. In advanced cases prostatic urethral obstruction can result in bladder dilatation and hydronephrosis with impairment of renal function. This is usually a gradual process and not associated with painful hydronephrosis. Local extension of tumour posteriorly into the rectum may in advanced cases cause rectal discomfort and difficulty with bowel motions, in extreme cases leading to large bowel obstruction.

Bone metastases may result in spinal cord compression or cauda equina compression due to encroachment on the spinal canal. Pressure on spinal nerve roots is also a well recognized problem causing neuropathic pain. Skull base infiltration is a recognized feature which may result in cranial nerve palsies.

Lymph node disease involving the pelvis and para-aortic chain may result in bilateral lower limb oedema and may itself cause ureteric obstruction and occasionally inferior vena cava obstruction.

Pain

Local disease is rarely associated with pain. Bone metastases are a prominent feature of prostate carcinoma and both local and scattered bone pain is therefore a common feature. Local bone pain may be a presenting feature and pathological fracture may occur. Para-aortic lymphadenopathy may be a cause of back pain.

Haemorrhage

Occasionally, prostatic carcinoma may present with haematuria or haematospermia. In locally advanced disease this may become a prominent problem due to local tumour growth within the urethra or invasion into the bladder base. Less commonly posterior extension into the rectum can result in rectal bleeding although a more common cause of bleeding in this group of patients is post-radiation proctitis following a course of radical radiotherapy to the prostate.

Other symptoms

Hypercalcaemia is seen relatively commonly in prostate cancer because of the high incidence of bone metastases. Prostatic outflow symptoms may predominate despite treatment with frequency, nocturia, and hesitancy causing considerable morbidity. Some patients require an indwelling catheter which itself may cause local pain, bladder irritation, and spasm. Renal failure resulting from ureteric obstruction by para-aortic nodes or chronic urethral obstruction may develop with associated nausea, diarrhoea, drowsiness, confusion, and itching. Extensive bone metastases may result in bone marrow failure with chronic anaemia, leucopenia, and thrombocytopenia.

Symptom management

Radiotherapy

This is used for radical treatment of localized prostatic tumours. The development of sophistocated radiotherapy techniques to shape the high dose regions away from the rectum (conformal radiotherapy) have enabled doses in excess of 90 Gy to be reached safely; standard treatment schedules currently aim to give up to 74 Gy. An alternative means of giving high dose radiotherapy to the prostate is using brachytherapy in which under guidance by a transrectal ultrasound probe radioactive seeds, typically iodine or palladium are placed inside the gland. Equivalent results to radical external beam radiotherapy and prostatectomy are reported for localized prostate cancer. Alongside the effect in controlling the underlying cancer, radiotherapy will result in good relief of prostatic outflow symptom as shrinkage of the gland occurs. Brachytherapy however, is frequently associated with a period of severe prostatitis and urethritis for several weeks or months following the procedure.

In advanced disease, local symptoms such as haematuria are also usefully treated with local radiotherapy delivering palliative doses such as 10 Gy in 1 fraction, 21 Gy in 3 fractions, or 30 Gy in 10 fractions.

Painful bone metastases respond well to local radiotherapy and for more widespread disease hemibody irradiation or radioisotope therapy may be indicated. Prostate cancer has been investigated extensively as a model for the use of radioisotope therapy, in particular strontium-89 [^{89}Sr] which is probably the treatment of choice now for widespread metastatic bone pain in this condition. A single outpatient injection of 150 MBq will result in pain relief in over 80 per cent of patients within 10–14 days with no immediate toxicity and usually only minor reduction in peripheral blood over the following 4–6 weeks. This treatment is, however, reserved for those patients who have relapsed after hormone treatment, androgen blockade being the most effective primary treatment for patients presenting with metastatic bone pain and where external beam treatment is not appropriate. An alternative to strontium is samarium [^{153}Sm] complexed with a phosphonate, EDMP, to target it at sites of bone remineralisation, also given as an intravenous injection with similar results.

Radiotherapy is indicated for spinal cord compression. Urgent investigations are essential for any patient with prostatic carcinoma who presents with neurological signs or symptoms; magnetic resonance imaging (MRI) is now the investigation of choice. Urgent local radiotherapy to an area of spinal canal involvement is indicated along with dexamethasone 4 mg six-hourly started immediately. Doses of 20–30 Gy in 5–10 fractions are usually given.

Skull base infiltration resulting in cranial nerve palsies will also respond well to radiotherapy with up to 80 per cent of patients regaining use of nerve function following doses of 20–30 Gy over 1–2 weeks. Para-aortic masses may benefit from local radiotherapy to relieve associated pain, particularly in hormone-resistant disease.

Key points: radiotherapy for prostate cancer

- High dose external beam or brachytherapy for radical treatment of localized disease.
- Low dose palliative treatment for bleeding, pain and obstructive symptoms in advanced disease.
- Palliative treatment for bone pain, spinal cord compression, skull base metastases.
- Wide field external beam or isotope (strontium or samarium) therapy for scattered bone pain.

Surgery

There is considerable debate as to the relative roles of radiotherapy and radical prostatectomy as treatment for early prostate cancer. Current evidence suggests both are effective with no clear difference emerging for local control rates in early (T1, T2) tumours. Surgery may have a greater incidence of impotence and urine outflow problems but radiotherapy will be associated with a higher incidence of bowel morbidity and urethral stricture. Brachytherapy may offer a compromise between toxicity and efficacy.

In the palliative setting, surgery may be of value for obstructive symptoms when transurethral resection of the prostate (TURP) can provide a rapid and simple means of relief for urethral and bladder obstruction. Where this is unsuccessful or whilst awaiting surgery urethral or suprapubic catheterization may be indicated. Local surgery may also be valuable for sites of haemorrhage in the urethra or bladder base. In pathological fracture internal fixation should always be considered when long bones are involved.

Hormone therapy

This has an established role in the management of metastatic prostate cancer and is also being increasingly used in the neoadjuvant setting for locally advanced or high grade prostate cancer alongside radical prostatectomy or radiotherapy. In the elderly patient unfit for radical radiotherapy or surgery and where there are equivocal staging tests they may be used as primary treatment alone.

Most prostate cancers are dependent upon androgen stimulation and treatment resulting in loss of the antigen drive will result in regression of tumour, a fall in serum prostate specific antigen (PSA), and symptomatic relief in over 80 per cent of patients. Treatment be with either an oral anti-androgen tablet such as bicalutamide, flutamide or cyproterone acetate or with an injection of gonadotrophin releasing hormone (GnRH) analogue such as goserelin or leuprorelin given subcutaneously on a monthly basis. If these GnRH agents are used the first month of treatment also requires an oral anti-androgen since they have an initial stimulatory effect which can cause a tumour and symptom flare. Long-term use of cyproterone is now contraindicated because of the rare complication of fulminant hepatic necrosis. An alternative approach, less popular today, but equally effective, is bilateral orchidectomy. A combination of GnRH and oral anti-androgen (total androgen blockade) is sometimes recommended as having higher response rates than either agent alone but this remains controversial, a meta-analysis demonstrating only borderline clinical significance. In metastatic disease there is no evidence that combination therapy is of greater value than either treatment used singly. Patients receiving anti-androgen therapy may have symptoms including hot flushes, apathy and listlessness, reduced libido, and impotence. Nausea may be associated with the oral anti-androgen tablets. It is claimed that potency can be retained by many men taking flutamide or the injection of GnRH analogues but objective assessments suggest that most men experience loss of sexual drive and impaired physical capacity. In patients where side effects are troublesome then intermittent androgen blockade is an option, although as yet, not formally compared to continuous treatment. In this approach, treatment is given until trough levels of PSA are reached and then discontinued, monitoring PSA until a significant rise is seen when anti-androgens are re-introduced. It has also been suggested that this may delay the emergence of hormone-resistant disease by maintaining a larger population of hormone-sensitive cells, but this is unproven.

There is no evidence that treatment of asymptomatic metastatic prostate cancer with anti-androgen therapy in asymptomatic men improves survival but early treatment may reduce the incidence of complications such as spinal cord compression in a small number. The decision as to when to introduce treatment is often difficult, particularly where it arises following radical treatment with only a slow rise in PSA levels but no detectable disease. As always it is a balance between possible benefits which are few in the asymtomatic patient and potential side effects, although often, the anxiety of knowing that relapse has occurred is sufficient for many patients to opt for active treatment at an early stage.

A major difficulty arises when patients relapse whilst receiving anti-androgen therapy. The median duration of response to any of the above primary anti-androgen manoeuvres is 18 months and most men relapse with hormone-resistant disease. Response rates to a second anti-androgen manoeuvre are rarely greater than 10 per cent. Similar response rates are achieved with corticosteroids. At relapse, therefore, a change in medication is rarely of value but many men are maintained on their anti-androgen therapy on the basis that there may still be a hormone-sensitive component to that disease and there is some evidence that this may be beneficial. More recently it has been claimed that a small number of men may exhibit a second response on withdrawal of anti-androgen therapy but this is controversial at present. The addition of a small dose of steroids or a progestogen such as megestrol or medroxyprogesterone may be of additional symptomatic benefit at relapse.

Chemotherapy

This has a very limited role in prostate cancer the majority of drugs being largely inactive. One trial has however shown a benefit in terms of improved quality of life in patients with symptomatic hormone resistant prostate cancer using mitozantrone with prednisolone. Superior results were seen when compared to prednisolone alone, and this has become a valuable addition to the treatment options as hormone resistance develops. There is however no impact of treatment on survival and it should therefore be selected for those patient with significant tumour-related symptoms.

Other treatment

Hypercalcaemia should be treated actively with hydration, frusemide, and intravenous bisphosphonate infusions such as clodronate or pamidronate. Persistent prostatic outflow problems may be best dealt with by an indwelling catheter and this is generally more successful than other urine collection devices such as the conveen. Some men find a urethral catheter difficult to tolerate with frequent bladder spasm and bypassing of the catheter in which case a suprapubic catheter may be considered a useful alternative.

Bone pain which persists despite hormone therapy and radiotherapy can present a major difficulty in advanced prostatic cancer and the management of this problem is discussed in Chapter 21.

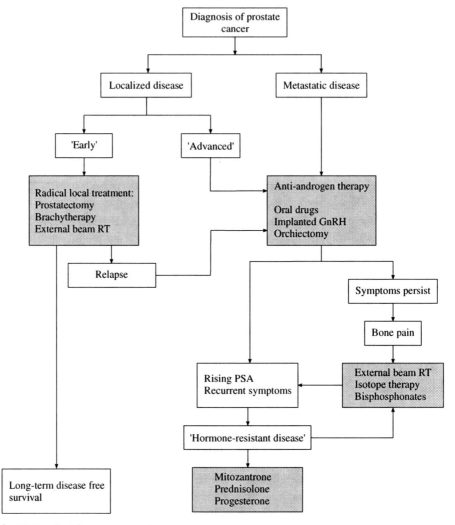

Fig. 10.2 Patient journey: prostate cancer.

Key points: systemic treatment for prostate cancer

◆ Metastatic disease, typically bone metastases will respond to androgen blockade in over 80 per cent.

◆ This may be achieved by oral anti-androgen drugs such as bicalutamide, cypro-terone or flutamide, injected gonadotrophin releasing hormone (GnRH) analogues such as goserelin and leuprorelin, or surgical orchidectomy.

◆ Relapse after hormone therapy rarely responds to alteration of the anti-androgen but steroids or progestogens may be of symptomatic value.

◆ Chemotherapy using mitozantrone with prednisolone may be of benefit in symptomatic hormone resistant disease.

Case History 10.2

An 80-year-old man with prostate cancer has been admitted to a hospice for symptom control. He had presented two and a half years earlier with bone pain and was found to have widespread bone metastases. His pain disappeared following a bilateral subcapsular orchidectomy but had returned in recent weeks. It responded to regular diclofenac and controlled release morphine 130 mg twice daily. Admission was requested because he had chronic diarrhoea and more recently, nausea and vomiting. He was noted to have a distended abdomen and a large irregular prostate was filling most of his rectum. His biochemistry, including his serum calcium, was normal.

It became clear that his diarrhoea was the passage of small amounts of liquid faeces and mucous up to eight times daily. The real problem was one of chronic constipation with incipient obstruction of the lower bowel by his large primary tumour arising from the prostate. The return of his bone pain suggested that his disease was becoming refractory to hormone treatment.

He was referred to the surgical team at the nearby hospital and subsequently transferred there to have a defunctioning colostomy. Palliative radiotherapy to the prostate was considered but decided against because he had good palliation from the surgery. However radiotherapy was given to sites of bone pain, enabling a reduction in his dose of morphine.

Practice points

◆ When the presentation of prostate cancer is through distant metastases, usually no treatment is indicated to the prostate.

◆ Hormone manipulation will induce tumour regression within the prostate as well as in the bones.

◆ Locally invasive prostatic tumour can cause pain, bleeding, rectal stenosis plus invasion into penis and bladder.

◆ Radiotherapy can offer useful palliation.

Renal cancer

The most common kidney malignancy is renal cell adenocarcinoma (hypernephroma). There are around 3500 cases of renal carcinoma annually in the United Kingdom.

Pathology and natural history

Renal cell adenocarcinomas arise from the parenchyma of the kidney and are distinct from transitional cell carcinomas which can develop throughout the urological tract including the renal pelvis. Typically they can progress to a considerable size before becoming clinically apparent when they will present with abdominal or loin pain or haematuria. Local invasion and extension into the renal vein is the typical pattern of growth with consequent blood-borne metastases which typically involve lung and bone but may be found at any site. Lymph node spread also occurs involving the para-aortic nodes but is not often a prominent clinical feature.

Prognosis

Renal cancer is typically a relatively slowly evolving tumour and even in the presence of metastases a patient may survive for several years. Tumours confined to the kidney are cured in over 50 per cent of cases with radical nephrectomy. Capsular invasion and involvement of the renal vein are poor prognostic features. A curious feature associated with renal cell carcinoma is that of spontaneous regression of metastases which is reported in around 7 per cent of patients who develop metastases. This usually involves lung metastases becoming progressively smaller with no active treatment.

Key points: renal cancer

- Usually adenocarcinomas which can grow to a large size before detection.
- Local infiltration and growth into renal vein occurs.
- Usually has a long natural history even with metastatic disease.
- Rare cases of spontaneous regression are documented.

Symptoms

Pain

Local pain in the abdomen or loin as the tumour invades the renal capsule and perinephric tissues can occur. In the occasional patient in whom para-aortic nodes are involved then progressive back pain may develop. Haematuria may result in clots presenting with severe abdominal pain. Bone metastases are relatively common in renal carcinoma and are typically lytic and vascular in nature. Because of their lytic nature they may be at high risk of pathological fracture.

Less frequently other metastatic sites may also result in pain including headache from cerebral metastases, pleuritic pain from peripheral lung metastases, and painful skin nodules.

Haemorrhage

Haematuria is a common feature in the presentation of renal cell carcinoma and may persist in advanced cases when the tumour is left *in situ*. Metastases are typically highly vascular. Intracerebral haemorrhage from a cerebral metastasis can occur, and haemorrhage into a lung or hepatic metastasis may result in acute pain.

Pressure symptoms

Local growth is usually by infiltration rather than causing obstruction. In advanced tumours growth along the renal vein into the inferior vena cava can result in obstruction to venous return from the lower limbs and pelvis with resulting distal oedema.

Other symptoms

Renal cell carcinoma may be associated with hypercalcaemia which may be seen even in the absence of extensive bone metastases due to the release of parathyroid hormone-like substance from the tumour. Polycythaemia occurs as a result of excess erythopoietin production from the kidney. This will result in typical features of confusion, blurred vision, plethora, and headache.

Symptom management

Surgery

The treatment of a localized primary renal cell carcinoma is radical surgery. This will be curative in 50 per cent of patients with localized disease, the remainder presenting at a later date with metastases. Surgery may also be indicated for solitary metastases in the lung or brain and even where there are a number of pulmonary metastases local resection may be contemplated in a patient having a long interval from primary treatment to the onset of metastases. In bone metastases, pathological fracture is an indication for internal fixation.

Radiotherapy

There is no role for radiotherapy in the radical treatment of renal cell carcinoma. In the case of advanced inoperable or metastatic disease, however, it may be of value given to the primary site for local pain and to stop haematuria. Normal kidney is very sensitive to radiation doses and beyond 15 Gy loss of renal function will occur. In advanced disease this is not usually a major concern but it is important to ensure that the contralateral kidney has good function before ablating the tumour-bearing kidney with radiation. An isotope nephrogram will establish this. Doses of 30–40 Gy in 10–15 fractions over 2–3 weeks are usually given although single doses of 8–10 Gy are effective for haematuria.

Local radiotherapy for bone metastases and symptomatic secondary deposits in other sites will be indicated. Post-operative radiotherapy to bones after internal fixation should also be considered in those patients having limited disease and a projected survival of more than a few weeks.

Chemotherapy

There is no proven role for chemotherapy in renal cell carcinoma used alone, however intensive chemotherapy regimes incorporating 5-FU with interferon have been developed and may result in small gains in survival for selected patients who can tolerate such intervention.

Hormone therapy

Treatment with progestogens such as megestrol or medroxyprogesterone acetate is often advocated for metastatic renal cell carcinoma. Whilst responses are occasionally seen renal carcinoma is not often hormone-sensitive and objective tumour regression is seen in only 10 per cent of patients. There may, however, be a non-specific advantage to progestogens in metastastic disease in improving the general well-being of the patient.

Biological therapy

Renal cell carcinoma is one of the few solid tumours in which responses to biological agents such as interferon and interleukin-2 (IL-2) have been described. Actual response rates are around 20–30 per cent. This treatment is usually reserved for patients with good performance status and only one or two sites of metastases in whom this approach may have some advantage. A randomized trial has shown a marginal survival advantage for patients receiving interferon when compared to progestogen in metastatic disease and comparison of interferon and interleukin with the combined schedules incorporating 5-FU is underway. There is however considerable morbidity associated with these schedules.

Other treatment

Hypercalcaemia will require treatment with intravenous fluids, frusemide and bisphosphonate infusions, as described elsewhere (p. 352). Polycythaemia, if symptomatic, will require intermittent venesection removing 1–2 units of blood through an antecubital vein to maintain the packed cell volume below 50 per cent. Treatment to the primary tumour with either surgery or, if inappropriate, radiotherapy may be of value in the control of recurrent polycythaemia and hypercalcaemia by suppressing production of the chemical agents driving the excess red cell production (and calcium mobilization in the case of hypercalcaemia). Arterial embolization is sometimes of value in reducing the viability of this vascular tumour in palliation of localized metastases.

Key points: management of renal cell cancer

◆ Half of the patients presenting with localized disease and undergoing radical nephrectomy will be cured, but the remainder will subsequently relapse with metastatic disease usually in lung and bones.

◆ Rarely, metastases may undergo spontaneous regression and around 10 per cent may respond to progestogens.

◆ More intensive treatment with combinations of interferon, interleukin and 5-FU is currently under investigation and may have small survival advantages for good performance status patients with only a small number of metastatic sites.

Case History 10.3

A woman of 63 has several episodes of haematuria and is treated for urinary tract infections. Some months later she develops upper lumbar backache. A plain X-ray of her spine at this point is reported to be normal but her pain persists. Eventually, after another episode of heavy haematuria she is sent to see a urologist. An isotope bone scan shows reduced uptake in L2 vertebra; a CT scan shows destruction of this vertebral body and a mass in the lower pole of her left kidney.

The urologist checks that she has a normal-functioning kidney on the other side and proceeds to a radical nephrectomy. Excision is complete and in view of this, she is given a fractionated course of radiotherapy to the lumbar spine as this is the only apparent site of metastatic disease.

After some initial improvement, her back pain persists. Eight months later she needs high doses of morphine. This controls pain at rest but she is experiencing severe pain on any activity.

An MR scan of her spine confirms residual tumour at the site of previous radiotherapy but no other spinal involvement. She is referred to a specialist spinal unit where she undergoes embolization of the vertebral tumour followed by surgical resection of the vertebral body and spinal stabilisation. She returns home three weeks later, after an intensive period of rehabilitation and is able to walk the dogs. She remains well for three years until she develops multiple pulmonary metastases.

Practice points

- Haematuria should be investigated.
- Purely lytic bone metastases do not show up as a hot spot (increased uptake) on a bone scan, therefore it can be missed.
- Renal carcinoma can follow an unpredictable course, with documented long-term survivals even with the metastatic spread. An aggressive treatment to primary and secondary sites may be justified.
- Tumours may be relatively resistant to radiotherapy.
- Tumours are often well-vascularized therefore surgical procedures are often combined with embolization.

Testicular cancer

Testicular tumours are relatively rare and typically affect young men aged 20–40, with around 1500 cases each year in the United Kingdom.

Pathology and natural history

The majority of testicular tumours are germ cell tumours, either seminomas or teratomas. A small number (around 7 per cent) are lymphoma and, rarely, tumours of the interstitial cells may arise. The natural history of germ cell testicular tumours is for lymphatic spread which is in most cases direct to the para-aortic lymph nodes with only 2–3 per cent having pelvic node involvement. Blood-borne dissemination is seen alongside this with involvement of lung, liver, and occasionally the central nervous system.

Prognosis

The prognosis for testicular tumours is good with even advanced cases being cured in over 90 per cent of cases due to the high chemosensitivity of germ cell tumours. Patients presenting with disease localized to the testes or with only early involvement of the para-aortic lymph nodes have cure rates approaching 100 per cent. Progressive advanced disease is therefore unusual. Few patients enter the realm of palliative medicine.

Treatment

Surgery

Inguinal orchidectomy is the treatment of choice at presentation with a testicular mass.

Radiotherapy

Post-operative radiotherapy to the para-aortic lymph nodes is recommended for testicular seminoma localized to the testes as a prophylactic measure. Radiotherapy is rarely used in other stages of testicular tumour.

Chemotherapy

These tumours are exquisitely sensitive to chemotherapy and drugs based upon cisplatin in combination with etoposide and bleomycin form the basis of most treatment schedules. Disease which has spread beyond the testis is usually treated in this way. Selected high risk patients with stage I testicular teratoma who have microscopic vascular invasion or an undifferentiated tumour will also receive adjuvant chemotherapy.

Key point

Testicular tumours are usually germ cell tumours (seminoma or teratoma). These are highly sensitive to radiotherapy or chemotherapy and cure is expected in most patients.

Carcinoma of the penis

This cancer is rare with 300 cases per year in the United Kingdom although it is much more common in other parts of the world where circumcision is not practised.

Pathology and natural history

The common penile carcinoma is a squamous carcinoma which invades the penile shaft locally and spreads by lymphatic invasion to the inguinal nodes and thence pelvic lymph nodes. Blood-borne dissemination occurs at a later stage typically involving lung.

Prognosis

The prognosis for localized disease is good but once lymph nodes are involved 5-year survival falls below 30 per cent.

Treatment

Surgery

Local excision for small tumours affecting the prepuce may be possible. For more advanced distal tumour sub-total amputation or complete amputation may be curative. Surgical treatment of involved lymph nodes is generally recommended. Lymphadenopathy may be reactive rather than malignant, however, and fine needle aspirate confirmation of metastatic involvement is required in all cases before progressing to lymph node dissection. For established metastases in mobile inguinal lymph nodes, groin dissection is the treatment of choice.

Radiotherapy

Local radiotherapy to the penile shaft by external beam or brachytherapy techniques is also highly successful and often chosen in preference to surgery to avoid amputation. Cure rates for small localized lesions treated with radiotherapy alone are similar to those following surgery. Radiotherapy may have a role for the treatment of groin nodes where there is residual disease following surgery or in the case of fixed glands which are inoperable. Post-radiation complications, however, with lymphedema of the lower limb are common when doses sufficient to control squamous carcinoma are delivered.

Chemotherapy

There is no established effective chemotherapy for penile carcinoma.

Key points

- Localized penile cancer may be cured by either local radiotherapy or amputation.
- Involvement of inguinal nodes is a poor prognostic feature and may herald more extensive node metastases or pulmonary metastases.
- In advanced disease local radiotherapy may provide palliation; chemotherapy has no role.

Chapter 11

Upper gastrointestinal tumours

Cancer of the oesophagus and stomach is particularly common in China and other parts of Asia including Japan, where it is the most common cause of death from malignancy. In the United Kingdom there are 5000 new cases of oesophageal cancer per year and 12 000 new cases of stomach cancer. Cancer of the pancreas affects around 6000 patients per year with a less marked geographical variation, being relatively rare in the developing world, and cancer of the bile duct and gall bladder is uncommon with fewer than 1000 cases per year in Britain.

Cancer of the oesophagus, stomach, and pancreas are all related to smoking. Oesophageal cancer is also related to high alcohol intake and other causes of chronic oesophageal irritation may predispose to malignant change including chronic gastro-oesophageal reflux and achalasia. The Plummer-Vinson or Patterson-Kelly-Brown syndrome is characterized by an oesophageal web which predisposes to oesophageal cancer typically seen in women and also includes iron deficiency anaemia and koilony-chias.

Whilst oesophageal cancer is not clearly diet-related, cancer of the stomach is related to ingested carcinogens; in particular, nitrosamines and diets rich in food which has been processed by smoking. Chronic mucosal conditions of the stomach also predispose to malignancy including pernicious anaemia and atrophic gastritis and there is also an increased incidence of gastrectomy. It is more common in deprived socio-economic groups and has a linkage to blood group A.

Cancer of the pancreas or bile ducts often has no apparent cause although in areas where the liver fluke, *Clonorchis sinensis*, is endemic, infection with this organism may predispose to bile duct cancer.

The natural history of these tumours is for local infiltration and spread via lymphatic drainage to regional lymph nodes within the mediastinum from the oesophagus and within the abdomen from the other sites. Drainage of abdominal lymphatics to the left supraclavicular lymph nodes results in a classical presentation with a palpable node in this region. In addition stomach characteristically spreads by transcoelomic seeding of cells across the peritoneal cavity giving rise to the well-known but relatively rare Krukenberg tumours – bilateral ovarian metastases from carcinoma of the stomach. Blood-borne metastases are also common. The pancreas, stomach, bile ducts, and lower oesophagus drain directly into the portal circulation and the liver is therefore the most common site for metastases; less frequently lung, brain, and bone metastases are seen.

The prognosis from all of these malignancies is poor with an overall 5-year survival of less than 10 per cent. The majority of long-term survivors will have the malignancy discovered incidentally, tumours in these regions once symptomatic having a high rate of local extension and metastasis.

In addition to the common squamous carcinoma (upper oesophagus) and adeno-carcinomas (elsewhere) described above, the stomach is a site for lymphoma and sarcoma, typically leiomyosarcoma.

Key points

- Cancers of the oesophagus and stomach are particularly common in China, Japan and the Far East.
- Cancer of the oesophagus, stomach and pancreas are all smoking-related.
- Cancers of the upper gastrointestinal tract infiltrate locally and are often dissem-inated at diagnosis; their prognosis in general is poor with <10 per cent long-term survivors.

Common symptoms

Pain

This is relatively unusual with cancer of the oesophagus and stomach apart from the discomfort of dysphagia. Cancer of the pancreas, however, is notorious for causing severe abdominal pain typically radiating through to the back. There may be a complex pain picture of both visceral and somatic nociceptive pain due to invasion of the retroperitoneal tissues. Segmental neuropathic pain may also complicate the situation as peripheral nerve damage ensues.

Discomfort may also be associated with ascites or hepatomegaly from metastatic disease.

Pressure

Cancer of the oesophagus typically presents with dysphagia which initially may be relatively minor, characteristically more marked for solids than fluids but ultimately progressing to severe restriction of nutritional intake and eventually complete dysphagia with inability to swallow even saliva. Similar events may follow a cancer of the fundus of the stomach and cardia as they involve the gastro-oesophageal junction. More distal stomach cancers will result in feelings of fullness, gastric distension, and ultimately gastric outflow obstruction with associated reflux and vomiting. Diffuse infiltration of the stomach (linitis plastica) also results in reduced gastric motility with early satiation and abdominal discomfort after food.

Both cancer of the pancreas and bile ducts may result in biliary obstruction presenting with obstructive jaundice and the very characteristic picture of painless jaundice and a palpable gall bladder due to distension from distal obstruction. The features of obstructive jaundice will include pale stools, dark urine, and itching.

Haemorrhage

Local haemorrhage from cancer of the oesophagus is relatively unusual but from the stomach may result in haematemesis which can be severe and even fatal. Neither pancreatic nor bile duct tumours tend to present with symptomatic bleeding, although extensive growth of a bile duct tumour into the duodenum can result in intermittent bleeding into the small bowel and the passage of melaena.

Other symptoms

Because of their effects on nutritional intake and digestion these tumours are frequently associated with profound weight loss and anorexia. Obstructive jaundice can be associated with severe and intractable pruritis. Gastric and pancreatic cancers are characteristically, but rarely, associated with superficial thrombophlebitis, typically of the lower limb. Diabetes mellitus may complicate pancreatic cancer and indeed may be a forerunner by some years of the diagnosis. In many cases, however, pancreatic islet function is well preserved despite advanced disease.

Key points

- Oesophageal and stomach cancers typically present with difficulty in swallowing, or gastric distension. Haemorrahge resulting in haematemesis or melaena is common in stomach cancer but not oesophageal.
- Severe central abdominal pain and back pain are cardinal features of locally advanced malignancy, particularly encountered in pancreatic cancer.
- Obstructive jaundice occurs with pancreatic cancer arising in the head of the gland and tumours of the bile ducts.

Management

Surgery

Curative treatment for cancer of the oesophagus depends primarily upon radical surgical excision. In selected series of localized tumours 5-year survival rates of up to 30 per cent are reported, although the overall survival in unselected surgical series is poor and equivalent to that in radical radiotherapy series at around 5 per cent long-term survival over 5 years. Pre-operative chemotherapy has been shown to improve the results of radial surgery in some, but not all, trials, and there are also advocates of pre-operative radiotherapy. Surgery for carcinoma of the oesophagus is a major procedure requiring a thoraco-abdominal procedure for lower and middle third tumours, the upper oesophagus being anastomosed to the stomach which is brought into the chest. For higher tumours then more complex surgery may be required to restore continuity of the oesophageal lumen using loops of small bowel or transposed colon. Patients therefore have to be medically fit to withstand such extensive surgery and this is reflected in the high surgical mortality rate from unselected surgical series of between 15–20 per cent. Careful selection to ensure that only patients with localized tumours undergo such procedures is required using CT, MRI, and transoesophageal ultrasound.

If the patient is not medically fit or the tumour too advanced either because of local infiltration or metastasis for radical surgery, it is still important to consider surgery as a means of optimal palliation to maintain swallowing. The simplest form of surgery is dilatation performed at oesophagoscopy which will relieve a malignant stricture but provide only temporary relief and may subsequently require repeated procedures. Local treatment to a proliferative tumour mass can be delivered using cryotherapy or laser therapy both of which have their advocates and may be successful in restoring swallowing where the lumen is narrowing. These may provide symptom relief for several months but again recurrence is inevitable as they do not eradicate completely the local site of tumour. A more permanent solution may be sought by combining one of these procedures with intubation passing a self-retaining tube or expandable stent as shown in Fig. 4.1 (p. 32), which can be placed in position through the site of obstruction. Intubation does, however, carry a morbidity with tubes becoming dislodged or blocking and with time tumour may recur around the tube and grow into the lumen of the tube. For many incurable patients, however, they provide rapid and successful relief of dysphagia.

Curative treatment for carcinoma of the stomach also requires radical surgery. Localized tumours may be subjected to radical excision by partial or total gastrectomy. Unfortunately, however, only about 15 per cent of patients presenting with stomach cancer are considered operable and even in this group the long-term survival is only around 20 per cent. Gastrectomy is associated with significant morbidity not only from the acute surgery but from the long-term effects of loss of gastric function resulting in diarrhoea, pernicious anaemia, vitamin deficiencies, dumping, and inability to tolerate large amounts of food. It should, therefore, be only undertaken after very careful assessment and staging to ensure that the tumour is localized and technically operable. Palliative surgery has a limited role in carcinoma of the stomach. Dysphagia is not typically a problem but local bleeding can be troublesome and may be an indication for palliative gastrectomy or laser therapy performed at gastroscopy.

Similarly, carcinoma of the pancreas is only cured by radical surgery which involves an extensive abdominal resection of the pancreas usually with the duodenum (Whipple's operation) but again this is relevant to only a small proportion of patients of whom only a few will be long-term survivors. For the majority of patients with carcinoma of

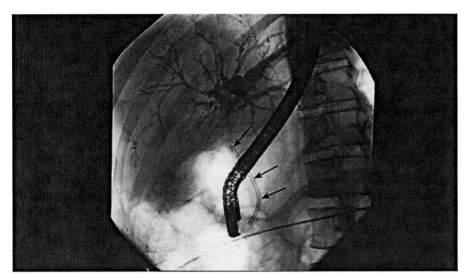

Fig. 11.1 X-ray showing fibre-optic endoscope in the second part of the duodenum and biliary stent in position (arrowed) having just been passed through the endoscope into the bile duct.

the pancreas the only other role of surgery is in relieving biliary obstruction. This may be achieved by retrograde stenting of the bile duct, the procedure being performed through a fibre-optic endoscope passed into the duodenum (ERPC) as shown in Fig. 11.1. Where stenting is technically impossible or unsuccessful, then bypass of the common bile duct, opening the gall bladder into the loop of the jejunum (choledo-chojejunostomy) is a worthwhile and effective means of preventing obstructive jaundice.

For a more proximal obstruction which may occur with carcinoma of the bile duct then percutaneous drainage of the dilated bile ducts under ultrasound control is of value and this may be followed by the passage of a stent to restore drainage into the duodenum.

Radiotherapy

Radical radiotherapy may be considered for carcinoma of the oesophagus in patients thought unfit for surgery but who none the less have localized tumours, or in those who refuse surgery. There may also be circumstances when tumours are technically inaccessible but still localized and amenable to radical treatment, for example when there is invasion of the adjacent mediastinal structures. Current techniques combine radiotherapy with chemotherapy, improved results having been shown when cisplatin and 5-FU is given at the beginning and end of a radical 5-week course of radiotherapy. Radical radiotherapy to the oesophagus is technically demanding and inevitably produces prolonged oesophagitis for which enteral nutritional support using a nasogastric tube or percutaneous gastrostomy may be required to support the patient through treatment. It should, therefore, only be considered for carefully selected patients.

Historically the results of radical radiotherapy for localized carcinoma of the oesophagus are no worse than surgery but the outlook was very poor with a 5-year survival of only 5 per cent. There is some evidence that combined chemoradiotherapy schedules have improved this survival rate in patients selected to withstand its greater morbidity.

In the palliative setting, radiotherapy for oesophageal cancer is highly successful at relieving dysphagia with reported response rates of between 70–80 per cent. It has been claimed that higher doses of around 50 Gy are better than lower doses but many centres prefer to give shorter low dose schedules particularly for the patient with advanced disease.

Oesophageal tumours are amenable to endoluminal therapy in which an afterloading catheter is passed through the oesophagus often within a nasogastric tube along which a radioactive source can be passed. The current common technique in modern centres uses a high dose rate afterloading machine with an iridium source of 1.6 mm diameter. This will pass down the afterloading catheter and rest against the tumour-bearing region of the oesophagus for a period of several minutes during which time it will deliver a high local dose to the surface epithelium and tumour (in a similar way to endobronchial treatment illustrated in Fig. 7.2, p. 72). The advantage of this technique is its simplicity requiring only a single outpatient procedure and the technical merit that it delivers a very high but localized dose to the area containing tumour with negligible doses to surrounding normal tissues. Response rates of 70–80 per cent are reported with this technique which in many centres has replaced external beam radiotherapy as palliative treatment for cancer of the oesophagus.

Palliative radiotherapy also has a role in the management of symptomatic metastases for example supraclavicular lymph nodes or bone metastases.

Key points

- Radical surgical excision is the best curative treatment for cancers of the stomach and pancreas.
- Radical chemoradiation and radical surgery are both effective for oesophageal cancers.
- Palliative surgery to relieve dysphagia (stenting) and obstructive jaundice (stenting or choledochojejunostomy) should be considered.

Management of dysphagia secondary to obstructing oesophageal cancer

The relative merits of radiotherapy and surgery for the patient with dysphagia secondary to oesophageal cancer are outlined in Table 11.1. Surgery undoubtedly has the advantage of rapid relief of dysphagia whilst external beam radiotherapy may take several weeks to achieve its maximal effect and indeed radiation oesophagitis may result in a transient deterioration before benefit ensues. There is some concern that the

Table 11.1 Comparison of radiotherapy and surgical techniques in obstructive dysphagia

Technique	Advantages	Disadvantages
Resection	Potentially curative Normal diet in >90%	Only for early disease Operative mortality high Later relapse common
Intubation or stent	Rapid response >90% improve procedure mortality <10%	No effect on tumour; may grow into tube Blockage with solids May become dislodged
Laser/cryotherapy	Rapid response 80% improve Little morbidity	Average response duration 6 weeks
External beam RT	>80% improve Tumour response seen 5–10% cure in early disease	Response slow (several weeks) Acute oesophagitis
Brachytherapy	>80% respond Response within 1 week Simple day case procedure Tumour growth restraint	Acute oesophagitis

duration of response to surgical measures is shorter but often this will be sufficient for the patient's lifespan, which is usually only a few months from diagnosis. For most patients immediate dilatation and if available laser or cryotherapy with intubation should be considered. Radiotherapy should be offered to those with a perceived prognosis of several months who require more prolonged tumour growth delay with a preference for brachytherapy unless radical treatment is contemplated for those with localized disease after staging. Where it is not technically possible to retain a tube, particularly in lower third tumours, or the patient's general condition is poor then primary palliative radiotherapy is entirely appropriate.

There are other treatments which may also be considered in difficult cases particularly where other treatments have failed. Local injection of oesophageal tumours has been advocated using formalin. Reports suggest that this may significantly impede tumour growth and if combined with oesophagoscopy and dilatation improve dysphagia.

For superficial oesophageal tumours photodynamic therapy is available in a few specialist centres. This relies on photosensitive protoporphyrins being administered systemically, taken up into the tumour which is then exposed to ultraviolet light. The subsequent activation of the porphyrins within the tumour cells results in a cytotoxic effect. The major limitation to this technique is the penetration of light which needs to be delivered through an endoscope and will only reach superficial tumour. It may, however, be a further useful adjunct to the palliative treatment of oesophageal cancer where available. Because the protoporphyrin has to be given systemically, the patient has to remain out of direct sunlight for several days whilst the substances clear from their other cells and exposed parts of the body must remain covered.

Radiotherapy has a very limited role in the treatment of cancer of the stomach. Occasionally it may be considered for a large tumour causing recurrent haemorrhage when doses of 20–30 Gy over 1–2 weeks are usually delivered in the hope of achieving haemostasis. In this respect radiotherapy is usually very successful but may be associated with significant side effects, in particular nausea and anorexia, because of the sensitivity of the stomach and adjacent liver to irradiation.

Radiotherapy has been advocated for those patients presenting with inoperable carcinoma of the pancreas. A number of studies have been reported using both radical radiation therapy alone and radiotherapy combined with concomitant chemotherapy using drugs such as 5-FU. Modest improvements in survival with the addition of chemotherapy are reported but in practice the overall outlook remains very poor and most patients with inoperable disease are also not suitable for radical radiotherapy at the time of presentation.

In the palliative setting, radiotherapy has been advocated for the pain associated with local infiltration from pancreatic carcinoma. Anecdotal reports suggest this is a useful procedure delivering short palliative courses of treatment to the area of the pancreas although pain relief is only partial and temporary.

Radiotherapy has a limited role for the treatment of carcinoma of the bile duct. In certain circumstances, however, where there is localized tumour within the bile duct causing obstruction and stents have been passed through the obstruction, a high dose rate afterloading catheter can be passed through the stent in the same way as described above for oesophageal cancer. This is used to direct an iridium source to rest within the bile duct and deliver a high localized dose of radiation to the lumen. This may prolong tumour regression and prevent further obstructive symptoms but will have no impact upon the overall natural history of the condition.

Chemotherapy

This treatment has a limited role in carcinoma of the oesophagus. It is used in primary treatment either in the neoadjuvant setting prior to radical surgery or postoperatively. There is a modest improvement in the results of radical treatment reported with this approach. The drugs used are usually combinations containing cisplatinum with one or two other drugs such as 5-FU, mitomycin C, or vindesine. It is also used to enhance the effects of radical radiotherapy, the standard regimen containing cisplatin and 5-FU.

In the palliative setting, chemotherapy has no role in the management of carcinoma of the oesophagus. In stomach cancer, trials continue evaluating the role of chemotherapy as an adjunct to primary radical surgery in the small number of patients for whom this is appropriate. For the majority, however, palliative treatment is the only option. Modest response rates are seen to chemotherapy with 5-FU-based schedules from which up to a third of patients may get some regression of their tumour. This may be associated with a transient improvement in symptoms.

Infusional chemotherapy may give improved response rates using a combination schedule, ECF, comprising epirubicin and cisplatinum given in single doses every 3 weeks together with a continuous infusion of 5-FU delivered through an infusion pump into an indwelling central line. Response rates of around 80 per cent are reported, with some patients achieving complete remission of their tumour. Despite this, however, a high rate of relapse is seen some months later but for many patients this offers a worthwhile respite from symptomatic disease.

Chemotherapy using 5-FU based schedules are used with radiotherapy in attempts at radical treatment for carcinoma of the pancreas and in the palliative setting both 5-FU based regimens and the newer drugs paclitaxel and gemcitabine have been shown to have modest activity and are of benefit to good performance status patients.

Cancers of the bile ducts are generally less sensitive to currently available chemotherapy and this is not generally included in their management.

Key points

+ 5-FU based chemotherapy, particularly by continuous in fusion may achieve high rates of response in advanced gastric cancer.
+ Gemcitabine or paclitaxel based chemotherapy may achieve palliation in pancreatic cancer.

Case History 11.1

Mrs T is a 69-year-old woman who has developed anorexia with marked weight loss in a period of 6 months. When she starts to have frequent vomiting, she seeks help. At endoscopy an extensive carcinoma of the stomach is discovered (linitis plastica). This is inoperable but there is a possible option of chemotherapy. During this period she remains on the hospital ward and is referred to the hospital palliative care team for advice on how to control her distressing nausea and vomiting. This proves to be difficult; while the background nausea responds, her frequent vomits continue. A trial of steroids make no difference.

Although her children have concerns, Mrs T decides to give chemotherapy a go. She is given a combination of mitomycin, epirubicin and 5-flurouracil. Improvement in her symptoms becomes apparent after the second course. She is later able to enjoy a small portion of birthday cake with the family. CT scan confirms that there has been some response so treatment continues. A few months later she develops ascites. No further chemotherapy is offered at this point but she has good relief of symptoms from drainage of the fluid.

Case History 11.1 (continued)

Practice points

- Prokinetic anti-emetic drugs may be ineffective when diffuse tumour infiltration is likely to disrupt normal peristalsis.
- Anorexia and vomiting may be due to tumour mass filling the lumen of the stomach.
- Chemotherapy can offer palliation of distressing symptoms and should not be dismissed as an option.
- Radiotherapy does not have a useful role in this situation and is not well tolerated at this site.

Other treatment

Nutritional support always presents major difficulties in patients with carcinoma of the oesophagus and stomach and to a lesser extent pancreas and gall bladder. The perceived need to eat to remain healthy often creates great stress and tension within relationships for the patient who is often neither hungry nor able to manage large amounts of food. It is important, therefore, to dispel such concepts and reassure both the patient and relatives that in general only a low level of nutrition and adequate hydration is required for comfort. Despite this there may be distressing symptoms because of the limitations in swallowing or abdominal fullness. In general, hydration can be maintained by non-invasive measures and ultimately simple oral hygiene and a subcutaneous infusion may be all that is required in the dying patient.

The role of other measures such as nasogastric intubation or percutaneous gastrostomy is limited. These may be essential for those patients requiring support during a period of intensive, potentially curative treatment. However, in the palliative setting they do not enhance symptom control in advanced disease and have no impact upon the natural history or survival of an individual. It is important, however, to identify the patient who may not have advanced cachexia and be distressed because of hunger for whom enteral feeding is important and may be justified despite advanced malignancy.

Gastric outflow obstruction will result in gastric distension and overflow vomiting. This is one situation where a nasogastric tube may make a major difference to the patient and should not be denied them. An alternative to this is a venting gastrostomy.

The pain from cancer of the pancreas can be intractable. The most successful treatment for this is intervention with a coeliac plexus block (see next section) and this should be available for such patients. In general this will be far more successful than other measures such as radiotherapy or palliative chemotherapy, and where pain is the primary symptom, it is the most appropriate manoeuvre.

Obstructive jaundice is best treated by surgical decompression either using a stent which may be introduced percutaneously or endoscopically, or by choledocho-jejunostomy. Patients with prolonged obstructive jaundice may have clotting deficiencies and their prothrombin time should always be checked before they are subjected to surgical procedures. This may be improved by the administration of vitamin K prior to intervention.

Intractable itching related to jaundice may be very difficult to control. Topical preparations are usually not effective and antihistamines have little effect. Cholestyramine will reduce the bile salt pool by chelation within the gut but is often unpalatable for the patient. The best solution is surgical relief of obstructive jaundice by decompression.

Key points

- Intensive nutritional support may be required for patients undergoing radical surgery or radiotherapy, but in the palliative setting it is rarely indicated.
- Nasogastic intubation is rarely indicated except where there is prolonged gastric distension.
- Pain from pancreatic cancer is best treated by a coeliac plexus block.

Coeliac plexus blocks

Visceral pain is mediated through sympathetic and parasympathetic nerve fibres. This explains why pain arising from pathology of internal organs may be poorly localized and associated with autonomic symptoms such as malaise, sweating and nausea.

A very successful example of neurolytic procedures in the management of cancer pain is the use of coeliac blocks. These can be used for pain arising from the pancreas, gall bladder and liver.

Pre-ganglionic sympathetic fibres from T5–T12 pass as splanchnic nerves to synapse in ganglia, which constitute the coeliac plexus. These lie bilaterally close to the first lumbar vertebra. Injection of alcohol in this vicinity will block pain arising from the upper abdominal viscera down to the transverse colon.

This may be performed at laparotomy, when an advanced pancreatic cancer is discovered, or by percutaneous injection using an image intensifier, under local anaesthetic.

Side effects of this procedure include hypotension, diarrhoea, impotence and para-plegia – the latter complication is rare, but may arise from injection into the vertebral arteries. For most patients this is an effective procedure for pain that is sometimes intractable. In some it may be necessary to combine with an intrathecal alcohol injec-tion to block coexistent somatic pain.

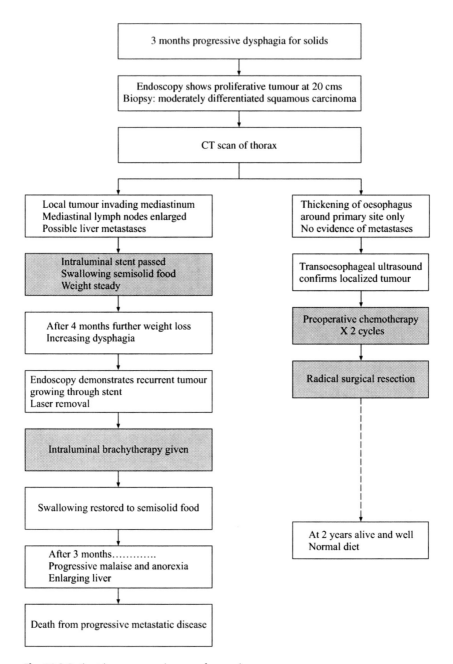

Fig. 11.2 Patient journey: carcinoma of oesophagus.

Case History 11.2

A 67-year-old man has had symptoms of reflux and heartburn for a few years. He now complains that he feels food stick at the level of his xiphisternum. When he is investigated, there appears to be a narrowing of his lower oesophagus. This turns out to be a carcinoma and he has a surgical resection. He makes an excellent recovery and all his symptoms resolve. 14 months later he develops severe palpitations and attends the accident and emergency department of his local hospital. He has a supraventricular tachycardia and is admitted. His chest X-ray shows an abnormal heart shadow and he has a CT scan. This demonstrates tumour involving the pericardium and also mediastinal lymphadenopathy. A CT scan of his abdomen is clear. He has a course of radiotherapy to his mediastinum and remains well for several months. He subsequently notices some skin nodules and an enlarged supraclavicular node. He has further palliative radiotherapy but is less well and is losing weight. He is later found to have liver metastases and deteriorates rapidly.

Practice points

- Chronic inflammation is an aetiological factor in oesophageal cancer.
- Patients with dysphagia are able to localize the level of obstruction with accuracy.
- When symptoms develop in someone with a recent cancer diagnosis – think of the cancer as a probable cause!
- The appearance of a supraclavicular node is often a marker of widespread dissemination.

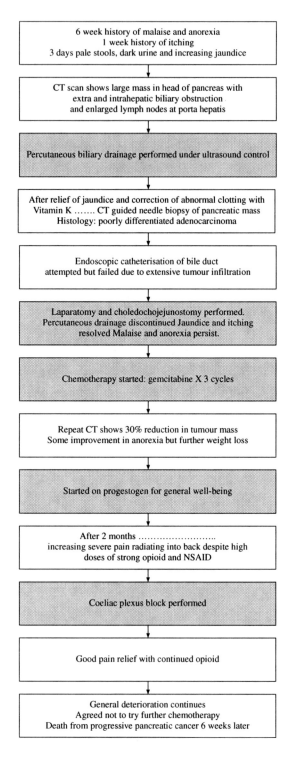

Fig. 11.3 Patient journey: carcinoma of pancreas.

Case History 11.3

A 53-year-old woman has a history of weight loss, epigastric pain radiating to the back, and latterly, nausea and vomiting. The vomiting happens every 2–3 days, when she fills a large bowl and then feels better. Her general practitioner is very concerned when he is called out to see her. He arranges for urgent admission to hospital.

A CT scan shows a mass in the body of the pancreas, and this is compressing the duodenal loop. The radiological diagnosis is of an advanced pancreatic cancer. A raised CA19 level supports this diagnosis.

A stent is passed by endoscopy into the duodenum and this relieves her vomiting. She has commenced regular morphine for her pain but this only helps to a bit and the doses are escalating. She is referred to a pain specialist who performs a coeliac plexus block with marked improvement in her pain. She is offered the option of entering a trial of chemotherapy but declines this and dies at home four months later.

Practice points

Cancers of the head of the pancreas may present with painless jaundice as they obstruct the common bile duct; those arising in the body may cause symptoms later.

- Intractable back pain usually indicates local invasion from the pancreas into retroperitoneal tissues and hence that the disease is inoperable.
- Intermittent, large volume vomits are strongly suggestive of gastric outlet obstruction.
- Stenting can relieve gastrointestinal and biliary obstructions.
- The value of palliative chemotherapy for advanced pancreatic cancer is still to be evaluated through clinical trials.

Chapter 12

Head and neck cancer

Aetiology

Head and neck cancer in its early stages confined to its site of origin will in many cases be cured by radical local treatment. In contrast advanced progressive disease presents a major challenge in symptom management. In Western nations it accounts for around 5 per cent of all cancer and is the cause of 2500 deaths annually in the United Kingdom.

The majority of tumours are squamous carcinomas arising from changes in the epithelium of the aerodigestive tract. This is exposed to a number of environmental factors that are potentially carcinogenic, especially smoking and heavy alcohol consumption which appear to have a synergistic effect on the risk of cancer development. These individuals may develop white patches of leukoplakia on the mucosal surfaces, which are associated with subsequent malignant transformation. Chronic trauma is another recognized factor, whether from ill-fitting dentures or broken teeth. The practice of chewing tobacco and betel among Asian people is a cause of high rates of oral cancer while early exposure to the Epstein–Barr virus in Chinese populations is implicated in the development of nasopharyngeal tumours.

Pathology and patterns of spread

Squamous carcinoma in accessible sites such as the mouth may present as a small, painless nodule which enlarges and subsequently ulcerates. There is invasion of the submucosal tissues and spread along myofascial planes until eventually cartilage and bone are invaded.

The head and neck tissues have a rich lymphatic drainage and so this is an important route of spread for cancer. The incidence of node involvement increases with the size of the primary tumour and there is also some variation with site, being very low in cancer of the true vocal cords but common with tumours in the oropharynx or nasopharynx. Involvement of the lymphatics leads to enlargement of the draining nodes; mid-line tumours especially those arising in tongue, epiglottis, or nasopharynx, will drain bilaterally and produce enlarged nodes on both sides of the neck. Patients may present with an enlarged cervical lymph node as the presenting symptom of an underlying head and neck cancer and on occasions depite an extensive search this may be the only detectable site of disease (see Chapter 19).

Lymphadenopathy may be reactive to adjacent ulceration and infection, but a firm painless node of 1 cm or more in size should be regarded with suspicion. Initially, a metastatic node is mobile on palpation against the superficial tissues but may subsequently become fixed by extracapsular spread. This is a serious development as it may preclude surgical clearance and cure. Involvement of the overlying skin ultimately leads to fungation. Metastatic spread may involve nodes throughout the cervical lymphatic chains from the base of skull to clavicle. In these situations patients develop facial oedema and restriction of movement. Other non-palpable nodes may also be involved, usually found on a staging scan or at surgery, for example those in the pre-auricular region (e.g. with tumours of the ear and parotid), or parapharyngeal nodes adjacent to the posterior pharyngeal wall. Whilst not being palpable they may cause local symptoms such as dysphagia or pain.

Distant metastases may arise in lung, liver, and bone in some patients, particularly if there is a locally advanced tumour or involvement of multiple lymph nodes. Squamous carcinoma of head and neck, including upper oesophagus, can occasionally be associated with hypercalcaemia.

In addition to the lining mucosa, malignant tumours also arise in salivary glands; most of these are adenocarcinomas or adenoid cystic carcinomas and occur most frequently in the parotid gland. Malignant transformation occurs in up to 10 per cent of patients with benign pleomorphic adenomas of the parotid, often some years after the initial diagnosis. Spread to lymph nodes and distant sites such as lung and bone occurs. Adenoid cystic tumours show characteristic spread along nerve sheaths which may result in neuropathic pain.

Other important cancers in adults include malignant melanoma, arising from the mucosa of mouth, nasal cavity, or within the orbit. Chemodectomas develop in the middle ear (glomus jugulare) and in association with the carotid sheath; these are highly vascular tumours which are usually benign. Localized plasmacytomas may occur in head and neck sites, such as nasal cavity or tonsil, without any evidence of multiple myeloma although this subsequently develops in up to a third of patients. Extranodal non-Hodgkin's lymphomas arise in the lymphoid tissues of Waldeyer's ring, especially the tonsil, and also the conjunctiva and orbit.

The population of adult patients with head and neck cancer includes many heavy smokers, alcoholics, and the elderly, which create additional problems in treatment. Most of those who are dying from head and neck cancers will have uncontrolled local disease whether or not metastases are present. Second primary tumours develop in 7–14 per cent of patients who have been treated for head and neck cancer. Of these, 50 per cent will be at another site in the head and neck and 30 per cent arise in lung or oesophagus. Sadly, the commonest cause of death among survivors of early laryngeal cancer is lung cancer and a number of successfully treated patients survive their head and neck cancer to die from other smoking-related illnesses. There is some evidence that giving retinoids to head and neck cancer patients may reduce the number of second primary cancers in this group although a greater impact would be made by alteration in smoking and alcohol intake.

Key points: head and neck cancer

- Major aetiological factors are smoking and alcohol exposure.
- Most cancers are squamous carcinomas arising from the mucosal surfaces.
- Salivary gland tumours may arise in both major glands and minor glands throughout the region and are commonly adenocarcinomas or adenoid cystic carcinomas.
- Spread is to cervical lymph nodes most commonly; blood borne metastases are relatively rare at presentation.

Management of early head and neck cancer

Head and neck cancer embraces a diverse range of malignancy arising from different sites, which are summarized in Table 12.1. The clinical problems and management are also diverse. Successful radical local treatment of head and neck cancer entails surgery, or radiotherapy, or often a combined approach. There is an increasing role for chemotherapy together with radiotherapy with improved local control rates in survival. Combination chemotherapy will be the initial treatment of choice for high grade non-Hodgkin's lymphomas, often followed by a course of radiotherapy.

The remainder of this chapter will focus on the management of patients with squamous carcinoma of the head and neck region.

Both surgery and radiotherapy aim to treat a volume of tissue containing tumour with a margin of normal tissue and usually the adjacent draining lymph nodes. In many patients with early cancers they may represent equally effective alternatives and there are advantages and disadvantages to both. Ideally, each individual should be jointly assessed by the oncologist and surgical specialist, who may be an ENT, plastic, maxillofacial, or dental surgeon.

The scope of surgery has been enhanced by modern techniques in reconstruction by which transfer of tissues from other sites can be successfully achieved using microvascular anastamoses. Surgical resection is usually the initial treatment of choice for tumours arising in the thyroid, major salivary glands, and anterior third of the tongue and for melanoma or soft tissue sarcoma as these respond less well to radiotherapy. Initial surgical intervention may also be needed if there is airway obstruction. Radiotherapy will be the treatment of choice for nasopharyngeal tumours.

Radiotherapy

This is the primary treatment for many early head and neck cancers as it avoids the loss of function and appearance caused by major surgery, and salvage is still possible if radiotherapy fails to control the disease. This may be of considerable importance for

Table 12.1 Classification of head and neck cancer by primary site

Site	Main histological types	Clinical problems
Oral cavity		
Lip, buccal mucosa,	Squamous carcinoma	Ulceration, pain, dental
Anterior 2/3 tongue	Salivary gland tumours	Difficulty chewing/swallowing
Floor of mouth, alveolus	Melanoma	Difficulty in articulation
Oropharynx[a]		
Tonsil, soft palate,	Squamous carcinoma	Otalgia, dysphagia
Posterior 1/3 tongue	Lymphoma	Trismus
Hypopharynx[a]		
Posterior pharyngeal wall,	Squamous carcinoma	Dysphagia, pooling of
pyriform fossa,		saliva
post-cricoid (pharyngo-		Hoarseness, otalgia
oesophageal junction)		
Nasopharynx[a, b]		
	Squamous carcinoma	Nasal obstruction & discharge
	(keratinizing, non-keratinizing,	Deafness, trismus, dysphagia
	or anaplastic)	Cranial nerve palsies, pain
Vocal cords	Squamous carcinoma	Hoarseness
Supraglottic[a]		Stridor, haemoptysis
Subglottic[a]		Dysphagia, otalgia
Nasal cavity and sinuses	Squamous carcinoma	Nasal obstruction, headache
Ethmoids, maxillary antrum	Adenocarcinoma	Blood-stained discharge
	Melanoma	Proptosis, diplopia
		Swollen cheek/palate, trismus
Ear		
Auditory canal, middle ear	Squamous carcinoma	Deafness, discharge, pain
	Chemodectoma (glomus jugulare)	Facial and other cranial
		Nerve palsies
Salivary glands[a, b]		
Parotid	Adenocarcinoma, adenoid cystic	Swelling, pain
Submental, submandibular	muco-epidermoid carcinoma	Trismus, dysphagia
Minor salivary glands	Squamous carcinoma	Facial and other CN palsies

[a] nodal involvement common

[b] associated with distant metastases

certain patients for example preservation of the larynx in a patient who has a profession in which the voice is essential. At any site, radical radiotherapy may be considered for tumour which is surgically inoperable because of size and anatomical constraints.

Radiotherapy has been greatly assisted by modern computerized tomographic (CT) scanning and magnetic resonance imaging (MRI), which define the extent of tumour spread and enable precise treatment planning with the aim of avoiding or shielding critical normal structures whilst covering the essential tumour volume. Immobilization shells are made for each patient to wear during every session to ensure reproducible positioning and accurate treatment. Brachytherapy techniques (see Chapter 5) are also valuable in the treatment of patients with accessible tumours, such as the tongue and floor of the mouth. These can be implanted with radioactive materials (e.g. iridium wires) or needles loaded with caesium. For the duration of the implant, usually a few days, a high dose is given in the immediate vicinity of the sources but normal tissues only a few centimetres away receive very little. This spares these tissues from the radiation side effects, in contrast to external beam treatments which encompass a much larger volume.

Radiotherapy is not given routinely following surgery but may be indicated if resection margins are close or incomplete or, if in the case of lymph node dissection there is extracapsular spread or multiple nodes were involved, when there is a high risk of local recurrence.

Side effects of radiotherapy

Acute effects develop during a course of radiotherapy and gradually settle over the following 4–6 weeks. The main side effect of any treatments involving the mouth or throat is a painful mucositis. Where this is visible, the mucosa looks raw and when severe develops a yellow, fibrinous exudate. The discomfort is compounded by an early reduction in saliva production. Swallowing becomes painful and difficult in patients who may already be malnourished because of poor diet or the effects of the tumour itself. Liquid food supplements are often indicated, either by mouth or nasogastric tube and more intensive nutritional support may be necessary for some.

Skin reactions occur where superficial tissues are included in the treatment volume. Temporary hair loss may occur in a few situations, such as from the back of the head when sinus cancers are irradiated due to the exit path of the beam.

Late effects develop from around 6 months onwards and are more significant as they represent irreversible changes and so symptoms persist and may worsen. A major problem for patients is a dry mouth due to reduced salivary flow, particularly when the parotid gland has been irradiated. This also leads to loss of taste and increased dental caries. Artificial saliva is not always acceptable to patients, but pilocarpine may be tried to improve the volume of saliva that can be produced. Regular dental checks and good oral hygiene are essential. Reduced mucosal secretion can also lead to persistent crusting of nasal passages. Sometimes, occlusion of lachrymal and salivary ducts occurs: treatment to tumour in the floor of the mouth can result in enlarged submandibular glands which are sometimes confused with metastatic nodes. Fibrosis around the temporomandibular joint causes trismus. Affected patients have difficulty in fully opening the mouth and so may have problems with feeding and oral hygiene.

High dose radiation leads to fibrosis of subcutaneous tissues and may cause stiffness and discomfort as when the anterior neck is treated, particularly after surgical dissection. The vascularity of tissues is reduced and so is the capacity for repair following injury whether surgery or trauma. In these situations, painful ulceration of soft tissues and necrosis of bone may develop which could require plastic surgery. Dental extraction can precipitate such problems and the dentist should be aware of any previous treatment to the oral cavity. Necrosis of the laryngeal cartilage is a recognized late complication of radiotherapy for cancer of the larynx. This is likely to occur in less than 5 per cent of patients but these will then require laryngectomy. Pharyngeal stricture may be a cause of swallowing difficulties in the absence of recurrent tumour.

Irradiation of the eye is always avoided unless there is no choice, for example, if a cancer of the maxillary sinus is invading the floor of the orbit. Cataracts can result from low doses and are inevitable with a dose of 15 Gy or more to the eye, but vision can be restored by cataract extraction. Other effects include radiation keratitis and secondary glaucoma. Inclusion of the eyeball in a high dose volume leads inevitably to blindness; the eye itself becomes closed and shrunken in the socket. Enucleation may be necessary if it is painful. Blindness can also result from damage to the optic nerve and chiasma. Great care is taken in treatment planning to ensure that the dose received by these and other vulnerable tissues such as brain and spinal cord does not exceed the limits of tolerance. Inclusion of the pituitary gland can result in hypopituitarism and when both lobes of the thyroid are treated hypothyroidism can develop, often not seen until several years after treatment.

Although some of these late radiation effects have serious consequences for the small number of patients who develop them, modern radiotherapy techniques aim to keep the radiation dose within safe limits to be sure of avoiding such complications.

Chemoradiation

Whilst chemotherapy alone has only modest effects in squamous head and neck cancer, and would not be considered as a primary treatment modality used alone, it has been shown that concurrent chemotherapy using cisplatin based drug schedules can improve results compared to radiation alone with overall gains of around 5 per cent in survival. In many centres this is now becoming part of routine management. In contrast no advantage has been shown for adjuvant chemotherapy used either before or after definitive local treatment although on occasions a very bulky tumour may be initially given chemotherapy in an attempt to either facilitate surgery or enable radiotherapy planning to be competed.

Management of metastatic lymph nodes

Surgical clearance of lymph nodes from the neck is performed electively as part of a radical local surgical resection where there is a high risk of subclinical node involvement and when there is palpable lymphatic spread at presentation. It will also be used when there is nodal recurrence after treatment to the primary. In the latter situation the success rate in controlling disease is about 50 per cent. Involvement of multiple nodes or invasion beyond the node capsule correlates with reduced local control and the development of distant metastases. Radiotherapy is given to the neck postoperatively in these circumstances to reduce the risk of relapse.

Radical node dissection includes removal of the sternomastoid muscle and internal jugular vein together with the lower pole of the parotid and sub-mandibular gland. As a consequence, the accessory nerve and mandibular branch of the facial nerve are also sacrificed. There may be complications of wound healing and occasionally, rupture of the carotid artery. As a longer-term consequence of this procedure, the patient may be conscious of disfigurement and will have a drooping lower lip. There is wasting of muscles around the shoulder with loss of function. The scar tissue in subcutaneous layers causes stiffness and discomfort and sometimes this includes pain secondary to nerve damage. In some situations, a functional node dissection may be performed with preservation of the lower parotid and nerves. A full block dissection cannot be carried out on both sides because it is necessary to have one internal jugular vein left intact.

Fixed nodes may indicate inoperability and radiotherapy is given in these situations. The nodal disease may be included in the primary treatment volume or in a separate field to treat the neck. Subsequent surgical salvage may still be possible for some patients who relapse after radiotherapy.

Results of treatment

Successful treatment depends upon effective control of the local disease (i.e. the primary tumour and any involved nodes). Obviously, the earlier the stage of the tumour at diagnosis, the better the outcome of treatment. An ulcer in the anterior mouth or persistent hoarseness usually leads the patient to seek prompt attention but unfortunately the opposite is true for a tumour of the base of tongue or pyriform fossa. Treatment of early oral and laryngeal cancers has a success rate of 80–90 per cent; in contrast locally advanced tumours will have only a 40 per cent long-term control rate falling to 15 per cent for tumours in the hypopharynx. The development of metastatic spread to lymph nodes significantly affects the prognosis for an individual patient and reduces the expected outlook for any stage by approximately 50 per cent.

Most recurrences of head and neck cancer occur within the first 2 years after initial treatment. Patients who remain apparently free of disease beyond this have a high chance of cure. However, late relapses are seen with some types such as cancers of thyroid, salivary glands, and nasopharynx.

Key points: treatment of head and neck cancer

- Radical treatment is with primary surgery or radical radiotherapy.
- Post-operative radiotherapy is indicated where there are incomplete or close resection margins.
- Neck nodes are managed by block dissection and where there are multiple levels or extracapsular extension post-operative radiotherapy.
- Results with radiotherapy are improved if cisplatin based chemotherapy is given concomittantly.

Problems associated with advanced disease

Pain

This is a significant problem for most patients with locally recurrent and advanced head and neck cancer. This reflects the rich sensory innervation of the tissues:

- *The trigeminal nerve* supplies the skin of face, forehead, and scalp anterior to the vertex; the orbit; nasal and oral cavities; the anterior part of the external ear and the dura.
- *The glossopharyngeal nerve* supplies the upper pharynx including tonsil and posterior third of tongue; eustachian tube and middle ear.
- *The vagus nerve* supplies larynx, lower pharynx, and upper oesophagus and also provides sensory innervation to the concha of the external ear, tympanic membrane, and external canal.
- *The second and third cervical nerves* supply the posterior scalp, skin over the angle of the jaw, and posterior pinna.

Neuropathic pain is commonly a result of nerve infiltration. It is a particular problem with adenoid cystic salivary gland cancers because of the tendency for them to spread by perineural invasion. The possibility of a neuropathic component should be considered especially where intense paroxysmal episodes of pain occur.

Referred pain may present a diagnostic challenge. Otalgia can be due to direct invasion of the ear but is also mediated via the vagal or glossopharyngeal nerves from the larynx or pharynx. Headache is caused by tumour invading the sinuses or extension into the anterior and middle cranial fossae while invasion of the base of skull produces pain in the temporal and occipital regions. A soft tissue mass in the neck or bone metastases in the upper cervical spine are further causes of occipital and neck pain.

In advanced cancer, several sensory nerves may be affected and disease is often bilateral, which limits the usefulness of specific neurolytic procedures.

Pain is also caused by tumour enlargement and associated tissue swelling in confined spaces; ulceration may be compounded by infection and direct invasion of nerve and bone may ensue.

Following treatment pain may arise because of fibrosis or rarely radionecrosis.

Difficulties in eating

The presence of infected, necrotic material from local tumour leads to unpleasant taste and breath which spoils the enjoyment of food and suppresses appetite. There may be loose or lost teeth and dentures may no longer fit. Progressing disease in the oral cavity and oropharynx may invade cheek muscles and fix the tongue so that food and saliva can no longer be propelled to the back of the throat and drooling occurs. Involvement of the retromolar area by tumour (as from tonsil or posterior tongue) or the parapharyngeal space (from parotid, nasopharynx) leads to trismus and great difficulty in opening the mouth for eating or even hygiene. The action of the superior constrictor muscles of the upper pharynx in swallowing may be impaired by direct invasion from the primary site or adjacent nodes. A tumour mass at any level in the pharynx or upper oesophagus will cause dysphagia by obstruction and sometimes this is caused by enlargement of a supraglottic tumour.

The neurological control of the involuntary stage of swallowing is disrupted by damage to the 10th, 11th, and 12th cranial nerves which can arise from invasion of the base of skull from the parotid, middle ear, and nasopharynx. Obstruction and impaired co-ordination lead to aspiration of food and secretions and ultimately to chest infections. This is a common terminal development in the weakened patient.

Following treatment, even if successful, symptoms may persist. Reduced salivation as a consequence of radiotherapy leaves the patient with a dry mouth and loss of taste. Laryngectomy patients have difficulty in clearing secretions as they cannot cough effectively. Reconstruction of the tongue and pharynx may leave residual problems with swallowing.

Issues surrounding feeding can be a dilemma in the care of such patients. At least a third who have advanced disease at diagnosis are severely malnourished; nutritional support is easier to justify if there is active treatment to be given. Patients with painful or difficult swallowing and inadequate intake may be given supplements through a fine-bore nasogastric tube if this can be passed. Alternative options include a pharyngostomy or percutaneous gastrostomy for feeding. These may be placed at laparoscopy or using endoscopic or radiological techniques.

It may be hard to assess the longer-term benefit of such procedures for patients who are beyond other active treatments and there may be professional concern at prolonging a distressing course of illness. Such decisions must involve careful consideration of patient comfort and choice; many individuals have little or no appetite and may choose not to be supported by feeding. At the same time measures are needed to prevent thirst and ensure that they receive drugs as needed for symptom control.

Case History 12.1

MR D was an ex-serviceman who had consumed a heavy intake of alcohol and had smoked heavily for a number of years. He developed a squamous carcinoma of his posterior tongue with fixed, enlarged lymph nodes in both sides of his upper neck. His disease was inoperable but it was possible to give him a course of radiotherapy. Unfortunately it became clear within three months of finishing treatment that he had residual tumour in his tongue. As the disease progressed, his tongue became fixed and swollen, affecting speech and swallowing. Palliative chemotherapy was offered to try to improve the situation for a while, but if this were to be embarked upon, he would need help with feeding. Nutritional support was given through a PEG (gastrostomy) and this made administration of drugs to help control some other problems much easier.

Case History 12.1 (continued)

He tolerated chemotherapy well and there was some reduction in the size of his tongue, and hence improvement in speech for a few weeks. However his cancer progressed quickly once treatment was stopped.

He wished to continue his gastrostomy feeds while at home, but decided himself against more treatment. Later on, solid tumour in his neck began to narrow his airway and cause stridor. He wanted to remain at home. Steroids made a transient improvement while he was commenced on a diamorphine and midazolam infusion to ease the distress of his breathing. Nebulised saline and oxygen, available at the bedside, also helped. Gastrostomy feeding had been discontinued by this time with the agreement of his family and he died peacefully a week later.

Practice points

- The best means of feeding and dealing with airway obstruction are frequent dilemmas in head and neck cancer. Interventions are justified to support the patient if further treatment is feasible and contemplated.
- More difficult decisions arise when no further treatment is an option. These are often influenced by the extent to which it is possible to improve the situation by symptom control and support; usually the individual patient is able to make a clear judgement on this.

Difficulties in communication

Problems in communication frequently add to the distress and isolation of the patient with advanced disease. Dysphonia is a major symptom of tumours involving larynx and also those that spread from the hypopharynx. Patients will be distressed by the sound of their voice and by the effort needed to make themselves understood. Some may already have undergone tracheostomy or laryngectomy; they will have a post-operative programme of rehabilitation and use pharyngeal speech, external vibration air in the upper tract, or amplification of whispers. In other patients valved tracheal cannulae may be used to preserve voice.

Speech and language therapists play an essential role in the pre- and post-operative management of these individuals. These professionals also offer valuable help in other patients who subsequently develop difficulties with speech or swallowing as a result of progressing disease. Other patients may have problems in articulation because of tumour involving the oral cavity, particularly where there is loss of mobility of the tongue. Deafness can cause additional problems particularly in the elderly person if there is blockage of eustachian tubes or the external auditory canal.

Obstruction of the airway itself presents further dilemmas in advanced stages. The patient may feel breathless at rest, there may be obvious stridor, and speech is an effort.

A tracheostomy is usually possible although there are occasional situations when extensive tumour in the anterior neck prevents this but as a result the patient will lose spontaneous speech, needing some means of occluding the stoma or a speaking tube to achieve speech. As with feeding, intervention in these situations requires careful assessment and again, some patients may decline this.

Other problems

* Visual disturbances may arise due to tumour involving the orbit or extending from the nasal sinuses which may cause proptosis with double vision; the latter may also arise from involvement of the 3rd–6th cranial nerve in the cavernous sinus, usually by tumour spreading from the nasopharynx. Pressure and damage to the optic nerve itself by retro-orbital disease will cause loss of vision.

* Neurological problems associated with cancer invading the neck include recurrent laryngeal and phrenic nerve palsy and Horner's syndrome.

* Cranial nerve lesions are commonly associated with tumour spreading through foramina in the skull base.

* Intracranial metastases are rare but direct extension into the anterior and middle cranial fossae may occur with tumour arising from the ethmoid and sphenoid sinuses, nasopharynx, and middle ear.

* Bleeding and discharge may occur from ulcerated surface tumour; deep invasion of the upper neck can occasionally cause a major haemorrhage from the carotid artery as a terminal event.

* Perhaps the hardest problem for people to live with is the disfigurement caused by the treatment, the disease, or both. Prostheses are widely used after major surgery to improve function and appearance: for example, radical surgery for cancer of the maxillary sinus may entail enucleation of the orbit and resection of the roof of the mouth and the patient will have a dental prosthesis and a false eye. They can sometimes be used to close off a fistula when a major cavity is caused by tumour at a late stage.

Management of advanced and incurable head and neck cancer

The consequences of uncontrolled head and neck cancer are so dire for the patient that radical, rather than palliative, treatment should be attempted both to give even a small chance of cure and also to achieve maximal palliation.

Surgical resection is sometimes undertaken for locally extensive disease with immediate palliation of a painful, ulcerating tumour. This may be followed by radiotherapy if there is a likelihood of residual disease. Such procedures submit the patient to major procedures followed by some weeks of rehabilitation and would not be justified in situations of borderline curability.

Tumour obstructing the pharynx or airway may need urgent intervention, possibly by laser resection or a tracheostomy even where radical resection is not possible.

Radiotherapy alone is the only option for many patients with advanced inoperable cancer. The results for late stage disease are poor but taking all sites, approach a 35 per cent, 5-year survival. Attempts have been made to improve the treatment results by a number of approaches. Combined radiotherapy with chemotherapy may improve response and control rates but at the cost of increased toxicity especially if both are given simultaneously. Another promising technique is to deliver the radiotherapy in smaller fractions, 2 or 3 times daily, over a shorter period of time – so-called accelerated hyperfractionation. This enhances the damage done to tumour cells without increasing late damage to normal tissues and may produce improved results in more advanced disease. Alternatively in the frail patient hypofraction delivering a small number of large fractions over a relatively short time will minimize hospital visits and still achieve significant tumour growth delay and shrinkage for palliation. Short courses may be given to prevent fungation of a lymph node mass in the neck or to the base of skull to prevent cranial nerve damage. Soft tissue recurrences may develop after surgery in the skin flaps or at a stoma, and these can be usefully treated.

In recurrent disease after high dose radical radiotherapy such treatment cannot be repeated to the same tissues as this would cause a high incidence of tissue damage. It is however sometimes possible to retreat small areas of tumour recurrence using palliative doses to keep the symptomatic disease in check; often single weekly treatments will be adequate and achieve useful regression and even healing of bleeding or ulcerated areas with acceptable side effects.

Chemotherapy, while not by itself curative in head and neck cancer, can be used in the palliation of advanced disease. Active drugs include methotrexate, cisplatin, and 5-fluorouracil (5-FU), each with a response rate of around 20 per cent. This can be increased by the use of combinations, but at the cost of increased toxicity. Particularly troublesome side effects for these patients are mucositis and nausea and vomiting, although the use of anti-emetics, such as ondansetron, will minimize the latter. Regional chemotherapy has been investigated as a means of reducing systemic toxicity; drugs are perfused via an indwelling catheter positioned in the external carotid artery. This can be used for unilateral, inoperable cancers and increased response rates are seen but without significant prolongation of survival.

In some difficult situations that appear to be hopeless, the decision may be to withhold any surgery or radiotherapy rather than add the problems of the procedure and side effects to the existing difficulties for the patient. When chemotherapy is given both patient and doctor must be very clear about the aims of treatment and the end-points. The situation should be re-evaluated after at most every 2–3 courses. Chemotherapy may lead to reduction in pain from a tumour mass, healing of ulceration, and improvement in function if, for example, the tongue is becoming fixed. There can undoubtedly be psychological benefits, especially in the younger patient with advanced disease. However, the results are short-lasting. Most studies show a median duration of response of 3–6 months and an overall median survival of 6–10 months.

Key points: advanced and incurable disease

- Pain is often neuropathic from direct infiltration of nerves.
- Nutritional problems are common.
- Communication may be difficult due to impaired speech or hearing difficulty.
- Radical treatment may still offer best palliation even in advanced disease.
- Palliative radiotherapy in advanced cancers can be used to treat symptoms associated with nodal disease, skin nodules and stomal recurrences, and bone metastases.
- Chemotherapy may also offer a means of achieving tumour shrinkage and palliation.
- The 'no treatment'option should always be discussed in the light of likely achievements and toxicity of treatment.

Case History 12.2

An 80-year-old lady, who was living alone, developed difficulty in swallowing. ENT investigation revealed that she had a 3 cm tumour in the post-cricoid region of the upper oesophagus. There was no evidence of lymph node involvement or distant spread so despite her age, it seemed reasonable to treat with radical radiotherapy. She remained in hospital for her treatment over 4 weeks; during the second half she developed painful mucositis so that swallowing was even more difficult. Oral intake was maintained via a fine bore nasogastric tube. At the end of her radiotherapy, the local hospice agreed to take her for ongoing care before she was able to return home.

In the week following transfer, her feeding tube slipped out and she refused to have it replaced. She still had been requiring regular morphine solution to help her pain, so this was continued as diamorphine injections. She became more withdrawn; at times she seemed distressed so occasional injections of sedative (midazolam) were administered. A visiting oncologist was concerned to learn that she was confined to bed and deteriorating.

The nursing team had not appreciated that her treatment was potentially curative and not palliative. In fact this lady had become low in mood and dehydrated; she was declining to take anything by mouth even though her swallowing had begun to improve.

She wished to remain at the hospice but accepted IV fluids. Her medication was reviewed and any sedative drugs were discontinued. Instead, there was an active program to mobilize her and encourage fluids. Although this took several more weeks, she eventually went home on a soft diet with regular monitoring by the community team.

Case History 12.2 (continued)

Practice points

- Age alone should not determine which cancer treatment (or none) is offered: radical treatment is usually justified for potentially curable disease.
- As hospices may offer intermediate supportive care, it is important to recognize the aims of recent or current cancer therapies and not make assumptions that there is advanced disease.

Chapter 13

Gynaecological cancer

Carcinoma of the cervix

Cancer of the cervix is the third most common cancer in women after breast and lung cancer. In the United Kingdom there are around 5000 cases each year accounting for around 20 per cent of cancers in women. Predisposing factors include early age of first intercourse, multiple sexual partners, low socioeconomic status, and smoking. There is increasing evidence that it is directly related to infection with human papilloma virus types 16 and 18, and this may account for the increased incidence in partners of men whose previous sexual partners have developed the disease.

The common cervical cancer is a squamous carcinoma; 5 per cent are adenocarcinomas arising from the endocervical glandular tissue. Distant metastases occur relatively late in the development of cervical cancer with local growth into the upper vagina and laterally into the pelvic tissue being the common routes of early direct spread. Lymph node involvement within the pelvis and subsequently para-aortic lymph node chain is also common once the tumour has escaped from the cervix being found in 50 per cent of patients presenting with stage 3 disease (defined as tumour which is fixed to pelvic side-wall or involving lower third of vagina).

In areas where there is an effective screening programme using cervical smears then early presentation of disease will predominate which is cured surgically with either a cone biopsy for in situ disease or hysterectomy for micro-invasive (stage IA) or early invasive (stage IB) cancer. In Europe and the United States around two-thirds of women will present with early stage surgically treatable carcinoma of the cervix, but in India and South America where the disease is much more common and there is no national screening programme, the majority of patients present with advanced inoperable disease.

Prognosis

Patients presenting with early localized disease treated with radical surgery have a 5-year cure rate of around 80 per cent. For more advanced disease spreading into the pelvic tissues or upper vagina this falls to around 50 per cent and if there is fixation to the pelvic side-wall or involvement of the lower vagina then 5-year survival of more than 30 per cent is unusual. Few patients presenting with distant metastases will survive for a period of years.

Common symptoms

Haemorrhage

The presenting symptoms of carcinoma of the cervix in those patients not detected by asymptomatic screening programmes are vaginal bleeding which may be spontaneous or provoked by intercourse. Advanced disease may present with continuous vaginal bleeding and often an associated offensive discharge from the necrotic tumour. Obstruction of the cervical canal can result in accumulation of altered blood (haemato-colpus) within the uterine cavity or infection (pyocolpus) within the uterine cavity. Locally advanced disease may infiltrate into the bladder base causing haematuria and posteriorly into the anterior rectal wall causing rectal bleeding. Recurrent disease following hysterectomy frequently results in a pelvic mass invading the vaginal vault which will bleed into the vagina presenting once again with vaginal bleeding.

Pain

The pain due to advanced carcinoma of the cervix can be severe and intractable. A progressive pelvic mass infiltrating the pelvic tissues and involving the lumbosacral plexus results in both local pain and neuropathic pain involving the lumbosacral segments. Pain from involved lymphadenopathy may also be a feature causing, in particular, back pain from para-aortic lymph nodes.

Bone metastases are rare in carcinoma of the cervix but nonetheless recognized and may present with bone pain.

Obstruction

Growth of tumour laterally from the cervix can involve the ureter and one well-recognized presentation of advanced cervical carcinoma is renal failure due to bilateral ureteric obstruction and hydronephrosis. Pelvic lymphadenopathy may result in oedema of the lower limbs.

Other symptoms

Involvement of the anterior vaginal wall may affect the urethra causing urinary frequency or dysuria. Invasion of the vesico-urethral angle can cause urgency and incontinence. Fistulae may form between the bladder and the vagina (vesico-vaginal), or the vagina and the rectum (recto-vaginal). These will result respectively in the passage of urine or faeces per vagina.

Key points: carcinoma of cervix

◆ The majority of women in Europe and the United States present with early disease and over 80 per cent will be cured by radical hysterectomy. The reverse is true in countries without established screening programmes.

- The common cervical cancer is squamous carcinoma.
- Commonly present with vaginal bleeding intermenstrual or post-coital, or in older women with post-menopausal bleeding.
- Advanced disease may present with pain from pelvic infiltration or renal failure due to ureteric obsrtuction.

Management

Radiotherapy

The treatment of choice for advanced inoperable carcinoma of the cervix is radiotherapy and there is increasing evidence that best results are achieved by combining radiotherapy with chemotherapy. The best combinations and sequencing have yet to be defined but the basis of chemoradiation in cancer of the cervix is to use cisplatin 40 mg/m^2 weekly during each of the external beam weeks of treatment. Disease localized to the pelvis but not involving the bladder or rectum (stage II or III) will be treated with a course of radical radiotherapy involving external beam treatment for 4–5 weeks followed by intracavitary treatment. This involves the insertion of applicators containing a radioisotope which are placed into the uterus and upper vagina. Delivering radiation in this way localizes the dose around the applicator and minimizes the exposure of crucial normal tissues such as the bladder and rectum to further radiation. It may be given by a low or medium dose rate system (using caesium) for which a patient will remain in a protected room on a radiotherapy ward for 2–3 days. Alternatively, a high dose rate afterloading system (using iridium) may be used with treatment given as an outpatient procedure lasting 15–20 minutes at a time but with a course of between 2 and 4 treatments during or following external beam radiotherapy. Both systems require the patient to have an examination under anaesthetic and uterine dilatation for insertion of the intra-uterine applicators. Accurate positioning of the applicators is vital in these techniques to avoid excessive doses to the bladder anteriorly or the rectum posteriorly; despite the greatest care however, major complications are occasionally seen following radical radiotherapy of this type for cervical cancer, with 2–3 per cent of women requiring operative intervention at a later date to remove or bypass areas of radiation damaged bowel. Less severe side effects occur in 10–15 per cent of survivors, often developing some years after treatment and usually taking the form of intermittent periods of diarrhoea due to changes in the rectum and sigmoid colon, haematuria from bladder taelangiectasia, and vaginal stenosis. Whilst these must be investigated to exclude other causes they are then best managed conservatively.

Palliative radiotherapy may be given for recurrent tumour at the vaginal vault after hysterectomy using intracavitary techniques using an intravaginal applicator, an example of which is shown in Fig. 13.1. It is rarely of value, however, to give further external

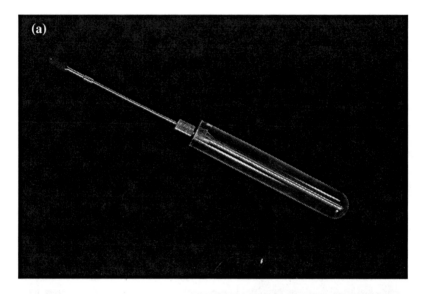

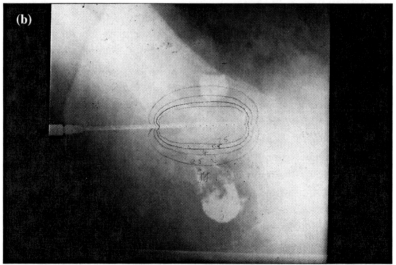

Fig. 13.1 Intravaginal high dose rate vaginal applicator (a) and X-ray after insertion (b) to show position relative to bladder and rectum.

beam radiotherapy to the pelvis if relapse occurs following a course of radical treatment and, indeed, it is potentially dangerous in that the tolerance radiation doses for the bladder and bowel will inevitably be exceeded.

The role of para-aortic node irradiation is controversial. In patients having documented involvement of para-aortic nodes this may be undertaken at the time of primary treatment in the hope of achieving long-term local control of disease in this site. It may, however, be argued in the case of asymptomatic para-aortic nodes that more distant metastases are very likely and the patient is therefore incurable.

Para-aortic node irradiation can therefore be withheld and offered palliatively should the patient develop discomfort from the progressive growth of disease in this site. There is no evidence that elective irradiation of enlarged para-aortic nodes at the time of primary presentation improves overall survival. However, there may be a small sub-group who have sub-clinical microscopic involvement detected at routine node biopsy during radical hysterectomy in whom para-aortic node irradiation will improve the chance of long-term disease control if not cure.

Relapse in para-aortic nodes with symptomatic disease may be usefully treated with local radiotherapy although involvement of a large abdominal volume will result in some associated gastrointestinal morbidity causing nausea, vomiting, and diarrhoea for a short period around the time of treatment. Because of the surrounding small bowel in this area doses are limited to around 45 Gy over 4–5 weeks and often more pragmatic palliative schedules will be given delivering 20–30 Gy over 1–2 weeks.

Locally advanced disease involving the bladder and rectum is generally considered beyond the scope of radical treatment. External beam radiotherapy to lower doses may be used to control local haemorrhage. There is always concern that tumour invasion into these organs may predispose to fistula formation which could be exacerbated by local treatment. In selected patients, however, high dose treatment may be considered accepting the risk of fistula formation and need for surgical bypass to allow healing if this occurs.

Where there is an established fistula in the face of advanced disease, radiotherapy is usually not indicated but may be considered if this is a result of limited local invasion from an otherwise localized tumour which could be appropriate for radical treatment. Healing of fistulae following radiotherapy is possible given a sufficient time period for re-epithelialization to occur provided the area is protected by either a colostomy for a recto-vaginal fistula or urinary diversion usually through a urinary catheter for a vesico-vaginal fistula.

Surgery

Radical surgery is the treatment of choice for early carcinoma of the cervix. This should take the form of a radical (Wertheim's) hysterectomy with removal of the uterus, fallopian tubes and ovaries, together with the parametrial tissue and upper vagina, and a pelvic lymph node dissection. Post-operative radiotherapy is usually given if there are involved lymph nodes or tumour is close to or present at a resection margin. Once the tumour has extended outside the cervix, however, surgery is rarely possible with adequate tumour clearance.

In advanced disease, surgery may have a limited role for the bypass of a recto-vaginal fistula with a colostomy. Colostomy may also be required if there is extensive rectal invasion and obstruction. Vesico-vaginal fistula is generally controlled with an indwelling catheter rather than direct surgical intervention.

The role of nephrostomy and ureteric stenting in renal failure due to advanced carcinoma of the cervix is controversial. In advanced incurable disease with poor prognosis it may be inappropriate but in other patients with limited disease it may enable recovery of renal function and allow radical treatment to be considered. It is important not to deny patients the opportunity of radical treatment simply on the basis of ureteric obstruction since between 30 per cent and 40 per cent will still have curable disease with radiotherapy if this is their initial presentation.

Pelvic exenteration involving removal of central pelvic organs including bladder and rectum may occasionally be indicated for very localized relapse. Such patients require very careful selection to ensure that they are not subjected to a major surgical procedure in the face of incurable disease.

Chemotherapy

Chemotherapy in the primary treatment of carcinoma of the cervix remains under investigation and concurrent chemoradiation for locally advanced disease is now considered by many as standard treatment. There is less support for chemotherapy in the adjuvant or neoadjuvant setting and this is not usually recommended.

Carcinoma of the cervix is however sensitive to chemotherapy in particular schedules such as cisplatin and methotrexate (PM), single agent cisplatin, or bleomycin, ifosfamide, and cisplatin (BIP). Response rates up to 70 per cent are reported and in advanced or metastatic disease chemotherapy may have an important role in palliation if symptoms are related to local tumour growth. Recurrent pelvic tumour following previous radiotherapy does not respond well to chemotherapy, however, and response rates for treating pelvic relapse after radiotherapy are in the region of 15 per cent with standard combinations.

Other treatment

Carcinoma of the cervix is not a hormone-sensitive tumour and such treatment has no defined role in its management. An important corollary of this, however, is that there is no contraindication to hormone replacement therapy in patients with advanced carcinoma of the cervix who may have ovarian ablation as a result of either surgery or radiotherapy, and this should be considered in all pre-menopausal women undergoing treatment.

Advanced pelvic disease may result in recurrent infections and foul discharge. This may be helped by antibiotic therapy, local application of metronidazole gel, and vaginal douching. Betadine pessaries may also be of value as an antiseptic in patients not sensitive to iodine.

Key points: carcinoma of cervix—management

- Early stage I and IIA cervical cancer is best treated by radical hysterectomy.
- Tumour which has spread outside the cervix will usually be treated with a course of radical radiotherapy comprising both external beam and intracavitary treatment together with chemotherapy using weekly cisplatin during the radiotherapy.

- Chemotherapy using cisplatin-based regimes has a limited role in palliation of advanced or recurrent disease.
- Pre-menopausal patients should be offered hormone replacement therapy.

Acute and late effects of pelvic radiotherapy for gynaecological cancers

Acute effects: these arise from large volume treatments which encompass the true pelvis and may extend up to the aortic bifurcation; lower border usually to pubic symphysis

- Nausea, less so vomiting
- Diarrhoea due to small bowel reaction (likely to be worse if previous surgery)
- Temporary loss of pubic hair
- Mild skin reaction in skin folds of groins, sacral cleft and vulva if field includes introitus
- Intracavitary treatments will also cause cystitis and proctitis

Late effects: develop after months to years following radiotherapy and may need surgical intervention

- Radiation-induced menopause
- Shortening and narrowing of vaginal canal
- Small bowel stenosis, may lead to obstruction
- Bleeding from rectum or bladder
- Cystovaginal or rectovaginal fistulae (high risk if advanced tumours treated)
- Lymphoedema (increased risk if radiotherapy given after nodal dissection)

Control and cure of cervical cancer by radiation necessitates delivery of a high dose to central pelvic tissues. Late radiation effects on normal tissues, especially rectum and bladder, are minimized by careful treatment planning. This includes assessment of the likely dose to adjacent tissues during brachytherapy. The risk of later complications is higher when pelvic radiotherapy follows surgery. These are covered in the discussion before consent to treatment and are also included in written information for these patients. This lessens the perception that late complications arise through negligence, which is rarely the case.

Problems may develop within 12 months of radiotherapy and sometimes several years later. Essentials of management include:

- Expert assessment to distinguish late tissue damage problems from those of active cancer.
- A multidisciplinary approach to address all physical and psychological problems and to agree realistic goals.

- Surgery, when needed, to be performed by teams who have experience in post-radiotherapy problems.
- Good communication and explanation of the problems with the patient, her carers and other professionals, especially primary care.

Table 13.1 Clinical problems that can arise as a result of late effects on normal tissues following pelvic radiotherapy

Reproductive tract: early menopause, infertility, vaginal stenosis, dyspareunia, discharge and fistulae
Bowel: stenosis, obstruction, bleeding, fistulae
Bladder: bleeding, contraction, fistulae
Other soft tissue/bone: pain, chronic sepsis, fistulae

Case History 13.1

Laura underwent a radical hysterectomy with pelvic node dissection for early cancer at the cervix. Excision appeared to be complete. She was put on hormone replacement therapy and after 4 months returned to work.

Twenty months later Laura complained of persistent backache which she attributed to her job, but became alarmed when both legs became swollen. She had also developed stabbing pain in the front of her left thigh. A CT scan showed enlarged para-aortic lymph nodes and also abnormalities in the lumbar vertebrae. A bone scan confirmed metastatic disease in the dorsal and mid lumbar spine and also sternum.

Laura was very shocked by the recurrence of her cancer and the news that any treatment offered would not be curative. Initially she was given radiotherapy to her dorsal and lumbar spine. Her pain improved with steroids, titration of opioid analgesics and the introduction of gabapentin for the neuropathic pain in her thigh. After further discussion she opted for chemotherapy with cisplatin. A repeat CT scan after two cycles showed reduction of the para-aortic disease so treatment was continued for a total of six courses.

Management of the lymphoedema involved massage and compression stockings and was carried out at the day unit of the local hospice. This proved to be a useful introduction to the team and facilities there. About eighteen months after her relapse, Laura suddenly became unwell with nausea and confusion. She was hypercalcaemic and this responded to intravenous fluids and bisphosphonates. However she was progressively declining. Further radiotherapy was given to enlarged supraclavicular lymph nodes. She had recurrent episodes of hypercalcaemia which eventually did not respond well to treatment and she died in the hospice.

Practice points

- Persistent back or pelvic pain with leg swelling following a diagnosis of cervical cancer is highly suspicious of recurrence.
- Chemotherapy can produce durable remissions in cervical cancer.
- Cervical cancer, as with other squamous carcinomas, can cause hypercalcaemia.

Case History 13.2

Susan was 29 when she was diagnosed with advanced cervical cancer. There had been problems with irregular bleeding and chronic pelvic pain for at least 6 months and she had lost nearly 2 stone in weight over this time. It was only when she became increasingly fatigued and nauseated that she went to see her GP.

She appeared pale and cachectic with suprapubic tenderness. On pelvic examination there was massive tumour filling the central pelvis and extending to the left side wall. Blood tests showed a haemoglobin of 6.8 g/L, urea 28 mmol/L and creatinine 450.

The likely cause of her renal failure was obstruction of the lower ureters by pelvic tumour. Ultrasound scanning showed hydronephrosis of both kidneys. Bilateral percutaneous nephrostomy tubes were placed by the radiologist; her renal function improved and she was given a blood transfusion.

Her MR scan demonstrated locally advanced cervical tumour with extensive pelvic lymphadenopathy tumour was invading the posterior vaginal wall. The treatment plan was a four week course of pelvic radiotherapy to try to control her locally advanced disease. She was felt to be too frail to contemplate chemotherapy. However considerable reduction in her pelvic tumour was achieved and bilateral ureteric stents were placed so that nephrostomy drainage was no longer needed.

Two months following radiotherapy she was distressed when she found that she was leaking faecal material through the vagina. Regression of tumour had lead to development of a rectovaginal fistula. Unfortunately she now had evidence of para-aortic lymph node involvement. A simple palliative colostomy was performed to manage this problem.

In hospital the complexities of Susan's problems had involved oncology, urology and surgical teams, together with input from the hospital palliative care team and social work. Good communication with primary care and community palliative care was essential so that the aims of treatment were understood and there was a rapid access to help when new problems arose. Susan remained frail but her physical symptoms were well controlled. Sensitive work and support enabled Susan and her partner to prepare their young children. She remained at home as she wished and died 5 months later from a probable pulmonary embolism.

Case History 13.2 (continued)

Practice points

- Renal failure due to obstruction by tumour at presentation should be treated actively when there is possible treatment to control the primary disease.
- Irradiation of stage IV tumours, with rectal and/or bladder invasion, is likely to lead to development of recto-vaginal or vesico-vaginal fistulae.

Carcinoma of the endometrium

Endometrial cancer has a similar incidence to that of cancer of the cervix but occurs predominantly in post-menopausal women with the majority of patients presenting with early disease. This is related to the fact that the usual initial symptom is post-menopausal bleeding which alerts patients to seek appropriate investigations.

The majority of endometrial carcinomas are adenocarcinomas arising from the glandular epithelium. There are other rare tumours of the uterus including uterine sarcomas and mixed mesodermal tumours which contain both sarcoma and epithelial cancer elements. Advanced cases spread from the endometrium into the cervix and laterally into the pelvic side walls. Involvement of the pelvic and para-aortic lymph nodes can occur and distant metastases are seen at a late stage of the disease typically to lung.

The prognosis for patients presenting with disease confined to the uterus (stage I) is good with over 85 per cent of patients expecting cure. Survival for more advanced cases follows the pattern of cervical cancer with around 40 per cent of women with disease confined within the pelvis (stage II and III) surviving 5 years. Distant metastases are incurable but women may survive several years with lung metastases which are often relatively indolent and slow-growing.

Common symptoms

Most women present with post-menopausal vaginal bleeding which may be continuous, intermittent, or only a single episode. It is also now recognized that endometrial hyperplasia and malignant change can be related to tamoxifen use and any vaginal bleeding in patients receiving tamoxifen for breast cancer should be actively investigated to exclude endometrial cancer. All such events should be investigated with endometrial sampling by hysteroscopy which has largely replaced dilatation and curettage (D&C) for diagnostic purposes. Endometrial tumours are not usually detected by cervical smear screening but more advanced cases can involve the cervix and in this instance the smears from the cervix will be positive.

Pain

Pain from endometrial carcinoma is relatively infrequent possibly because advanced disease invading deep into the pelvis is not often seen. If this does occur, however, deep pelvic pain often with a neuropathic component similar to that seen with other pelvic tumours will occur.

Pressure

Local pelvic tumour may cause ureteric obstruction but again this is relatively infrequent, the tumour usually being contained within the uterus at presentation. Lymphadenopathy can occur and distal limb oedema may develop as a result.

Other symptoms

Metastases from endometrial cancer are relatively infrequent but when they do occur they are commonly found in lungs causing cough and dyspnoea, intra-abdominally causing ascites, and in bone with local pain. One characteristic but rare site for recurrence is at the urethral orifice with a tumour nodule arising from spread through vaginal submucosal lymphatics. This may cause local discomfort, dysuria, and surface bleeding.

Management

Surgery

The mainstay of treatment for disease localized to the uterus is hysterectomy which may be followed by post-operative radiotherapy if there is deep invasion of the uterine wall (myometrium) or the tumour is other than well-differentiated.

Radiotherapy

This may be given as the sole treatment with similar results to surgery. Patients with endometrial cancer are often elderly, obese, and medically unfit and in these patients primary radical radiotherapy may be offered. This will follow a similar pattern to that of carcinoma of the cervix with external beam treatment followed by intra-uterine treatment; when the tumour is localized to the uterine muscle intracavitary treatment alone may be adequate. Post-operative radiotherapy is given to the pelvis and vaginal vault following hysterectomy in those tumours which are moderately or poorly differentiated and those invading deeply into the uterine wall. For the intermediate group of tumours where the inner half of the uterine wall is invaded but the tumour is well differentiated then vaginal vault irradiation alone using intravaginal applicators as illustrated in Fig. 13.1, is indicated. Intravaginal radiotherapy may also be indicated for recurrence at the vaginal vault and sub-urethral nodules may be controlled by an interstitial implant even where previous external beam and intravaginal radiotherapy has been given.

Chemotherapy

Whilst there are modest response rates to drugs such as adriamycin and cisplatin, chemotherapy has a limited role in metastatic endometrial cancer, the toxicity of such treatment often outweighing any potential benefit in this relatively elderly and often medically compromised group of patients.

Hormone therapy

Endometrial cancer is a hormone-dependent tumour. Its aetiology is linked to high levels of circulating oestrogen stimulating the endometrium. It is sensitive to both progestogen and gonadotrophin releasing hormone analogues (GnRH) such as goserelin or leuprorelin. Response rates of up to 40 per cent with medroxyprogesterone or megestrol are reported and similar response rates with the GnRH analogues are also seen. Since such treatments have relatively low toxicity they are usually worthwhile in advanced and metastatic disease. There is no evidence that adjuvant hormone treatment given after primary surgery is of value in improving survival.

Since this tumour is generally considered oestrogen-dependent, hormone replacement therapy containing oestrogen has been deemed inadvisable in the immediate period after treatment for endometrial carcinoma. There is however no clinical evidence to suggest that it would cause recurrence which would not otherwise occur, and judicious use of local oestrogen for vaginal dryness and where generalized symptoms are severe then low dose systemic oestradiol may be considered with little real risk. Occasionally there is a quandary in women who subsequently develop breast cancer for whom tamoxifen may be indicated. If there is thought to be any significant risk of residual endometrial cancer then a safer option is to use progestogens as first-line hormone treatment for breast cancer in this group of women.

Key points

- The majority of endometrial cancers present with disease confined to the uterus and are cured by radical surgery and post-operative radiotherapy.
- Endometrial cancers are frequently oestrogen-dependent, and tamoxifen should be avoided after a diagnosis of endometrial cancer at least until the early high risk period for relapse has passed.
- Endometrial cancers may respond to progestogens (e.g. medroxyprogesterone or megestrol), and gonadotrophin releasing hormone (GnRH) analogues (e.g. leuprorelin or goserelin), both of which are indicated for symptomatic recurrent or metastatic disease.

The morbidity from serious late effects is monitored and fortunately very low; when it occurs, surgical diversion of bowel and urinary tract may be necessary. These are also needed to manage fistulae. Multidisciplinary teamwork is essential to jointly manage such problems and provides support to the individual who may be cured but left with difficult problems as a result of treatment.

Vaginal occlusion may be avoided by regular use of dilators following treatment. Hormone replacement therapy is usually prescribed except for those with endometrial cancers.

Note that bowel obstruction in a patient who has had previous pelvic surgery and/or radiotherapy may be due to adhesions or a section of narrowed bowel due to fibrosis. A laparotomy should be performed especially if there is no other evidence of active malignancy.

Carcinoma of the ovary

Ovarian cancer commonly presents with advanced disease as reflected by the fact that the incidence of around 5000 new cases each year and there are 4000 deaths from ovary cancer per year.

There are a wide range of ovarian neoplasms but the common ovarian cancer is an adenocarcinoma frequently arising within a cyst and therefore termed a cystadeno-carcinoma. These may be of different types, either producing large amounts of mucous (mucous cystadenocarcinoma) or containing non-mucinous fluid and papillary cellu-lar growth (serous cystadenocarcinoma). Other rare tumours found within the ovary include malignant teratomas, squamous carcinomas, and mixed mesodermal tumours. It is important to distinguish malignant tumours from benign tumours such as fibro-mas, benign teratomas, and benign cystadenomas. There is also a group of tumours which, although cytologically classified as carcinomas, do not show evidence of invasion and these are termed as being 'borderline' malignancy. Although their initial overall prognosis is better, they are often particularly resistant to treatment if this is required at a later date for progressive intra-abdominal disease.

The natural history of ovarian carcinoma is to grow locally within the ovary before spreading within the pelvis and abdominal cavity. Bilateral tumours are seen in up to 30 per cent of cases. These may represent spread from one ovary to the other or synchronous primary tumour development. Multiple peritoneal seeding is a common feature due to transcoelomic spread across the peritoneal cavity. The greater omentum is frequently involved at an early stage of transcoelomic dissemination and when infil-trated forms a characteristic 'omental cake' as shown in Fig. 13.2. Multiple tumour nod-ules may also be found studded over small bowel wall. Peritoneal disease is often associated with gross ascites. There may be a reactive pleural effusion, a condition known as Meig's syndrome, or tumour may actually involve the pleural cavity, distinguished by an exudative pleural effusion as opposed to a transudate when reactive.

Distant metastases outside the abdomino-pelvic cavity from ovarian carcinoma occur at a later stage. They may be seen in many sites including the lung, liver, and rarely, bones.

Common symptoms

Pain

Persistent abdominal discomfort is a major feature of ovarian cancer. Initially, this is usually only vague discomfort and abdominal distension may be present for some

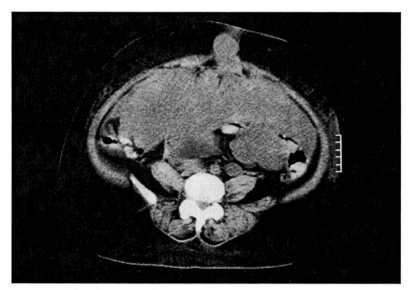

Fig. 13.2 Abdominal CT scan demonstrating 'omental cake' of tumour with associated skin nodule (Sister Joseph's nodule) and ascites.

months prior to presentation later leading to more severe abdominal pain, as the bowel becomes increasingly affected by tumour nodules. The vague nature of the initial symptoms associated with ovarian carcinoma often results in a late diagnosis.

A common complication of widespread intra-abdominal disease is sub-acute small bowel obstruction with associated colicky abdominal pain. Abdominal pain may also develop as the tumour infiltrates the abdominal wall. Pelvic pain from a local ovarian mass may occur and with advanced disease lumbosacral nerve involvement may also be a feature with neuropathic pain.

Pressure

Extensive intra-abdominal seedlings will result in ascites and distension of the abdomen. They may also result in areas of bowel obstruction or form a focus for rotation of the bowel (volvulus) which is a further cause for obstruction. Renal tract obstruction in ovarian cancer is less common than other pelvic carcinomas.

Haemorrhage

Vaginal bleeding may be a feature of ovarian carcinoma but is relatively unusual in the primary presentation. One unusual but well-recognized exception is the granulosa cell tumour which produces oestrogens resulting in hyperstimulation of the uterus and even on rare occasions a co-existing endometrial cancer. Recurrent pelvic disease following surgery may well present with vaginal nodules or a mass at the vaginal vault which will bleed locally. Metastatic nodules may cause haemorrhage into the bowel. Haemorrhage into an ovarian cyst may occur resulting in acute pain.

Other symptoms

Transperitoneal spread along the broad ligament may result in a fungating tumour nodule at the umbilicus. This is known as a Sister Joseph's nodule and is shown in Fig. 13.2.

Dyspnoea may result from an accumulating pleural effusion or gross ascites. Pulmonary metastases may also be seen. Lymph node spread is recognized. Initially, pelvic nodes will be involved with spread up the para-aortic chain which may cause pelvic and back pain. The drainage of abdominal nodes is into the left supraclavicular lymph nodes which may become enlarged and associated with local discomfort.

Key points: ovary cancer

♦ The majority of cancers present with advanced stage disease.

♦ The common type is an adenocarcinoma but several subtypes exist; rae tumours include germ cell tumours, fibromas and granulosa cell tumours; metastases typically from stomach or breast are also seen.

♦ Presentation is often with only vague symptoms of abdominal distension and discomfort, sometimes labelled 'irritable bowel' until advanced disease has developed.

Management

The primary treatment of an ovarian carcinoma involves, wherever possible, radical surgery with total abdominal hysterectomy, bilateral salpingo-oophorectomy and omentectomy, together with pelvic and para-aortic node biopsy, and careful examination of the peritoneal surfaces including the sub-diaphragmatic region. In ovarian cancer localized to the ovary this surgery alone may be curative (stage I disease). In more advanced disease maximum surgical debulking improves prognosis and should usually be attempted.

In recurrent disease, surgery will have a limited role. In general, surgical management of bowel obstruction secondary to ovarian carcinoma is discouraged since most patients will have multiple levels of obstruction throughout the small bowel which cannot be addressed by resection. However, it is important to note that one surgical series has demonstrated that almost one-third of patients undergoing surgery with ovarian cancer and sub-acute bowel obstruction had a non-malignant cause for their bowel obstruction.

Surgical management of ascites in resistant cases where this is a predominant symptom may be of value with the insertion of a peritoneal shunt draining the ascites into a large vein (e.g. the Le Veen shunt), which runs from the superior vena cava to the peritoneal cavity. These shunts, however, may in themselves present difficulties with blockage if the ascitic fluid is proteinaceous and viscous.

Chemotherapy

This has a major role in the management of advanced carcinoma of the ovary. There remains debate as to the optimum drug schedule but most patients will receive a platinum-based drug, either cisplatin or carboplatin, given at 3–4 weekly intervals for 5–6 courses. In many cases this will be given in combination with a taxane, usually paclitaxel, although there remains considerable controversy as to the best use of taxanes in ovarian cancer.

All patients presenting with disease which has escaped from the ovary whether in the form of free cells within ascitic fluid (stage IC) or advanced macroscopic disease (stage III and IV) will generally receive platinum-based chemotherapy. Response rates of around 60–70 per cent are to be expected, with 30–40 per cent of patients achieving complete remission (i.e. the absence of any detectable disease at the end of treatment), a major factor in achieving this being the bulk of residual disease after primary surgery. There is also some evidence that even patients with earlier stage I tumours will benefit from initial chemotherapy, and in many centres the policy now is for all patients to receive 5 or 6 cycles of platinum-based chemotherapy after maximal surgical debulking.

Cisplatin may cause peripheral neuropathy and tinnitus, both of which should be monitored during treatment in addition to renal clearance which is also affected. Carboplatin may result in bone marrow depression, the most common manifestation of which is thrombocytopenia, but neutropenia may also occur. Paclitaxel also causes peripheral neuropathy and more profound bone marrow depression is usually seen with combination chemotherapy; in addition, the use of paclitaxel results in unavoidable but reversible alopecia.

Despite the success of first-line chemotherapy over 50 per cent of patients will relapse. Second-line chemotherapy is rarely as effective as initial treatment and in some circumstances may not be appropriate. In general, patients relapsing at more than one year after initial treatment with a cisplatin-based chemotherapy schedule can expect similar rates of response to re-treatment and should be challenged with a further cisplatin-based chemotherapy regime. Patients relapsing in a shorter time have a poor prognosis. Options for further chemotherapy include single agent alkylating drugs such as intravenous cyclophosphamide or oral chlorambucil, or more intensive schedules using alternating taxane/platin regimens or anthracycline containing schedules. Other active drugs include etoposide (with cisplatin), topotecan, altretamine and gemcitabine. Many of these patients enter phase II studies evaluating experimental new drugs or new combinations. For many other patients further chemotherapy is inappropriate.

Ultimately, over 80 per cent of patients with advanced disease either fail to respond or subsequently relapse. There is therefore considerable interest in evaluating further consolidation therapy after initial chemotherapy has achieved a response. Trials have shown that there is no advantage to continuing beyond 5 or 6 courses of standard chemotherapy. In patients who have achieved a complete remission at this point there are trials of high dose consolidation chemotherapy using peripheral stem cell support or intraperitoneal monoclonal antibody therapy. In patients who still have residual disease after standard chemotherapy there may be a role for further laparotomy with surgical removal of the residual tumour, particularly in those patients who may have presented with initially unresectable disease.

Radiotherapy

Today, radiotherapy has little if any role in the management of primary ovarian carcinoma. There are, however, still advocates for pelvic irradiation after surgical removal of disease limited to the pelvis. In some centres this remains standard treatment, but in most cases, chemotherapy will be given and radiotherapy reserved for palliation.

Radiotherapy may be of value when given to residual or recurrent pelvic masses of tumour, particularly when these are symptomatic due to local infiltration or haemorrhage. Vaginal bleeding from pelvic tumour eroding the vault can be usefully treated with local intra-cavitary vaginal radiotherapy applications and doses of only 4–8 Gy in 1 or 2 treatments will arrest haemorrhage for most patients.

In the past, complex techniques for abdomino-pelvic irradiation to treat peritoneal disease have been described but these are rarely considered now as effective chemotherapy is available. Intraperitoneal treatment with radioactive isotopes such as phosphorus [^{32}P] or gold [^{198}Au] has also been advocated. Its major limitation is the problem of even distribution within the peritoneal cavity and in general these techniques have fallen into dis-repute. A further development of this is the use of targeted monoclonal antibodies to epithelial ovarian cancer cells within the peritoneal cavity linked to yttrium-90 or iodine-131. Currently, such techniques remain research tools, their main potential application being in the eradication of minimal residual disease as discussed above.

As in other metastatic diseases local radiotherapy for bone and brain metastases from ovarian carcinoma should always be considered when simple effective relief is required. A specific indication encountered in ovary cancer is the development of a fungating umbilical nodule which may respond well to superficial radiotherapy.

Hormone therapy

In general, ovarian cancer is not considered to be a hormone-sensitive tumour and this is not an effective treatment modality. The limited data available suggest that hormone replacement therapy has no adverse effects following ovarian ablation for carcinoma and should be considered when patients have symptoms from oestrogen withdrawal.

Other treatment

Advanced ovarian carcinoma commonly causes symptoms due to the effect of multiple peritoneal seedlings with repeated episodes of sub-acute intestinal obstruction. In general these are best managed conservatively and there are now well-established protocols for this in palliative medicine. High dose dexamethasone 4 mg six-hourly, given intravenously or intramuscularly, may be of value and in persistant cases subcutaneous infusions of octreotide or hyoscine butylbromide can reduce both colic and volume of secretions which also reduces vomiting. In general, surgery should be avoided as most patients will have multiple levels of obstruction that is not amenable to surgical correction but is important to recognize that in some patients obstruction may be due to adhesions or a volvulus, and readily corrected by surgery. This is particularly the case in patients without known intra-abdominal tumour who should be investigated further and if necessary submitted to laparatomy.

Persistent ascites may cause troublesome symptoms. Repeated paracentesis is uncomfortable and may result in loculation of the fluid and decreasing success at subsequent attempts despite ultrasound guidance. Protein depletion may occur due to loss in the ascitic fluid and is not corrected by albumin or plasma protein infusions in this setting. The role of a venous shunt is discussed above. Introduction of drugs such as bleomycin into the peritoneal cavity, which has been in vogue in the past, has not been shown to carry significant advantages and is not recommended. An alternative to the venous shunt is an indwelling Tenkopf catheter through which serial paracentesis can be performed. This can be inserted using a minor surgical procedure and may be of value in persistent cases. There may, however, be complications associated with infection and peritonitis.

Patients with persistent obstructive bowel symptoms may present with dehydration and malnutrition. Oral supplementation will be unsuccessful due to the reduced gastrointestinal motility. For the patient presenting with a primary diagnosis having not previously received chemotherapy, then there is every reason to consider active intravenous rehydration, nutritional supplements and if necessary total parenteral nutrition (TPN) to enable her to proceed through definitive treatment with a real possibility of, if not cure, a good response and period of remission. The situation is clearly different when recurrent intestinal symptoms are a herald of relapse and the terminal phase of the illness. In this situation then balanced judgement will need to be reached in discussion with the patient and her family as to what the future may hold and the role of nutrition and hydration in her comfort. Whilst intial intravenous rehydration may well be needed, simpler less intrusive and restrictive means of maintaining hydration should be considered using subcutaneous or oral routes.

Key points: ovary cancer management

- Initial treatment is radical surgical debulking with total abdominal hysterectomy and bilateral salpingo-oophorectomy, omentectomy, peritoneal washings and para-aortic node sampling.
- Post-operatively most patients will receive cisplatin-based chemotherapy, often with the addition of paclitaxel.

- At relapse second-line chemotherapy may be useful.
- The most common complication of advanced ovarian cancer is sub-acute intestinal obstruction. This may respond to further chemotherapy if possible (see above) and it is important to exclude 'benign' surgically correctable causes. In many, however conservative management with opioids, laxatives, anti-emetics and antispasmodics is more appropriate.

Case History 13.3

Over the preceding two years, Mrs D had complained of bloating and intermittent abdominal pain. She was seen by a gastroenterologist and a diagnosis of irritable bowel syndrome had been made. It was not until she developed persistent and increasing abdominal swelling that she returned to her GP. He examined her and found unequivocal signs of ascites and a probable pelvic mass. Ultrasound scanning confirmed the fluid with an ovarian tumour mass. A raised serum Ca 125 level suggested that this was ovarian cancer.

At laparotomy there were extensive tumour deposits over the peritoneum, mesentery and bowel loops. A total hysterectomy, bilateral oophorectomy and omentectomy were performed with debulking of other tumour deposits. Once recovered, Mrs D embarked upon 6 months of chemotherapy. This was tolerated well and she was encouraged by the fall in tumour markers to normal.

She remained well for nearly two years but then the Ca 125 began to increase. This coincided with bouts of colic and vomiting. Another CT scan confirmed extensive intraperitoneal relapse. The surgical team did not think that surgical relief of her small bowel obstruction would be possible. At this point she was on an oncology ward with an IV infusion, nasogastric tube in place and a subcutaneous infusion of cyclizine and diamorphine – although distressed by her relapse, physical symptoms were under control. She and her husband were anxious that further treatment would be given.

Her initial good response and prolonged remission following chemotherapy suggested that second line treatment offered a reasonable chance of a worthwhile response, which might relieve the obstruction. Mrs D was keen to proceed but at this point had eaten virtually nothing for 3 weeks. It was decided to embark on total parenteral nutrition to support her through treatment.

She remained in hospital for a further 10 weeks. After 3 courses of chemotherapy there was no clinical improvement and she remained in obstruction. It was impossible to control vomiting without her nasogastric tube in place, so a venting gastostomy was performed. Mrs D did not want to continue chemotherapy and was determined to get home. A frank discussion with her took place together with her husband. Her goal was to see the wedding of her grandchild in another three months; however her oral intake remained negligible and withdrawal of feeding would

Case History 13.3 (continued)

probably lead to an earlier death than would otherwise occur. While accepting her poor outlook, Mrs D was clear that her current quality of life, in spite of her difficulties, was worth maintaining.

Funding to continue TPN was negotiated and she went home. The situation was monitored by the GP and oncology team; she achieved her wish to attend the wedding. Subsequently Mrs D deteriorated rapidly but elected to remain at home and died a few days later.

Practice points

- Good responses to second-line chemotherapy are seen in ovarian cancer, especially if there has been a disease-free interval of 6 months or more.
- When chemotherapy is contemplated in patients who are obstructed and not candidates for surgery, nutritional support with TPN is justifiable.
- Use of TPN outside active treatment is more contentious, but some patients are likely to die from starvation before they do so from malignancy . . . analogous to complete dysphagia in head and neck cancer.
- The degree to which distressing symptoms such as pain or nausea can be controlled should be considered before embarking on other interventions.

Carcinoma of the vulva

Vulval cancer is uncommon and typically affects elderly patients often with a long previous history of skin dystrophy around the vulva. The majority of cancers in this region are squamous carcinomas although, rarely, a basal cell carcinoma or melanoma may appear.

It will usually present as a lump readily palpable in this region and lymph node spread to inguinal lymph nodes occurs relatively early. More distant metastases are unusual except with advanced local disease.

Prognosis

The prognosis is dependent upon the extent of local disease. Disease confined to the vulva can usually be cured by radical excision. Once inguinal nodes are involved there is a higher likelihood of distant metastases and the 5-year survival is around 40 per cent.

Common symptoms

Haemorrhage

Local bleeding is not uncommon from a superficial tumour within the vulval region. This must be distinguished from haematuria or bleeding from a higher vaginal source. There is usually an obvious lesion on inspection.

Pressure symptoms

Inguinal lymphadenopathy may result in distal limb oedema.

Pain

Local pain from vulval carcinoma is relatively unusual unless very advanced. In these cases it may infiltrate the underlying perineal tissues and even pubic bone.

Other symptoms

Advanced cases may present with a necrotic fungating tumour at the introitus. Rarely, urinary outflow may be affected and fistulae into bladder or bowel can develop. Subcutaneous spread can result in multiple skin nodules around the perineal area.

Management

Surgery

This is the treatment of choice. Wide local excision by radical vulvectomy should be performed for localized disease. When inguinal lymph nodes are involved then lymph node dissection is recommended to achieve local control of disease in the groins. This should, however, be preceded by a CT evaluation of pelvic nodes since radical local surgery will be inappropriate if inguinal nodes herald extensive pelvic node involvement.

Radiotherapy

In advanced cases, recurrence after surgery or in the elderly infirm patient, local radiotherapy may be given to the vulval region. The perineum is typically very sensitive to radiation and severe skin desquamation may result from treatment requiring a prolonged period of nursing before healing occurs. Combinations of chemotherapy such as 5-FU and mitomycin C with radiotherapy are being evaluated and may give better local control rates although with the price of more acute skin reaction and toxicity.

Local radiotherapy to inoperable nodes in the inguinal region may result in significant regression, prevent fungation, and improve distal oedema. Doses of 20–30 Gy over 1–2 weeks are usually given with which radiation associated lymphoedema should not be expected.

Chemotherapy

Vulval carcinoma has only modest sensitivity to chemotherapy and this has no role in its primary management as the sole therapy. Advanced disease usually takes the form of local tumour with inguinal lymphadenopathy best dealt with by surgery or radiotherapy. In recurrent disease, chemotherapy is not usually considered but drugs such as 5-FU and cisplatin may produce useful response and should be considered where there are severe local symptoms. The toxicity from such regimes which will include nausea, mucositis, and possible diarrhoea, should however be balanced against potential gains in this group of often frail, elderly patients.

> ## Key points: vulval cancer
>
> ♦ Vulval cancer is rare and usually affects older age groups.
> ♦ Radical surgical excision is curative for localized disease.
> ♦ Local control may also be achieved by radical radiotherapy.
> ♦ In advanced disease, palliation may also be achieved with local radiotherapy to the primary site or inguinal nodes. Chemotherapy using cisplatin with mitomycin C or 5-FU may also produce useful responses.

Carcinoma of the vagina

Vaginal cancer is rare and typically occurs in elderly patients associated with chronic irritation secondary to pessary use. A further rare group of patients are those related to maternal use of stilboestrol when characteristic clear cell vaginal adenocarcinomas have been found in the female offspring as they reach their teens and early twenties.

Common symptoms

Typically, vaginal tumours present with bleeding and discharge. This may be spontaneous or related to local trauma such as intercourse. Local irritation due to discharge may be present but pain is rarely a major feature.

Management

Primary treatment with radical surgery is usually advocated. Radiotherapy may give similar local control rates and will be considered for older patients and those with disease spreading beyond the vagina. For advanced and recurrent disease, local radiotherapy may be of value. Discharge and bleeding can be controlled with local intravaginal treatments using applicators, as shown in Fig. 13.1, with only one or two applications usually providing good symptom control.

Chemotherapy is not usually considered for vaginal carcinoma.

Choriocarcinoma

This is rare and the management is concentrated in a small number of specialized centres. It arises as malignant transformation within the placental tissues during pregnancy and presents with persistent vaginal bleeding after pregnancy, persisting high levels of human chorionic gonadotrophin in blood or urine, and the presence of a pelvic mass. Early blood-borne dissemination is typical and many patients present with the features of metastases such as haemoptysis (lung metastases), headache or fits (cerebral metastases), bone pain, and weight loss.

Management

Choriocarcinoma is highly sensitive to chemotherapy. Depending upon tumour extent either single agent methotrexate or more complex combination schedules will be used. Response rates approach 100 per cent and even in patients presenting with very advanced disease over 80 per cent will be cured.

Palliative treatment will rarely be needed for persistent local tumour or metastases. Local radiotherapy is of value for vaginal bleeding, bone metastases, and cerebral metastases, delivering a standard palliative schedule varying between single doses of 8–10 Gy and 20–30 Gy in 1–2 weeks. Surgery has little role in this disease.

There is concern that hormone therapy immediately after the treatment may provoke relapse and patients are advised to avoid oral contraception and hormone replacement therapy for 6 months following completion of chemotherapy. Further pregnancy without complications is well recognized after successful treatment.

Chapter 14

Central nervous system tumours

Primary tumours of the central nervous system (CNS) are relatively uncommon and indeed overall cerebral metastases are more common than primary intracerebral tumours. They form a relatively high proportion of childhood tumours, accounting for around 30 per cent of malignancy in those under the age of 15. Overall, 80 per cent of tumours in the CNS will occur within the brain and the remaining 20 per cent within the spinal cord.

In children, the common intracranial tumours are low grade astrocytomas, medulloblastoma, and ependymoma, whilst in adults the common tumours are high grade astrocytomas. Less common tumours include oligodendrogliomas, pinealomas, germ cell tumours, and meningioma. Lymphoma may also affect the brain or spinal cord as the primary site. Tumours of the pituitary gland are not uncommon, being either developmental, as in craniopharyngioma, or benign adenomas arising from the pituitary cells.

Tumours of the CNS are unusual in that with few exceptions they behave as benign tumours with local growth but without distant metastasis or in many cases even local infiltration. Localized seedling through the cerebrospinal fluid circulation is recognized specifically with ependymoma, medulloblastoma, and germ cell tumours; very rarely these also produce distant metastases.

The prognosis for tumours of the CNS depends upon their type and extent. In general, tumours which can be excised completely have a better prognosis than those where sub-total excision only is possible. Surgical intervention is, however, often limited by the anatomical constraints within the brain and spinal cord and the risk of producing major neurological deficits. Cure rates approaching 50 per cent are seen with low grade astrocytoma and medulloblastoma whereas, in contrast, high grade astrocytomas are invariably fatal with few patients surviving more than two years from diagnosis with a grade IV glioblastoma. The prognosis for other tumours falls between these two extremes.

Key points

- CNS tumours account for 30 per cent of childhood tumours but are relatively rare in adults when brain metastases are the most common problem.
- CNS tumours typically are non-metastatic, but seedlings through the CSF can occur in medulloblastome, ependymoma and germ cell tumours.
- Low grade gliomas, medulloblastomas and ependymomas are cured in around 50 per cent.
- High grade gliomas (glioblastoma multiforme) are universally fatal.

Common symptoms

Neurological deficits

Neurological disability is obviously a major feature of tumours within the nervous system. Very large tumours may arise within silent areas of the brain such as the frontal lobe with few effects, but very small tumours close to motor or sensory cortices can result in major problems. Confusion and emotional lability may be seen and epileptic events both focal and generalized are common. Fortunately, major disturbances in personality and higher cerebral function are rare. There may, however, be significant developmental effects upon intelligence and behaviour following treatment for childhood brain tumours.

Pain

Tumour growth within the cranium can result in raised intracranial pressure and associated headache. Typically this is persistent, occurring through the night as well as during the day, worse on movement, coughing, bending, and straining. It may wake the patient at night and is usually generalized across the head. Neuropathic pain may also result from tumour within or around the spinal cord. Damage to upper motor neurones will result in increased tone in those muscle groups supplied. This may result in painful muscle spasm and clonus.

Haemorrhage

External bleeding is not a feature seen with intracranial tumours. Haemorrhage within the tumour may occur however and this can result in sudden changes in neurological condition or acute headache.

Other symptoms

In addition to the constellation of neurological symptoms that may arise, some tumours may affect hormone function particularly those around the hypothalamus and the pituitary. Hypopituitarism may present in a number of ways including loss of gonadotrophin, resulting in altered menstruation, hypothyroidism, and hypo-adrenalism. There may also be effects on the posterior pituitary resulting in diabetes insipidus. In contrast, certain pituitary adenomas may be functional producing excess amounts of hormone which can present as acromegaly (growth hormone) or Cushing's syndrome (ACTH). Hyperprolactinaemia may cause amenorrhoea and infertility.

Visual disturbance may occur because of damage to the optic chiasm, optic radiations, or visual cortex in the occipital region. Pressure around the optic chiasm will result in bitemporal field loss, involvement of one or other optic tract, homonymous hemianopia, and involvement of the occipital cortex results in a characteristic perceptive loss (cortical blindness).

Obstruction to the flow of cerebrospinal fluid will cause hydrocephalus. This may arise due to tumours around the mid brain and posterior fossa restricting cerebrospinal fluid (CSF) flow through the aquaduct and fourth ventricle into the subarachnoid space which results in an obstructive hydrocephalus causing distension of the third and lateral ventricles within the cortex. Less frequently, obstruction around the base of the skull will result in a communicating hydrocephalus preventing flow of CSF caudally into the subarachnoid space in the spine, but with flow maintained from the fourth ventricle to the subarachnoid space around the cerebral cortex. Hydrocephalus may cause headache and gait disturbance. If it develops acutely then global neurological deterioration may be seen. It should always be considered in patients with tumours of the posterior fossa and those who already have a CSF shunt in place which can become blocked.

Cranial nerve palsies arise from tumours of the brain stem and posterior fossa as they leave the brain and pass through the skull, particularly around the cavernous sinus and orbital fissures. Meningeal disease can affect multiple cranial nerves affecting their outflow paths.

Tumours of the spinal cord will produce symptoms affecting the limbs; above T1 the upper and lower limbs will be affected, below this level only the lower limbs. Weakness and sensory loss below the level of the affected spinal segment will be seen. Disturbance of bladder and bowel function will also occur. At the levels of the tumour flaccid lower motor neurone weakness will predominate and below this spastic weakness with increased tone and clonus will develop. Patients with primary brain tumours and immobility are at increased risk of postural oedema of the limbs and thrombosis.

Key points

- Headache, neurological defects and fits are the common presenting symptoms of cerebral tumours.
- Pituitary tumours may cause bitemporal visual loss and endocrine disturbances.
- Functioning pituitary tumours may cause acromegaly (growth hormone), Cushings syndrome (ACTH) or infertility (prolactin).
- Many patients with non-functioning primary brain tumours become Cushingoid due to prolonged use of exogenous steroids to control cerebral oedema.
- Hydrocephalus occurs when CSF flow is obstructed and presents as headache and general deterioration in gait and other neurological function.
- Postural oedema and thromboses may arise as secondary complications in patients with CNS tumours who are immobile.

Management

Diagnosis

The demonstration of CNS tumours is usually clear on CT or MR scanning, the latter being particularly good at showing tumours in the posterior fossa of the skull, brain stem and spinal cord.

Surgery

The role of surgery in the management of tumours of the central nervous system is three-fold.

Diagnosis The histological diagnosis is important in view of the wide variety of tumours which can be found within the CNS. It may also have important implications with regard to treatment in distinguishing between a germ cell tumour or lymphoma and a high grade astrocytoma. Open biopsy or stereotactic needle biopsy may be performed prior to radical excision or if the tumour is in an inoperable site stereotactic needle biopsy is usually possible. Similar principles apply to the spinal cord as to the brain.

Excision of a tumour is generally desirable unless it is exquisitely sensitive to other modalities of treatment as is the case for germ cell tumours and lymphoma which respond to chemoradiotherapy. Whilst complete excision is desirable sub-total excision is generally associated with a better prognosis than no debulking at all. However, there must be a balance between the maximal tumour removal and the risk of post-operative neurological deficit.

Palliative surgical manoeuvres may also be of value. In particular, the insertion of a ventriculoperitoneal shunt allowing drainage of CSF above a level of obstruction causing hydrocephalus. This involves a plastic drain tube being passed from above the obstruction subcutaneously down to the peritoneal cavity. Occasionally a permanent internal shunt may be inserted through the aquaduct from the third to fourth ventricle as an alternative. Large cystic tumours may also benefit from surgical drainage to reduce raised intracranial pressure and neurological deficits due to distortion of adjacent nervous tissue.

Radiotherapy

For many tumours, radiotherapy will be an important part of the primary management. Many tumours of the CNS are sensitive to radiation but surrounding normal brain tissue is also affected and the doses required for tumour control are close to or may even exceed those which normal brain can tolerate. Spinal cord is even more critical with respect to radiation tolerance, radiation myelitis and paraplegia being a substantial risk when doses of 50 Gy in 5 weeks are exceeded; a similar dose limit applies to the optic chiasm. Cerebral cortex will tolerate 60 Gy in 6 weeks to a limited volume.

Whilst these doses may be sufficient for primary treatment, difficulties arise in recurrent tumours requiring retreatment. Some recovery of tolerance with time is seen, perhaps as much as 40 per cent after 1 year allowing for additional radiation to be given; a general rule is to use small fraction sizes of 1.5 Gy or less in this scenario to further minimize the risks of late radiation-induced CNS damage. Where recurrence is localized to an area <5 cm diameter then stereotactic radiotherapy may be preferred to minimize the high dose region of treatment. The side effects of CNS irradiation are shown in Table 14.1.

In low grade astrocytoma, medulloblastoma and low grade ependymoma, radiotherapy following maximal surgical debulking can result in a significant cure rate of around 50 per cent and should always be considered. In other tumours including oligodendroglioma, meningioma, and pituitary tumours, local radiotherapy is of value where complete surgical excision is not possible and long-term survival in a significant proportion can be expected.

In high grade astrocytoma radiotherapy may double the duration of survival but this in practice will equate to an improvement from a mean of 5–6 months to a mean of 10–12 months. There is therefore often debate as to whether patients benefit from such treatment particularly when a course of radiotherapy to the brain will take 4–6 weeks of treatment time. Randomized trials by the UK Medical Research Council have demonstrated that a dose of 60 Gy over 6 weeks is optimal for symptom control and

Table 14.1 Side effects of CNS irradiation

Side effect	Management
Acute	
Increased intracranial pressure	Steroids
Increased weakness	Steroids
Headache	Analgesics
Vomiting	Antiemetics
Alopecia	Wig provision
Scalp skin erythema and desquamation	Aqueous or 0.5 per cent hydrocortisone cream
Fatigue	Reassurance
Intermediate	
'Somnolence syndrome' typically around 6 weeks, profound sleepiness self limiting over 2 to 3 weeks	Reassurance
Late	
Cerebral necrosis (may be difficult to distinguish from recurrent tumour)	Steroids
Cataract	Removal

improved survival in selected patients who have good performance status, minimal neurological deficits, who present with fits only, and are aged under 65. For poor prognosis patients who do not have these features then shorter, and more pragmatic courses of radiotherapy may be appropriate. In general, patients under 65 years who are ambulant and self-caring will benefit from radiotherapy whilst older patients and those who are non-ambulant are unlikely to derive a clinically significant benefit from treatment.

Primary tumours of the spinal cord will be managed in the same way as primary brain tumours except for the important consideration that tolerance to radiation in the spinal cord is less than in the brain. Doses of more than 40–50 Gy over 4–5 weeks carry a significant probability of late spinal cord damage with transverse myelitis and major neurological disability.

In tumours where there is a high probability of CSF seeding, in particular medulloblastoma, ependymoma, pinealoma, germ cell tumours, and lymphoma then craniospinal irradiation may be considered. This involves complex radiation techniques to deliver doses of 30–35 Gy over 4 weeks to the whole craniospinal axis, followed by boost doses of 15–20 Gy to the site of the primary tumour or known metastases.

In the palliative setting, radiotherapy will have been included in the primary treatment of many patients and will therefore have a limited role. In untreated patients relapsing after surgery alone or chemotherapy, it should always be considered as a means of preventing progressive neurological deficits and controlling raised intracranial pressure from progressive tumour growth. Retreatment may be considered for a limited area where there has been a long period free from disease after initial treatment, but will inevitably carry risks of later radiation-induced neurological damage.

Case History 14.1

David, a 49-year-old advertising executive, had been bothered by frequent throbbing headaches, usually in the morning which he had attributed to stress. Recently he had been unsteady when walking and his boss had raised concerns about a possible problem with alcohol. Things became worse as he developed persistent nausea and vertigo. He collapsed at work and was admitted to the local hospital, where he was found to be ataxic.

An urgent CT scan showed low density lesion in the middle of the posterior fossa which was enhanced following injection of contrast. In addition there was dilation of the ventricles suggesting obstruction to the CSF. Appearances were of a tumour, either a primary glioma or a metastasis. David was a smoker but there had been no other symptoms or weight loss; his chest X-ray and CT scan of chest and abdomen were clear. He underwent craniotomy and with subtotal excision of his tumour and at the same time a shunt was inserted to relieve the hydrocephalus. Pathology was a grade 2 astrocytoma and he was referred for post-operative radiotherapy. This treated a small volume of his brain but caused permanent hair loss at the back of his head. Apart from this, he made a full recovery and returned to work in his previous post.

One Bank Holiday weekend he suddenly became confused at home and had a fit. The on call doctor told the family that the tumour had recurred and wanted to admit him to the hospice. However, as there was no bed available, David was sent into hospital where the neurosurgical team saw him. The problem was found to be a blocked shunt, which was dealt with. There was no evidence of recurrent tumour on his scan.

Practice points

- Low grade gliomas have a much better prognosis than high grade tumours.
- When a patient with a CSF shunt in situ deteriorates suddenly, consider possibility of shunt blockage and seek neurosurgical advice.

Chemotherapy

For germ cell tumours and lymphoma, chemotherapy has an important part to play in primary treatment using combination chemotherapy as detailed in the relevant chapters. This will often be supplemented by radiotherapy to sites of local disease. For other primary tumours the indications for chemotherapy are less clear. In general primary tumours of the CNS are not particularly sensitive to chemotherapy. This may partly reflect intrinsic resistance but also the limitations of many drugs to pass from the peripheral circulation in the vascular compartment into the CSF and nervous tissue. This 'blood–brain barrier' may, however, be disrupted in many tumours in contrast to the normal nervous tissue. In medulloblastoma there is some evidence that for poor prognosis patients, chemotherapy using drugs such as vincristine, procarbazine, and methotrexate may prolong survival. Its use in high grade astrocytomas is more controversial but there is some evidence that small gains in survival may be achieved using drugs such as procarbazine, CCNU, and vincristine (PCV). In practice it is estimated that only about one-third of patients who relapse with high grade (grade III or IV) gliomas after initial therapy receive chemotherapy, typically PCV, with an improvement in survival of between 1 and 3 months. Temozolamide is a relatively new drug given orally which is recommended for second line treatment in recurrent high grade glioma; responses or disease stabilisation are seen in 30–40 per cent of patients with an improvement in quality of life shown before further progression ensues.

Key points

♦ Surgery is the most important treatment in CNS tumours for diagnosis and primary treatment.

♦ Radiotherapy is limited by the tolerance of surrounding brain and spinal cord to radiation but will be given to many patients where surgery is incomplete or technically not possible.

♦ Chemotherapy has an important role in germ cell tumours and CNS lymphoma; in other CNS tumours it has a much more limited role.

♦ Palliative treatment of recurrent high grade glioma with PCV and temozolamide may improve quality of life.

♦ Reirradiation should also be considered in recurrent tumours one year or more from original treatment.

Other treatment

Raised intracranial pressure may be a difficult problem because of progressive tumour growth or hydrocephalus within the skull. Since the skull is a closed box, expansion of the tumour can only occur by displacement of surrounding structures and increasing pressure. This will result in headache and ultimately brainstem compression with slowing of the pulse, respiratory depression, and if this persists, death. Most patients with intracranial tumours present with persisting headache and on examination signs at the retina of papilloedema due to raised intracranial pressure. A CT scan or MRI scan will demonstrate extensive oedema around a tumour and displacement of mid-line structures as a result of the increased pressure.

Initial management of raised intracranial pressure is with high dose steroids. Dexamethasone 4 mg, 6-hourly is usually prescribed although equivalent doses of prednisolone are equally effective. There is some controversy as to the optimal dose of steroids in this setting and in metastatic disease a lower dose of 4 mg twice daily has been shown to be as effective with fewer steroid-induced side-effects compared to the standard dose of 16 mg. In severe cases where rapid reduction of raised intracranial pressure is required then an intravenous infusion of 10 per cent mannitol, giving 200 ml over 30–60 min is indicated. This acts as an osmotic diuretic and draws water into the vascular compartment from the extracellular space where cerebral oedema develops. Mannitol may be repeated on a 6-hourly basis in severe intractable cases but the response is usually only temporary and ultimately any initial improvement is lost unless more definitive measures such as the use of steroids, surgical decompression, or radiotherapy can be pursued. Many patients with intracranial tumour require prolonged periods of steroids and reach a threshold dose, below which cerebral oedema develops and symptoms return. This may result in a need for long-term steroid use with its associated side effects in particular weight gain, fluid retention, cushingoid facies, and proximal myopathy.

Key points

◆ Steroid dose should be the lowest needed for clinical effect.

◆ Dexamethasone causes less fluid retention and being more potent requires fewer tablets for the same effect; it may however cause more psychomimetic effects with hallucinations.

◆ Even low doses of dexamethasone used for several months will result in weight gain, peripheral oedema and Cushingoid facies and body changes; these will not resolve quickly even if stopped completely.

◆ Patients with pre-existing heart disease may be pushed into frank heart failure with steroids; this will usually respond to steroids.

◆ Urinalysis for sugar should be checked occasionally to detect unmasking of glucose intolerance.

◆ Omeprazole, lansoprazole or misoprostol should be used for prophylaxis in patients with a history of, or symptoms of, dyspepsia.

In the acute presentation of a tumour, dramatic measures including high dose steroids, mannitol, and urgent neurosurgery may be justified. For recurrent progressive tumour, however, surgical intervention is rarely of value and progressive intracranial hypertension may occur despite steroids, resulting ultimately in the patient's death. In this setting management should aim to minimize symptoms from headache and vomiting with the judicious use of opioid analgesics and anti-emetics.

Epileptic attacks are common with any intracranial lesion. These may be focal in nature affecting the periphery of a limb and then spreading more centrally or may be generalized grand mal seizures. Transient absent attacks may also occur. Prophylactic anticonvulsant treatment should be used to prevent recurrent fits in patients who have a subsequent seizure after initial presentation. It is important to inform patients who have had a fit of any legal restrictions this may impose on them (e.g. in the United Kingdom they are not permitted to drive for at least one year after the fit). For many patients with high grade astrocytomas this will mean that they will never resume driving for the remainder of their lifespan. Occasionally, tumours of the basal ganglia may result in abnormal dystonic movements, either myoclonic or choreoathatoid in nature. These can be difficult to control but small doses of tetra-benazine may be of value.

Upper motor neurone weakness either due to tumour within the motor pathways of the brain or spinal cord can result in painful spastic legs with associated clonic spasm. This may be helped with small doses of diazepam 2 mg, 6 to 8 hourly or baclofen 5 mg, 8-hourly increasing to a maximum of 100 mg daily. Nausea and sedation can, however, be a problem with baclofen at high doses.

Patients with indwelling ventricular peritoneal shunts may develop blockage of the shunt with recurrence of headache and drowsiness as hydrocephalus develops. This should always be considered when symptoms change over a short period in such patients and urgent scans obtained to detect ventricular dilatation. Surgical correction of a blocked shunt is required. Infection may become a problem with an indwelling shunt. This may also arise where there is an open access to the cerebrospinal fluid which may be from tumour or surgical intervention causing leakage into the nasal cavity (rhinorrhoea) or through the auditory canal (otorrhoea). Such patients are at continued risk of infection, and symptoms and signs of meningism should be investigated carefully and if necessary appropriate high dose broad-spectrum antibiotics started.

Rising intracranial pressure may cause bulging of a craniotomy scar and even leakage of CSF by this route, providing another potential conduit for infection.

Key points

- Raised intracranial pressure should be treated initially with high dose dexamethasone.
- Where there is rapid deterioration, despite steroids before primary definitive treatment (surgery or radiotherapy) has been possible then intravenous mannitol may be required.
- Ventriculoperitoneal shunts are used for hydrocephalus but may be complicated by infection or blockage requiring surgical revision.
- Anti-epileptics and antispasmodic drugs also have an important role in these patients.

Case History 14.2

A 17-year-old boy presented with a grand mal seizure and left hemiparesis. Subsequent investigations reveal a right-sided parietal lobe tumour that is partially resected. The pathology is a grade 3 astrocytoma and he undergoes radiotherapy.

He returns to normal life and embarks on a university course. In the second term, he has a fit and is left with left sided weakness. CT scan shows recurrent tumour. He returns home to live with his parents. He is seen at the oncology centre and is keen to try further treatment.

He embarks on chemotherapy with temozolomide but has a poor response. By now he needs to use a wheelchair to get around. With some persuasion he has respite stays at the near-by hospice. He finds that this is better than he expected and it gives his parents a break. He has been on dexamethasone 8 mg since his recurrence and this has been increased further with some improvement in his hemiparesis.

Eight months later he is an in-patient at the hospice with little prospect of returning home; his mother has also been seriously ill. He has been on dexamethasone 24 mg for a number of months. However he has now become extremely obese and refuses visits from his previous friends. A hoist is required to enable him to use a commode and he has a painful spine and sore abdominal striae. As he deteriorates further, no increase in steroid is made. He lapses peacefully into a comatose state and dies two weeks later.

Practice points

- Recurrence or progression of intracerebral tumour is usually associated with repetition of the presenting symptoms.
- Palliative chemotherapy may be useful and reduce the steroid requirements.
- Careful judgement is needed about the value of escalating doses of steroids when no other active treatment is an option. Side effects of high doses, of long duration, may extend survival at high cost.

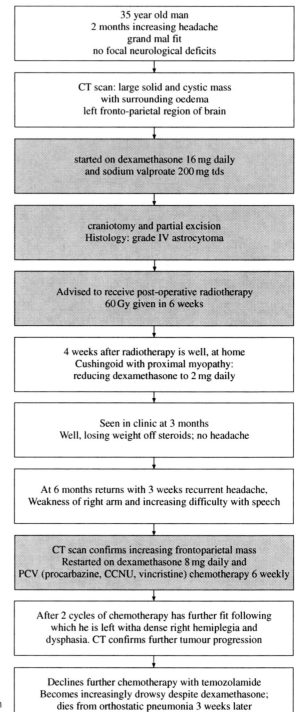

Fig. 14.1 Patient journey: High grade glioma.

Chapter 15

Lymphomas

Lymphomas comprise a wide range of disease from very indolent low grade lymphomas to highly aggressive conditions such as lymphoblastic lymphoma. The classification of lymphoma is complex in detail but relatively simple in principle.

The definition of different subtypes of lymphoma is a rapidly changing field becoming increasingly dependent upon immunophenotyping to define different prognostic groups within each major class of tumour. The current classification is the WHO-REAL classification shown in Table 15.1 which seeks to define clinicopathological entities rather than pure variations in cell morphology. However in the practice of palliative medicine the broad distinctions between early and advanced Hodgkin's disease and aggressive and non-aggressive non-Hodgkin's lymphoma remain valid and useful in the management of a patient with advanced symptomatic disease.

In practice the management of lymphomas still depends upon the broad categories of Hodgkins and non-Hodgkins lymphoma. Non-Hodgkins lymphoma may be low grade (including follicular lymphoma and marginal zone lymphomas) or high grade (most commonly diffuse large cell) in its behaviour. Burketts lymphoma and lymphoblastic lymphomas are particularly aggressive forms, whilst the MALT lymphomas and splenic marginal cell lymphoma may be very indolent.

Hodgkin's disease

This disease represents one large group of lymphomas, around 40 per cent of the total, with approximately 2000 cases per year in the United Kingdom. It is a disease of young adults with a second peak of incidence in the 60–70 age group. It is also seen occasionally in childhood.

Pathology and natural history

Hodgkin's disease is diagnosed by its characteristic appearance when looked at microscopically. The pathognomonic cell type is called a Reed–Sternberg cell which is typically a large binucleate mirror image cell found within a varying background of cells infiltrating the area of involvement, usually a lymph node. Other large Hodgkin's cells may also be seen with the characteristic cell marker CD30. Sub-classification of Hodgkin's disease is based not on these cells but the associated cell infiltrate which may be predominantly lymphocytes (lymphocyte-predominant), contain mixed cells including plasma cells, histiocytes, and eosinophils alongside other lymphocytes (mixed cellularity) or it may be

Table 15.1 Simplified WHO-REAL classification of non-Hodgkin's lymphoma

B-cell neoplasms	T-cell neoplasms
I: Precursor B-cell neoplasm	I: Precursor T-cell neoplasm
Precursor B-lymphoblastic leukaemia/lymphoma	Precursor T-lymphoblastic lymphoma/leukaemia
II: Peripheral B-cell neoplasms	II: Peripheral T-cell neoplasms
Small lymphocytic lymphoma/chronic lymphocytic lymphoma	T-cell CLL/prolymphocytic leukaemia
Lymphoplasmacytic lymphoma	Large granular lymphocytic leukaemia
Mantle cell lymphoma	Mycosis fungoides/Sezary syndrome
Follicular lymphoma	Peripheral T-cell lymphomas, unspecified
Marginal zone lymphoma including MALT (mucosa associated lymphoid tissue)	Angioimmunoblastic T-cell lymphoma
Splenic marginal zone lymphoma	Angiocentric lymphoma
Hairy cell leukaemia	Intestinal T-cell lymphoma
Plasma cell myeloma	Adult T-cell lymphoma/leukaemia
Diffuse large B-cell lymphoma	Anaplastic large cell lymphoma
Burkitts lymphoma	

relatively acellular (lymphocyte-depleted). A further sub-classification is into nodular sclerosing Hodgkin's disease, the most common form seen, in which the background cellular appearance is broken into separate nodules by fibrous bands. In general, the prognosis for lymphocyte-predominant Hodgkin's disease is better than for mixed cellularity which in turn is better than lymphocyte-depleted. The most common form of Hodgkin's is lymphocyte-predominant; lymphocyte-depleted is very rare.

The natural history of Hodgkin's disease is to remain predominantly within the lymph node chains spreading in a contiguous fashion from one site to the adjacent node chain. It most commonly arises from lymph nodes in the neck, spreading to axillary or mediastinal nodes and then to para-aortic nodes. Hodgkin's disease may also involve extra nodal tissues in particular the spleen, liver, and lungs. Primary extranodal Hodgkin's disease is rare.

Staging

Since the management of lymphomas depends critically upon its staging this is described in Table 15.2.

Prognosis

The overall prognosis for Hodgkin's disease is relatively good with most patients ultimately cured and overall survival rates of over 90 per cent. Extensive involvement of extra-nodal tissues is a relatively poor prognostic sign as is lymphocyte-depleted histology. An

Table 15.2 Simplified Ann Arbour staging for lymphoma

Stage 1	A single lymph node site involved
	If an extranodal site, e.g. tonsil, this will be designated stage IE
Stage II	More than 1 lymph site, but confined to one side of the diaphragm
Stage III	Lymphoma on both sides of the diaphragm
	If the spleen is involved this will be designated stage IIIS
Stage IV	Involvement of major organs, e.g. bone marrow, lung, liver, CNS
Each stage may be designated 'A' or 'B' as follows:	
A	Absence of 'B' symptoms
B	Presence of 1 or more 'B' symptoms (see p. 204)

international prognostic index, the Hasenclever index, has now been defined based on the presence or absence of seven prognostic features as shown in Table 15.3.

There is undoubtedly an incidence of second malignancy in patients with Hodgkin's disease. This appears most common in those having had splenectomy which can be part of the management, and those who receive combined treatment with chemotherapy and radiotherapy. In the first few years there is a risk of a new leukaemia or lymphoma, and there appears to be an on-going risk thereafter for an increased incidence of solid tumours which approaches 20 per cent in patients living for 15–20 years after diagnosis, and may yet rise beyond this. Young women having mediastinal, axillary or low neck irradiation before the age of 25 years may have up to a 30 per cent risk of later breast cancer.

Common symptoms

Pain

Lymph node masses in Hodgkin's disease are usually pain-free presenting as large rubbery nodes in the neck. Occasionally they may press upon nerve roots causing neuropathic pain; para-aortic nodes may cause back pain and intra-abdominal nodes may result in a tender abdominal mass or intermittent colicky pain if the bowel is affected. There is a characteristic but rare symptom in Hodgkin's disease of alcohol-related pain in affected lymph nodes in which patients report severe discomfort when alcohol is taken.

Table 15.3 International prognostic index for Hodgkins disease: poor prognostic factors

Age >45
Male sex
Stage IV disease
Serum albumen <40 g/L
Haemoglobin <10.5 g/dl
Total white cell count >15 × 10^9/L
Lymphocyte count <0.6 × 10^9/L

Hepatosplenomegaly, if massive, can be painful both due to local distension of the organ and its capsule and to associated abdominal fullness.

Pressure

Lymph node masses from Hodgkin's disease may cause pressure symptoms in the site they arise.

- Limb oedema may occur from axillary or inguinal lymphadenopathy.
- Dysphagia and venous obstruction (superior vena caval obstruction, SVCO) from mediastinal lymphadenopathy.
- Lung collapse from mediastinal and tracheobronchial lymphadenopathy.
- Hydronephrosis from para-aortic and pelvic lymphadenopathy.

Haemorrhage

This is a rare symptom in Hodgkin's disease in the absence of bone marrow infiltration and thrombocytopenia. Typically, lymphoma nodes do not ulcerate until they reach a very advanced stage.

Other symptoms

Lymphomas are characteristically associated with a constellation of symptoms designated 'B' symptoms. These are:

- Fever more than 38°C
- Weight loss more than 10 per cent
- Night sweats

Itching and pain in affected nodes on drinking alcohol are other characteristic symptoms of Hodgkin's disease though relatively rare. When present it is severe, generalized, and often intractable. Splenomegaly may cause local pain and hypersplenism with associated pancytopenia. This may result in symptoms of anaemia, low white count with predisposition to infection, and thrombocytopenia with bleeding.

Key points: Hodgkins disease

- Relatively rare occuring in young adults and >60 years.
- Characteristic histological appearances confirmed by presence of CD30 positive malignant cells.
- Typically, presents with painless node enlargement spreading to adjacent node sites in a stepwise pattern.
- Symptoms may include fevers, night sweats, weight loss, itching and alcohol intolerance.

Management

Surgery

Surgery has a limited role in Hodgkin's disease:

Diagnosis: because of the complex pathology of lymphomas open biopsies are preferred to obtain a suitable amount of tissue for careful assessment and specialist immunohistochemistry to be performed.

Splenectomy has in the past been a routine part of Hodgkin's disease management with a staging laparotomy. This procedure has now largely been replaced by CT scanning to stage the abdomen and pelvis. Occasionally, splenectomy may still be performed where this appears to be a sole site of residual disease or in advanced disease where a massive spleen is symptomatic.

It is important where managing patients with splenectomy to be aware of their increased risk of infection, in particular pneumonococcal and meningococcal infection. Current recommendations are for patients who have had splenectomy to receive immunization with anti-pneumococcal, anti-meningococcal, and anti-haemophilus influenzae injections together with long-term prophylactic penicillin V 250 mg twice daily or erythromycin in patients allergic to penicillin. Infective episodes in these patients should be treated aggressively with broad-spectrum antibiotics at an early stage.

Hydronephrosis, particularly at presentation, should be treated aggressively with nephrostomy and intra-ureteric stenting to restore renal drainage. This should be considered appropriate in all patients where it is possible to relieve the underlying cause of obstruction either by chemotherapy or local radiotherapy to a lymph node mass. In more advanced disease where such treatments have already failed then relief of renal obstruction may no longer be considered appropriate.

Radiotherapy

Hodgkin's disease is a highly radiosensitive tumour requiring doses of less than 40 Gy to eradicate the disease from involved sites. Hodgkin's disease may remain radiosensitive even in patients with advanced disease who have failed successive chemotherapy treatments. It can therefore be of considerable value not only in the definitive management of early disease localized to one or two node groups (stage I or II) but also for symptomatic lymph node masses in disseminated disease.

In the palliative setting, symptomatic lymph node masses will respond to doses of 20–30 Gy which can be given over 1–2 weeks. Painful hepatic or splenic infiltration no longer sensitive to chemotherapy will also respond to low dose radiation with doses of 10 Gy or less often effective and associated with minimal side effects.

Chemotherapy

This is the mainstay of treatment for Hodgkin's disease other than that localized to one or two node groups and in all cases where there are systemic symptoms at presentation (i.e. stages Ib, IIb, III, and IV). Chemotherapy for Hodgkin's disease involves combinations of drugs of which ABVD (adriamycin, bleomycin, vinblastine, DTIC) is recognized as the international gold standard. Newer schedules under evaluation give chemotherapy on a weekly basis to increase the intensity of drug delivery, usually with involved field radiotherapy to initial bulky sites at the end of chemotherapy. These schedules include Stanford V and BEACOPP. Bone marrow support with colony stimulating factors (GCSF) is often required during such treatment and many patients experience neutropenia which may be complicated by fever and on occasions neutropenic sepsis. All schedules appear to have an equivalent response rate with over 80 per cent having good initial regression of their disease.

Patients relapsing after primary chemotherapy with the above schedules or who fail to achieve complete remission with such schedules may be considered for more intensive chemotherapy unless the residual or recurrent disease is very localized when radiotherapy may be appropriate. This will take the form of high dose chemotherapy requiring bone marrow support using either an autologous bone marrow transplant or more commonly previously 'harvested' peripheral blood progenitor cells (stem cells) which are subsequently re-infused after high dose chemotherapy. The high dose chemotherapy schedules comprise either high dose cyclophosphamide or combinations such as BEAM (BCNU, etoposide, cytosine arabinoside, melphalan). Such procedures require hospitalization and isolation because of the risk of infection during the period of bone marrow ablation and whilst waiting for its recovery. This may mean periods of 3–4 weeks during which the patient requires intensive supportive therapy with blood product transfusions, intravenous antibiotics, and antifungal drugs. Salvage rates using such schedules approach 60 per cent but there is a procedure related mortality of around 5 per cent. This rises with age and in general such procedures are not considered for patients over the age of 65.

In patients relapsing after high dose chemotherapy or those for whom it is felt inappropriate because of age or general condition, the outlook is poor. Localized disease may occasionally be salvaged by radiotherapy. Second-line chemotherapy may be given using a combination to which the patient has not previously been exposed. Other approaches are to use gentle intermittent oral chemotherapy such as chlorambucil which may be given in combination with weekly injections of vincristine or vinblastine. High dose steroids may be of value in the short term to attain periods of symptom relief. There is however, a small group of patients who are recognized as having 'chronic relapsing Hodgkin's disease' who may survive for many years with repeated courses of chemotherapy and radiotherapy.

Other treatment

Steroids are of value for many of the symptoms associated with advanced Hodgkin's disease. In particular painful lymph node masses and the intractable itching which can be associated with Hodgkin's disease may be helped. Doses of prednisolone 60–80 mg should be used initially, or dexamethasone 8–12 mg daily. These should, however, be reduced over a period of several weeks to a lower maintenance dose to avoid excessive steroid side effects. Itching may respond to local measures although these are often unsuccessful. Topical steroid creams or crotamiton cream (Eurax) may be successful. Anti-histamine drugs such as chlorpheniramine or hydroxyzine are not usually effective although there are anecdotal reports of cimetidine working in this situation.

Fevers and night sweats may herald recurrence of Hodgkin's disease and be a difficult problem with advanced disease. Steroids offer the best solution when chemotherapy is no longer an option. It may be difficult to distinguish concurrent infection to which patients with advanced Hodgkin's disease are also prone and the possibility of tuberculosis should always be borne in mind.

Hypersplenism or bone marrow involvement from advanced disease may result in symptomatic anaemia for which blood transfusion should always be considered. This should be on the basis of symptoms such as effort dyspnoea and fatigue rather than specific haemoglobin levels although most patients whose haemoglobin falls below 8 g/dl will become symptomatic and require transfusion.

Key points: management of Hodgkins disease

- Most patients are cured of Hodgkin's disease using modern combination chemotherapy and radiotherapy.
- Standard combination chemotherapy is ABVD (adriamycin, bleomycin, vinblastine, dacarbazine).
- There is a significant incidence of second malignancy in this group of patients approaching 20 per cent after 15 years.
- Splenectomy is no longer performed routinely but if undertaken, patients require precautions against infection include anti-pneumococcal (Pneumovax), anti-haemophilus influenzae, and anti-meningococcal vaccines together with prophylactic continuous oral penicillin.

Non-Hodgkin's lymphoma

Overall, non-Hodgkin's lymphoma is approximately three times more common than Hodgkin's disease with around 5000 cases per year in the United Kingdom. It occurs at all ages but increases in incidence with age; the overall incidence is increasing. Non-Hodgkin's lymphoma (NHL) covers a much broader group of disease than Hodgkin's disease. Two main types are identified with very different clinical patterns, low grade and high grade NHL.

The low grade type is an indolent disease with a course usually over many years culminating in either chemotherapy-resistant progressive low grade lymphoma or transformation to a high grade lymphoma. In contrast, high grade lymphoma is usually an aggressive malignancy which left untreated or, if unresponsive to chemotherapy, is rapidly fatal.

A further feature of NHL, distinct from Hodgkin's disease, is the common involvement of extranodal tissues which may be present in up to half of all patients. Primary lymphoma may arise in any site, the most common being the head and neck region involving Waldeyer's ring (tonsil, posterior tongue, and nasopharynx), gastrointestinal tract, skin, and central nervous system.

Non-Hodgkin's lymphoma can arise in any distribution. Typically, multiple sites of lymph nodes are involved which may be widespread throughout the body and the step-wise pattern seen in Hodgkin's disease is unusual in NHL. Bone marrow involvement is common particularly in low grade disease. Involvement of the central nervous system may occur and is particularly recognized in high grade diffuse large cell lymphomas with the highest incidence related to those arising in testis, tonsil, and nasal sinuses and where there is bone marrow involvement.

Non-Hodgkin's lymphoma is typically very sensitive to initial treatment. In low grade NHL the cycle is one of intermittent periods of remission and relapse with no evidence that intensive treatment is of any value. Intermittent gentle chemotherapy or local radiotherapy is usually delivered and patients will survive for many years in this pattern of disease. Ultimately, either resistance develops or transformation occurs with an incidence of around 15 per cent after 5 years. The average survival for low grade NHL is between 8 and 10 years with many patients surviving beyond 15 years. Since this is a disease which develops in middle age and beyond, many patients will die from other causes.

In contrast, high grade NHL, whilst usually responding to initial treatment, will follow a rapid relentless path with death occurring within a short time unless a complete remission can be achieved. On average around 40 per cent of patients will be cured of their high grade NHL, the majority of the remainder die within 2 years of diagnosis. Inevitably, the outlook is related to tumour stage, patients with localized disease affecting only one lymph node area having survival rates around 85 per cent whilst those with widespread disease and particularly where there is lung, liver, or bone marrow infiltration having less than 30 per cent chance of long-term survival.

Common symptoms

The symptoms of lymphadenopathy are similar to those of Hodgkin's disease.

Pain

This is a rare accompaniment of non-Hodgkin's lymphoma. It may arise because of rapid expansion of the liver or spleen and occasionally large lymph node masses may be uncomfortable. Backache may be a feature of para-aortic lymphadenopathy.

Pressure

Lymph node masses will cause obstruction resulting in dysphagia in the mediastinum, bronchial obstruction causing cough, and possible lung collapse. Ureteric obstruction will cause hydronephrosis, which if bilateral will ultimately result in renal failure and may be associated with local loin pain. Groin or axillary lymphadenopathy may result in lower or upper limb oedema respectively.

Extranodal lymphoma arising in the head and neck region may cause local symptoms of nasal or sinus obstruction and, rarely, the airway or swallowing mechanism may be affected. Gastrointestinal lymphoma may present with an acute abdominal crisis either due to perforation, obstruction, or haemorrhage or alternatively with chronic gastro-intestinal symptoms and malabsorption. There is an increased incidence in patients with gluten enteropathy and it may present as a deterioration in these patients. Central nervous system (CNS) symptoms may arise because of pressure on peripheral nerves, cauda equina, spinal cord, or cranial nerves. Intrinsic CNS lymphoma is rare but recognized and is of increased incidence in patients with HIV infection.

Haemorrhage

This may arise from mucosal lymphomas within the head and neck region, gastro-intestinal tract or more rarely the bladder. As a rule, however, ulceration of the mucosa is a late event in lymphoma which tends to develop submucosally. Thrombocytopenia secondary to marrow infiltration may also predispose to spontaneous bleeding, typically epistaxis, haematuria, menorrhagia, or rectal bleeding. Haemolysis may also be a feature of some non-Hodgkin's lymphomas and should be remembered as an alternative cause of falling haemoglobin in these patients.

Other symptoms

As with Hodgkin's disease there are characteristic 'B' symptoms:

- Fever more than 38°C
- Weight loss more than 10 per cent
- Night sweats

Itching may be a feature of non-Hodgkin's lymphoma either as a paraneoplastic phenomenon or directly related to primary skin lymphoma. Primary skin lymphoma may take the form of diffuse infiltration resulting in a maculopapular rash or the characteristic mycosis fungoides with widespread skin infiltration and desquamation.

Key points: non-Hodgkin's lymphoma

- More common than Hodgkin's disease with incidence increasing with age.
- Extranodal sites and bone marrow involvement are common.
- Low grade disease indolent with long natural history over many years and median survival of 8 to 10 years.
- High grade non-Hodgkin's lymphoma is an aggressive malignant condition requiring intensive combination chemotherapy and has only a 40 per cent chance of cure.

Management

Low grade lymphoma

This is usually treated with intermittent chemotherapy using either simple oral chemotherapy with alkylating agents such as chlorambucil or cyclophosphamide or intermittent injected chemotherapy such as CVP (cyclophosphamide, vincristine, prednisolone). Fludarabine is an alternative drug which is also highly effective in low grade lymphoma and can also be given orally. It may be more active in combination with an anthracycline and steroids, e.g. FMD (fludarabine, mitozantrone, dexamethasone). These chemotherapy agents are generally associated with few acute side effects although all have effects on the bone marrow, most profoundly seen with fludarabine, and careful surveillance of the blood count is required during their use. Fludarabine also has major effects upon the immune system and patients receiving it are usually given prophylactic cotrimoxazole (Septrin) because of the increased risk of pneumocystis pneumoniae infection and should have irradiated blood products if they require a blood transfusion to avoid the risk of a transfusion versus host reaction which is usually fatal.

Many patients receive several course of chemotherapy as above, over a period of several years with periods of remission punctuated by relapse and further treatment. In general the response rates become lower and the duration of response shorter with each relapse. An initial response rate of over 80 per cent with chlorambucil is to be expected which falls to around 50 per cent by the time of a second or third relapse and the median duration of response falls from 30 months to around 12 months.

When the disease is no longer responsive to the initial treatment then alternative drugs will be used so that a patient failing to respond to chlorambucil will usually receive fludarabine or CVP. When these measures are no longer effective then more intensive chemotherapy such as that used in high grade disease containing antracycline drugs, such as adriamycin, will be used (see below).

A further new treatment option is now available with immunotherapy using rituximab. This is a monoclonal antibody targetted against a cell marker CD20 which is on the surface of B lymphocytes. It is given as an intravenous infusion weekly for 4 weeks and in relapsed chemotherapy resistant disease there is a response rate of over 50 per cent. A further development of this approach is to tag the anti-CD20 antibody with a radioactive isotope as a means of delivering targetted radiotherapy. The role of rituximab in first line treatment for both low grade and high grade B-cell lymphomas is also under evaluation with early results to suggest that it may well improve results of primary chemotherapy also.

Key points: low grade lymphoma management

- Except for localized stage I disease when radiotherapy is indicated, treatment with chemotherapy does not alter survival and should be given for symptoms or impending organ damage.

- Low grade non-Hodgkin's lymphoma is usually treated with intermittent oral chemotherapy such as chlorambucil or fludarabine.
- Patients receiving fludarabine are at increased risk of opportunist infection: they will receive prophylactic cotrimoxazole and should, even after chemotherapy has finished receive irradiated blood products.
- Rituximab offers a further treatment intervention when conventional chemotherapy is ineffective.
- In relapsed low grade disease the possibility of transformation to high grade disease should always be considered, and relapse after more than 18 months or rapidly progressive disease are indications for rebiopsy. If confirmed, this requires intensive combination chemotherapy as for *de novo* high grade disease.

Case History 15.1

An 86-year-old lady with a low grade lymphoma has been on intermittent chlorambucil for the past 4 years. She is not on any treatment at present but has multiple enlarged lymph nodes. She does not like blood tests and is reluctant to go back to hospital so her GP keeps an eye on her.

A little while after this he refers her to a hospice for respite stay. It appears that although she feels generally well, she has developed swelling of her left leg. This has become slowly worse and is now affecting her mobility. The clinical picture is of lymphoedema secondary to enlarged inguinal lymph nodes and these are likely to fungate in the near future. There is no swelling of the other leg.

Her oncologist is asked if he will call in to review her. He does so and suggests a short course of radiotherapy over 5 days, while she remains at the hospice and travels to the centre each day. She agrees to this.

The treatment does not make her ill and the only after effects are a mild skin reaction with some soreness and reddening, which resolves over a further 2–3 weeks. During this time her lymph nodes reduce in size as does the swelling of her leg. She mobilizes well and returns to live independently at home.

Practice points

- As the name implies, low grade NHL may be an indolent condition for several years.
- Systemic symptoms may arise from marrow infiltration or autoimmune problems such as haemolytic anaemia.
- Enlarged lymph nodes may cause symptoms due to pressure or obstruction and localized radiotherapy is an effective means of local palliation.

High grade lymphoma

The standard chemotherapy for high grade non-Hodgkin's lymphoma is CHOP (cyclophosphamide, adriamycin, vincristine, prednisolone). This is given intravenously with oral prednisolone every 3 weeks provided the blood count recovers between cycles. Between 6 and 8 cycles are usually delivered in primary treatment and response rates of around 80 per cent are to be expected. Alternative approaches to CHOP use weekly schedules of alternating drugs such as adriamycin, cyclophosphamide and etoposide on week 1 with bleomycin, vincristine, methotrexate on week 2 (PACEBOM) using oral steroids throughout. There is no evidence that these regimes are more effective than CHOP. Variations exist for all these schedules, for example, substituting alternative anthracyclines such as idarubicin or mitozantrone for Adriamycin. Response to intravenous chemotherapy in both Hodgkin's and non-Hodgkin's lymphoma, as shown in Fig. 15.1, may be rapid with palpable masses disappearing within a few days, and even in advanced disease, dramatic responses both objectively and symptomatically can be achieved.

Patients who respond only partially to CHOP may be offered further treatment with high dose chemotherapy using schedules such as high dose cyclophosphamide or BEAM (BCNU, etoposide, cytosine arabinoside, melphalan). This requires intense supportive treatment and the use of peripheral blood stem cells, as described below.

For patients who relapse following standard chemotherapy, further chemotherapy will usually be offered using drugs similar to their initial treatment or alternative schedules such as ESHAP (etoposide, cisplatin, cystosine arabinoside, methyl prednisolone). Patients who are shown to have disease still responsive to chemotherapy will then be considered for high dose chemotherapy with peripheral blood stem cell support. The results of this approach in patients with disease which does not respond to a challenge with standard chemotherapy are very poor and do not justify the morbidity and mortality of the procedure. In contrast, in those with responsive disease between 40 and 50 per cent may go on to be salvaged with long-term survival.

The technique of high dose chemotherapy requiring peripheral blood stem cell support is becoming increasingly common. In general it is applicable only to patients under the age of 65 years, beyond which the mortality of the procedure increases. The principle of this approach is to give very high dose chemotherapy, sometimes in conjunction with the total body irradiation to completely eradicate residual lymphoma. This inevitably causes complete ablation of normal bone marrow and the procedure can only be performed if some form of bone marrow rescue is available. In the past this has been with autologous bone marrow (ABMT) having taken and stored bone marrow from the patient prior to high dose chemotherapy and re-infusing these. The more modern technique uses mobilization of peripheral blood stem cells by chemotherapy such as cyclophosphamide followed by injections of colony stimulating factor (GCSF or GmCSF). The circulating peripheral progenitor cells which are released from the marrow are then isolated and removed from the circulation by plasmaphoresis. This technique has largely replaced ABMT. The progenitor cells are stored in liquid nitrogen

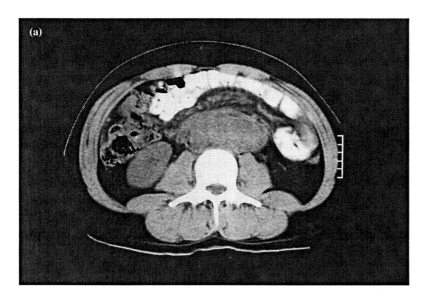

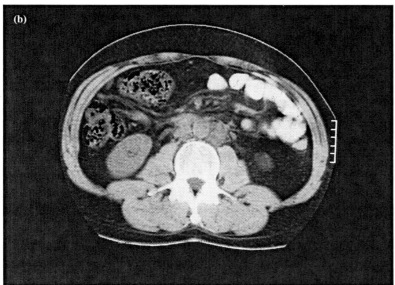

Fig. 15.1 Response of enlarged para-aortic nodes from non-Hodgkins lymphoma before (a) and after (b) one cycle of chemotherapy.

to preserve them and then re-infused following high dose chemotherapy. Regeneration of the bone marrow then follows but there is a period of around 20 days when the patient is pancytopenic and at considerable risk of opportunist infection and neutropenic sepsis. Intensive antibiotic and blood product support is required during this period which is usually spent in single room isolation. In experienced units, however, procedure-related mortality is below 5 per cent.

Although now well established in relapsed high grade lymphoma, there remains some controversy as to whether high dose chemotherapy should be used in primary treatment or only at relapse and the position is even less clear with low grade lymphoma unless transformation to high grade lymphoma has occurred. Some low grade lymphoma patients may be selected for high dose chemotherapy but the evidence for this being beneficial is still uncertain.

In patients with chemotherapy-resistant disease or those who are outside the age range suitable for high dose chemotherapy then the options for further treatment are limited. High dose steroids often provide useful reprieves when disease is symptomatic. Disease stabilization may sometimes be achieved using oral chemotherapy such as cyclophosphamide, chlorambucil, or etoposide and sometimes weekly or fortnightly injections of vincristine or vinblastine will provide a further short remission. These agents have the benefit of low toxicity in the patient with advanced disease.

Radiotherapy

Primary radiotherapy is only used in non-Hodgkin's lymphoma for small volume stage I disease involving one nodal area. Radiotherapy may be used for residual disease following primary chemotherapy particularly in those patients who are too old or otherwise unfit for consolidation with high dose chemotherapy, and also for sites of bulky or residual disease after high dose chemotherapy. Low doses compared to those required for solid tumours are effective with durable control achieved after 30 Gy.

For extranodal sites such as the head and neck region, primary treatment with planned chemotherapy followed by radiotherapy is usually given. A similar approach to CNS lymphoma is usually adopted where cranial or cranio-spinal irradiation, (i.e. treatment of the entire brain and spinal canal), will often be required. For local and symptomatic skin lymphoma, radiotherapy using superficial X-rays or electrons will provide good palliation. For widespread skin lymphoma there are techniques available in some centres for whole body electron therapy which again can provide useful palliation although often this is only short-term with relapse within a few months. The rare lymphomas affecting the conjunctiva and orbit may also be treated successfully with local radiotherapy.

In relapsed disease, radiotherapy can often provide valuable palliation for symptomatic node masses and resistance to chemotherapy does not predict for a response to radiation. In fact it is unusual for lymphoma to be resistant to radiation even in advanced disease, its main limit being the distribution of disease and dose which can be safely delivered without excessive toxicity and normal tissue damage.

For widespread disease in patients resistant to chemotherapy wide field radiation techniques (hemibody irradiation) may have considerable benefit, see Chapter 5. Response rates of 70–80 per cent are seen with corresponding benefit in terms of symptom relief to the patient although this may be short-lived with further relapse some months later. The use of these techniques does not exclude more localized radiotherapy to a bulky node mass. Where there is disease above and below the diaphragm sequential hemibody irradiation can be considered with a gap of 4–6 weeks between treatments to allow bone marrow recovery.

Surgery

This has a limited role in the management of non-Hodgkin's lymphoma beyond the initial diagnostic biopsy. Occasionally ureteric stenting may be required to overcome obstruction from para-aortic lymphadenopathy and certainly in initial presentation should always be considered in view of the high response rate to treatment. In more advanced disease it may be considered inappropriate. Spinal cord compression secondary to lymphoma is generally best managed with needle biopsy to establish the diagnosis and a combination of chemotherapy and radiotherapy, rather than spinal surgery, unless there is a significant spinal instability.

Other treatment

Because lymphoma is generally very sensitive to treatment, certainly in the early stages, rapid tumour lysis may be seen. Because of this, patients should be actively hydrated and treated with allopurinol to prevent excess breakdown of cell products to uric acid which will otherwise cause both joint pain and nephropathy. In the later stages where less significant responses are to be expected this may be less important but should always be considered in these tumours. As with Hodgkin's disease the itching associated with non-Hodgkin's lymphoma can be intractable. Steroids may be of value as may topical anti-pruritic drugs such as crotamiton (Eurax).

Key points: management of non-Hodgkin's lymphoma

- High grade lymphoma is treated with combination chemotherapy such as CHOP (cyclophosphamide, adriamycin, vincristine, prednisolone).
- In relapsed high grade disease if there is further response to chemotherapy then high dose chemotherapy using peripheral stem cell support should be considered in patients <65 years.
- In chemoresistant disease high dose therapy this has no role and the outlook is very poor.
- Symptomatic disease unresponsive to chemotherapy should always be considered for local radiotherapy.
- Immunotherapy with anti-CD20 drugs is a further treatment option in relapsed disease and may improve results when given with CHOP in first-line management.

Case History 15.2

Carol is a 40-year-old woman with a rapidly enlarging lump in her upper neck and is noted to have swelling tonsil on that side. Pathology of the tonsil is a high grade non-Hodgkin's lymphoma. Further staging investigations reveal and enlarged mediastinal and abdominal nodes and there is evidence of bone marrow involvement. She is also experiencing drenching sweats and intermittent fever.

She is admitted to hospital in pain from the pressure of the increasing mass in her neck. This is bad enough to require strong opioid analgesics. Carol starts chemotherapy and the regimen includes high dose steroids. Within 48 h there is a noticeable reduction in the neck mass and the pain improves rapidly. By discharge a few days later she no longer requires strong analgesics; the pyrexia and sweats are diminished. She goes on to complete the scheduled chemotherapy although requires a re-admission on several occasions because of neutropenic sepsis. Treatment achieves complete remission on repeat investigations and she undergoes radiotherapy to her head and neck.

Twelve months later she develops a persistent cough and has relapsed with pulmonary deposits as well as recurrent lymphadenopathy. Further chemotherapy is commenced but this time she struggles with a period of prolonged marrow suppression and remains in a side room for several weeks. During this time, she complains of persistent pain in one side of her chest and back. X-Rays are unhelpful and while a bone scan is awaited, the nursing staff notice a rash. She has developed herpes zoster and receives acyclovir for this.

Unfortunately the lymphoma is clearly not responding well to the treatment this time and she is not suitable for more intensive treatment supported by autologous transplant. A few weeks later Carol becomes confused and drowsy. Although CT brain scan shows no abnormality, there are lymphoma cells present in the CSF at lumbar puncture. An MRI scan shows multiple small cerebral deposits. There is little response to steroids but her symptoms improve following intrathecal methotrexate and she has palliative cranial irradiation. This enables her to go home and spend some time with her family. She develops further drowsiness and headache some weeks later, but Carol and her family opt for her to remain at home and she does not wish for further treatment.

Practice points

- Lymphoma should be considered in the presentation of a young adult with an enlarged neck node.
- Tumour responses to chemotherapy or radiotherapy are often dramatic; progression on relapse can also be rapid.
- Patients with lymphoma, especially on chemotherapy, are susceptible to infection. Exposure to herpes zoster can lead to severe, generalized chicken pox.

Key points: management of relapsed/progressive HD/NHL

- A positive outlook, with high cure rates, is often emphasized at diagnosis of Hodgkins disease, so failure to achieve this can be especially hard for the patient and family to accept.

- Active management with sequential chemotherapy may control the disease and suppress B symptoms for some time. Patients may be receiving treatment and attending hospital frequently throughout the course of the illness and into the terminal stage. It is important that contact with community professionals is maintained.

- Radiotherapy for localized symptomatic sites offers very useful palliation; side effects are usually mild as relatively low doses can be used.

- Patients with lymphoma are prone to opportunistic infections such as candida, herpes simplex and zoster. These should be treated actively at the earliest manifestation.

- Steroids are useful to control B symptoms. Thalidomide can be tried to suppress itch.

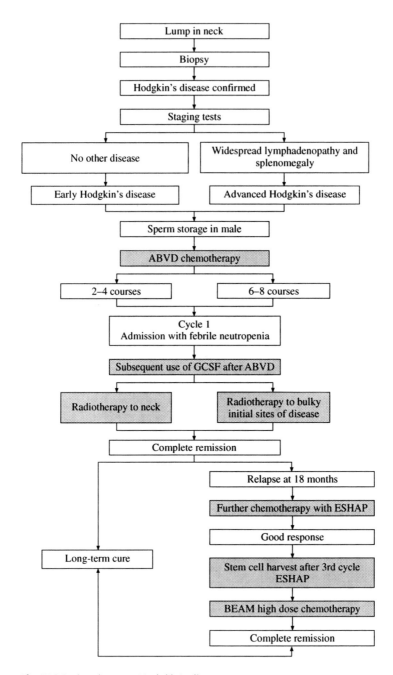

Fig 15.2 Patient journey: Hodgkin's disease.

Chapter 16

Leukaemia and myeloma

Acute leukaemia

Acute leukaemia occurs in two main forms either acute lymphoblastic (ALL) or acute myeloid leukaemia (AML) within which there are several subtypes. ALL is more common than AML. It is particularly common in children under the age of 5 although it may also be seen in young adults. It accounts for approximately one-third of malignant conditions in childhood. Both forms of acute leukaemia represent neoplastic proliferation of immature cells within the bone marrow, either of the lymphoblastic series (ALL) or the myeloblastic series (AML). The proliferating clone of malignant cells replaces normal bone marrow, resulting in bone marrow failure. This produces symptoms of anaemia, infection due to low white blood cell count, and bleeding from thrombocytopenia. Leukaemic infiltration of other tissues may also occur, in particular the liver and spleen may be involved, peripheral lymphadenopathy is common and ALL has a high incidence of central nervous system involvement.

Prognosis

In general the prognosis for acute leukaemia is better in childhood than for adults. ALL has a better prognosis than AML with around 70 per cent of children being cured compared to only 40 per cent with AML. In adults long-term survival rates are approximately half those in children.

Common symptoms

The common symptoms are due to bone marrow failure. This results in:

♦ Anaemia causing fatigue and effort dyspnoea.
♦ Leucopenia causing an increased incidence of infection.
♦ Thromocytopenia causing purpura and bleeding, in particular epistaxis, rectal bleeding, haematuria, and dysfunctional uterine bleeding.

Pain

This may arise due to bone marrow infiltration causing scattered bone pain. Headache may arise because of central nervous system infiltration and nerve root pain from spinal meningitic infiltration.

Pressure

These symptoms are unusual as leukaemic deposits rarely form large tumour masses but infiltrate tissues locally. Diffuse meningeal thickening may cause nerve root and cranial nerve symptoms from nerve compression and occasionally diffuse meningeal thickening may result in obstruction of cerebrospinal flow and hydrocephalus.

Other symptoms

Central nervous system involvement may cause scattered neurological signs. In males, testicular infiltration is a recognized phenomenon in ALL causing local pain and swelling. Gum hypertrophy and bleeding is a feature of myelomonocytic and monoblastic subtypes of AML.

Key points

- ◆ Acute leukaemias may be lymphoblastic (ALL) or myeloblastic (AML).
- ◆ Symptoms are typically due to bone marrow failure with anaemia, infections, purpura and bleeding.
- ◆ The diagnosis is usually confirmed on a peripheral blood film and bone marrow sample.
- ◆ Rarer manifestations include CNS involvement and testicular infiltration.

Management

Chemotherapy is the mainstay of treatment for acute leukaemia and prolonged intensive schedules incorporating a period of remission induction followed by consolidation and thereafter maintainence therapy is the usual pattern. In general, ALL will go into remission with relatively simple schedules including vincristine and prednisolone whilst AML requires more toxic drugs such as doxorubicin, cytosine arabinoside, and thioguanine. Consolidation therapy in ALL will include central nervous system treatment with intrathecal injections of methotrexate. In the past, radiotherapy to the brain has been given but long-term sequelae from this in children have led to its exclusion wherever possible. Maintainence therapy in ALL will continue for 2–3 years using methotrexate and mercaptopurine. There is no value in maintainence treatment beyond 6 months in AML. High risk patients and those relapsing and going into a second remission will often proceed to bone marrow transplantation with high dose chemotherapy and total body irradiation. This may be either in the form of marrow from a matched donor (allograft) or from the patient themselves (autograft). Increasingly autografts are being replaced by the use of peripheral blood progenitor cell infusions (PBPC) which can be collected by plasmaphoresis after stimulation of bone marrow with chemotherapy exposure followed by daily granulocyte colony stimulating factor injections (GCSF or GmCSF).

Relapse after initial remission will usually be treated with further induction chemotherapy similar to that chosen initially. If a second remission is obtained then consolidation with high dose chemotherapy and bone marrow transplantation will be considered if not previously performed. Relapse following bone marrow transplantation is usually not salvageable but further periods of remission may be obtained using permutations of the drugs previously used.

Radiotherapy

This treatment has only a limited role in the management of acute leukaemia. For established central nervous system disease, cranial irradiation or craniospinal irradiation may be indicated. Leukaemia is usually highly sensitive to radiation and doses of 18–20 Gy are generally sufficient to control the disease. Rarely, isolated bone lesions may be painful and may require low dose radiation and similarly localized lymph nodes masses or splenomegaly in end-stage disease may benefit from local irradiation to prevent pain or in the case of lymph nodes masses obstructive symptoms and fungation.

Other treatment

Anaemia and thrombocytopenia will require blood product support by way of blood and platelet transfusion. White cell tranfusions are not usually indicated but careful management of the neutropenic patient is required with urgent treatment of febrile episodes using high dose intravenous broad-septrum antibiotics such as ceftazidime 2 g 8-hourly or combinations of gentamicin and ticarcillin. Persistent haemorrhage may be a difficult problem in the patient with end-stage acute leukaemia and ultimately the cause of death often as a result of intracranial haemorrhage. Platelet transfusions should be given when the platelet count falls below 5000×10^9/L or at higher levels when there is spontaneous haemorrhage. The efficacy of platelet transfusions, however, is short-lived and most are consumed within 24 h. Repeated transfusions will also increase the likelihood of immune incompatibility and increased systemic reactions such as fever and rigors with the transfusion together with accelerated consumption of platelets once transfused. Anti-fibrinolytic agents such as tranexamic acid may be of value for actual bleeding but will often make little or no impact. Patients having frequent transfusions may have febrile reactions during the transfusion. These may be overcome by administering intravenous hydrocortisone 100 mg and chlorpheniramine 8 mg but if persistent or associated with rigors the transfusion should be terminated and serum taken to be returned with the blood for further cross-matching. In this group of patients, hydrocortisone and chlorpheniramine are often given prophylactically when the transfusion is started in an attempt to reduce the likelihood of a major transfusion reaction. These patients will require frequent infusions and intravenous drugs. This is often facilitated by the insertion of a central catheter such as a Hickman line, see Chapter 5.

Rapid lysis of leukaemic cells often occurs during treatment because of their extreme sensitivity to both drugs and radiation. This may release high levels of uric acid into the circulation and both gout and tumour lysis syndrome are potential dangers. These can be prevented by ensuring good hydration of the patient prior to treatment and also using allopurinol 300 mg daily to block uric acid production. Acute gout if it develops is treated with non-steroidal anti-inflammatory drugs.

Key points

- Induction, consolidation and maintainence are the three phases of acute leukaemia management.
- Most patients will go into initial remission with relatively simple combination chemotherapy.
- ALL will require 2 to 3 years maintainence treatment including CNS prophylaxis with intrethecal chemotherapy.
- AML does not benefit from >6 months initial treatment.
- Marrow ablative chemotherapy with marrow transplant will be required for younger high risk patients and those who relapse.

Graft versus host reaction (GVH)

This is a condition which develops following allogenic bone marrow transplantation. It represents a reaction of the transplanted foreign cells against the host patient. This can result in a wide constellation of signs and symptoms typically involving the gut causing diarrhoea, the skin with a characteristic rash, and the liver causing hepatic dysfunction. Treatment of acute GVH will require high dose steroids and often the addition of other immunosuppresant drugs such as azathioprine. Chronic GVH may require continued steroid therapy and low dose methotrexate. There is some evidence that a low level of graft versus host disease can improve the results of bone marrow transplantation but acute GVH is a serious life-threatening medical condition. It is not seen after autologous transplants or PBPC bone marrow support as these use cells of the patient themselves with no immunological mismatch.

Itching, although a recognized symptom of many malignant conditions, can be prominent in leukaemia and leukaemic skin infiltrates are well recognized. These will respond to systemic therapy for the leukaemia, but in advanced relapsed disease this may no longer be possible. Topical steroid cream and systemic steroids may be of value. Conventional anti-histamines are often prescribed but frequently are unsuccessful. Cimetidine is also advocated in intractable cases and topical anti-pruritic agents such as crotamiton (Eurax) may also be of value where steroid creams fail.

Chronic leukaemia

This type of leukaemia also exists in two major forms, chronic lymphocytic leukaemia (CLL) and chronic myeloid leukaemia (CML), representing neoplastic proliferations of the two different cell lines in the bone marrow; CML is also referred to as chronic granulocytic leukaemia (CGL), the two terms are interchangeable. Chronic myeloid leukaemia typically causes massive splenomegaly and there can also be associated lymphadenopathy. Chronic lymphocytic leukaemia typically results in widespread lymphadenopathy with associated hepato-splenomegaly but rarely the very large spleen is seen with CML. These leukaemias are rare in children and typically affect middle-aged and elderly adults. Both conditions may result in bone marrow failure with associated anaemia, neutropenia, and thrombocytopenia.

The natural history of CML is ultimately to transform into an acute leukaemia which may be an acute lymphoblastic or acute myeloblastic leukaemia. There is a characteristic cell marker in CML, the Philadelphia chromosome, representing chromosomal translocation in the cells from chromosome 22 to chromosome 9, present in around 80 per cent of cases. The presence of the Philadelphia chromosome in a picture of acute leukaemia will confirm that this represents a transformed chronic myeloid leukaemia, even if the chronic phase has not been recognized, although usually the clinical course is obvious developing 3–4 years after the initial diagnosis of CML. The outlook for the acute leukaemic phase of CML is poor. This type of transformation is not seen in CLL which has a longer and more predictable natural history.

Mean survival in CML is between 3 and 4 years with most patients dying in the acute leukaemic phase of the illness. In contrast, median survival in CLL is around 8 years with many patients surviving well beyond this and dying from other causes, since this is often a disease of the elderly.

Common symptoms

In both chronic leukaemias (CLL and CML), bone marrow failure may occur resulting in symptoms of:

- Anaemia causing fatigue and shortness of breath. In CLL this may be exacerbated by a characteristic autoimmune haemolytic anaemia associated with cold agglutinins.
- Leucopenia causing an increase in infection.
- Thrombocytopenia causing haemorrhage such as haematuria, epistaxis, and uterine bleeding.

Pain

Massive splenomegaly in CML may result in left-sided abdominal pain particularly where there is rapid growth of the spleen. Intrasplenic haemorrhage or infarction may also occur resulting in an acute exacerbation of pain in this region. Minor trauma may result in splenic rupture precipitating massive haemorrhage requiring emergency splenectomy. Bone pain may occur due to widespread bone marrow involvement or localized bone deposits.

Pressure symptoms

Pressure may arise from massive splenomegaly in CML or diffuse lymphadenopathy in either form of chronic leukaemia. This can cause dysphagia and bronchial obstruction in the mediastinum, ureteric obstruction and renal failure in the abdomen, and limb oedema from axillary or inguinal nodes.

Other symptoms

Fever and night sweats may occur due to the high metabolic activity associated with bone marrow proliferation. High circulating levels of white cells which may exceed $100 \times 10^9/L$ may cause hyperviscosity with associated headaches, confusion, and visual disturbance. This may also cause, on treatment, rapid cell breakdown and tumour lysis syndrome resulting in hyperuricaemia and gout with painful joints in addition to widespread metabolic disturbance. Itching is also a feature of chronic leukaemia and this is often generalized and intractable.

Key points

- CML (CGL) and CLL are diseases of patients typically >60 years.
- Characteristic peripheral blood and bone marrow findings will confirm the diagnosis.
- Extensive peripheral lymphadenopathy may be seen in CLL.
- Massive splenomegaly is a feature of CML which may be painful and cause pancytopenia.

Treatment

Chemotherapy

Both forms of chronic leukaemia respond well to simple oral chemotherapy. In CML, busulphan or hydroxyurea are the drugs of choice. A new drug for the treatment of CML, working through inhibition of the abl-kinase enzyme pathway, imatinib mesylate, appears highly active and may replace alkylating agents in the future. Patients with CML will ultimately develop a blast crisis, analogous to an acute leukaemia, and will be treated as such with treatment as described previously, although the results are not as good as *de novo* acute leukaemia.

In CLL, other alkylating agents such as chlorambucil or cyclophosphamide are often chosen. The new purine analogue drugs such as cladribine and fludarabine are also highly active in CLL and are alternative options either initially or when resistance to alkylating agents has evolved. In relapsed patients re-introduction of the initial oral chemotherapy is often successful. In CLL, sequential relapses will be treated with re-exposure to chlorambucil or cyclophosphamide and when these fail drugs such as fludarabine or cladribine were introduced. Occasionally, combination chemotherapy such as CVP (cyclophosphamide, vincristine, prednisolone) or CHOP (cyclosphosphamide, adriamycin, vincristine, prednisolone) will be used. Ultimately patients with CLL become resistant to chemotherapy. In these patients intermittent high dose steroids may be of value for a short time.

Immunotherapy

Rituximab is a monoclonal antibody targeted against the B-cell surface protein CD20 which is now available for further treatment of patients with CLL. In relapsed disease after chemotherapy, response rates of >50 per cent are seen and its role in earlier treatment is under evaluation. Its mode of cell killing is uncertain after binding to the CD20 receptor, but it is specific for that cell population and as a result has no effect on bone marrow and peripheral blood count. It may occasionally cause generalized host immune reactions and rarely acute respiratory failure has been reported.

Interferon prolongs survival when given to patients with CML once they have achieved initial remission but has no proven value in CLL.

Radiotherapy

This has a limited role in the management of chronic leukaemia. Its main value is in the shrinkage of symptomatic lymph node masses. Relatively low doses of 30–40 Gy over 2–4 weeks will achieve durable remission and will be effective even in chemotherapy-resistant disease. Massive splenomegaly will also respond to splenic irradiation and low doses of only 3–5 Gy delivered over 1–2 weeks will be sufficient to cause significant shrinkage and symptom relief. There is often considerable tumour lysis with such treatment and patients should be well-hydrated and receive allopurinol during this period.

Local radiotherapy for painful bone lesions is always of value, delivering single doses of 8–10 Gy to the site of pain. In advanced disease there may also be extranodal infiltration. Symptomatic sites may include the lymphoid tissue within Waldeyer's ring (nasopharynx, tonsil, posterior tongue), the orbit, and paranasal sinuses. Local radiation to these sites will achieve control of chemotherapy-resistant disease and relief of symptoms.

Surgery

Splenectomy may be considered for patients with massive splenomegaly who have a prognosis of more than a few months. Surgical excision of lymph node masses is rarely of great value.

Other treatment

Bone marrow failure will require blood transfusion and platelet transfusion where symptoms arise. Blood transfusion is rarely indicated with haemoglobin levels greater than 10 g/dl and in patients with chronic anaemia levels of 8–9 g/dl may be well tolerated without major impacts upon quality of life. The indications for blood transfusion in these situations, particularly with advanced chemotherapy-resistant disease, are therefore purely for symptom relief and should not be influenced unduly by the level of haemoglobin. Patients who have received fludarabine should always receive irradiated blood products because of the risk of a transfusion versus host reaction.

Platelet transfusion is indicated for patients with spontaneous haemorrhage or if the absolute platelet level is less than $5000 \times 10^9/L$, prophylactic platelet administration is recommended. Neutropenia should be monitored closely and febrile episodes treated energetically with intravenous broad-spectrum antibiotics. Acute gout should be treated prophylactically with allopurinol and with non-steroid anti-inflammatory drugs if it develops.

Itching may be a feature of chronic leukaemia. Topical treatment with steroid creams and systemic treatment with steroids is indicated. Anti-histamine preparations may occasionally be of value as may topical anti-pruritic drugs such as crotamiton (Eurax).

Key points

- Both CLL and CML will respond well initially to simple oral alkylating agents.
- CLL is a chronic disease requiring intermittent treatment, rotating through the various treatment options which include chlorambucil, cyclophosphamide, fludarabine, cladribine, CHOP, rituximab and radiotherapy.
- CML will enter remission which is prolonged by the use of interferon; it will later transform into a blast crisis requiring treatment for acute leukaemia with a poor prognosis.

Myeloma

Multiple myeloma represents the most malignant end of a spectrum of disease arising due to neoplastic transformation of plasma cell lines in the bone marrow. The benign form of this, benign paraproteinaemia, may be a forerunner of subsequent multiple myeloma as may the localized form of myeloma in which a single site of plasma cell proliferation occurs forming a tumour mass, termed a 'plasmacytoma'. Up to 70 per cent of patients presenting with apparently localized plasmacytoma, however, ultimately develop multiple myeloma in which there is widespread involvement of the bone marrow with malignant cell proliferation taking up more than 20 per cent of the bone marrow.

This is associated with multiple bone lesions typically osteolytic and the presence of high levels of circulating abnormal immunoglobulin-like proteins, the paraproteins. High paraprotein levels can result in renal failure and hyperviscosity. Multiple bone lesions result in hypercalcaemia. Associated bone marrow failure occurs because of the proliferation of plasma cell lines, resulting in anaemia and an increased tendency to infection.

Prognosis

The outlook for myeloma in general is poor. Cure is virtually never seen and the median duration of survival is around 3 years depending upon the stage and severity at presentation. Poor prognostic features are haemoglobin less than 10, urea greater than 10, raised serum β_2-microglobulin and poor performance status. These figures, however, hide the fact that there is a group of patients with indolent disease ('smouldering myeloma') who may have low grade symptom-free disease for several years before entering a more aggressive phase. A small number of long-term survivors are now recorded who may have achieved a cure following intensive chemotherapy and bone marrow transplantation.

Pain

This is a common feature of multiple myeloma usually related to multiple sites of bone infiltration and erosion. The lesions are typically lytic with the accompanying risk of pathological fracture and vertebral collapse. Generalized osteoporotic changes may also be seen alongside lytic changes. There may be associated neurological symptoms with neuropathic root pain at sites of vertebral damage.

Other symptoms

Hypercalcaemia occurs in up to two-thirds of patients at some point in the course of their disease. This will manifest by confusion, thirst, polyuria, constipation, and bone pains. Renal failure may cause confusion, drowsiness, thirst, polyuria, nausea, anorexia, and diarrhoea. A rare complication of myeloma is amyloid formation which in the bowel may also cause malabsorption and diarrhoea. High levels of paraprotein can result in hyperviscosity causing headache, drowsiness, confusion, and visual disturbance. The results of bone marrow failure may cause symptoms of anaemia with fatigue and breathlessness, leucopenia with a high risk of infections, and thrombocytopenia with purpura and bleeding disorders.

Key points

- Myeloma will present with features of the classic triad: bone marrow failure, renal failure and bone pain.
- Dehydration and infection are common inpatients presenting with myeloma.

- Complications of bone disease in particular hypercalcaemia, pathological fracture and spinal cord compression are also common presentations.
- Diagnosis is based on >30 per cent plasma cells in bone marrow with an associated serum paraprotein, Bence Jones proteinuria and multiple lytic lesions on skeletal X-ray survey.
- Solitary plasmacytomas are seen in both soft tissue and bone; 70 per cent of the latter will eventually develop multiple myeloma.

Management

Chemotherapy

This mode of treatment has a major role in multiple myeloma, and in the initial phases of the disease most patients will respond. The options for chemotherapy in myeloma are:

- Oral alkylating agent (e.g. melphalan or cyclophosphamide) given for 1 week every month.
- Combination chemotherapy such as ABCM (adriamycin and BCNU injections alternating 3-weekly with oral cyclophosphamide and melphalan).
- High dose steroid-based schedules such as VAD (vincristine, adriamycin, dexamethasone) or VAMP in which methyl prednisolone is substituted for dexamethasone.

The choice of chemotherapy will depend upon both the stage of myeloma and the condition of the patient. Myeloma is frequently encountered in elderly patients who will not tolerate intensive combination chemotherapy. There is conflicting evidence as to the relative efficacy of oral alkylating agents and combination chemotherapy. Current analyses suggest that for a low grade myeloma with normal haemoglobin, normal renal function and good performance status an oral alkylating agent may be as good as more intensive treatment. This form of treatment is also better tolerated in the elderly patient which is an important consideration in a disease in which over half of patients will be over 65 years. For the younger patient with aggressive disease, combination chemotherapy using ABCM or VAD may have advantages.

Some patients may be selected to proceed to high dose chemotherapy with peripheral blood stem cell support or autologous bone marrow transplantation. There is evidence that such procedures may prolong the duration of first remission but more long-term data are required support the claim that patients may be cured from this approach. It is only appropriate for patients under the age of 60 because of the procedure related mortality and morbidity though only very few selected patients will be considered for these options.

Most patients will enter some degree of remission. Response in myeloma is typically defined by attainment of a 'plateau phase' when there has been a stable paraprotein level for a period of 3 consecutive months. The rate of attainment of plateau phase does not appear to be important and indeed there is some evidence to suggest that patients reaching this stage rapidly also relapse very quickly.

Relapse at some stage is inevitable and at this point further treatment may be considered. This may take the form of either re-challenge with oral alkylating agents if this was the initial treatment or the use of a combination schedule. There is some evidence that in relapse high dose dexamethasone alone (40 mg/m^2 for 4 consecutive days) is as effective as schedules containing cytotoxic drugs. High dose steroid schedules have the advantage of improving general well-being and energy levels but in these doses may be associated with considerable fluid retention, and in the elderly problems with hypertension and cardiac failure. They therefore need careful monitoring.

Alpha-interferon has been advocated in myeloma as a means of prolonging the plateau phase and delaying relapse. Current evidence regarding interferon in myeloma is contradictory, and it is uncertain whether this is of value at present. In the palliative setting with established relapse there is no role for interferon.

Bisphosphonates

A reduction in 'bone events' measured by pathological fracture and spinal cord compression rates, or the need for local radiotherapy for bone pain, has been shown with the use of adjuvant bisphosphonates, either in the form of intermittent intravenous pamidronate or oral clodronate. It is likely that these will be replaced by more potent oral bisphosphonates in the future. These drugs may also play an important role in the management of symptomatic bone pain.

Radiotherapy

Irradiation is of great value in the management of local bone pain from myeloma. Single doses of 8–10 Gy are usually effective and may be repeated if pain recurs with on each occasion a probability of response of around 80 per cent. Multiple sites of bone pain present a more difficult problem and myeloma is one of the conditions in which hemibody irradiation can be of considerable value. Doses of 6 Gy mid-plane dose to the upper half body (usually defined above the umbilicus) and 8 Gy mid-plane dose to the lower half body will result in pain relief for over 80 per cent of patients within a few days of treatment. This is maintained for most until their death. Sequential hemibody irradiation treating the upper half followed by the lower half with a break of 4–6 weeks to allow bone marrow recovery is also an effective treatment modality and should be considered in patients who have relapsed after chemotherapy and have chemotherapy-resistant disease on re-challenge. Useful further remissions can be obtained with this technique although as with all myeloma treatment later relapse is inevitable. Hemibody irradiation can be given despite previous local radiotherapy and similarly local radiotherapy to persistent sites of pain after hemibody irradiation can also be given.

Pathological fracture is also common in myeloma due to the lytic nature of the bone disease. Where internal fixation is not possible then local radiotherapy may help pain and enable bone healing although extensive areas of vertebral collapse or rib fractures will often present a major challenge to achieve good pain control due to the mechanical component of pain in these circumstances.

Surgery

This has a very limited role in myeloma. The major indication is in the case of actual or impending pathological fracture, which is relatively common in this disease characterized by extensive lytic bone disease. Internal fixation of fractures involving long bones is the treatment of choice and in selected patients with localized vertebral collapse and spinal instability spinal surgery and stabilization should be considered. Prophylactic pinning should also be considered in active patients who have large lytic lesions involving long bones. Recognized criteria for high risk lesions include those where there is >50 per cent cortical destruction (seen on any one of two perpendicular X-ray views), lesions >2.5 cm in diameter associated with pain, and areas of diffuse lytic infiltration.

Other treatment

Hypercalcaemia should be managed aggressively with rehydration aiming to give 3–4 litres of fluid per day together with frusemide to encourage diuresis and calcium excretion. Thiazide diuretics should be avoided as they reduce urinary calcium excretion. Bisphosphonate infusions using either pamidronate, 30–90 mg or clodronate, 1500 mg should follow this. The patient should be encouraged to remain well hydrated thereafter although relapses of hypercalcaemia are very common and there is some evidence that intermittent clodronate or pamidronate infusions can be of value repeated at 3–4 weekly intervals.

Renal failure will be treated conservatively with appropriate fluid balance restriction unless dehydrated. This may create difficulties where hypercalcaemia is present. Dialysis is rarely indicated but may be considered in the patient presenting with deteriorating renal failure prior to chemotherapy.

Hyperuricaemia is a feature of myeloma and associated gout may occur. This should be treated with allopurinol and non-steroidal anti-inflammatory drugs in the acute phase.

Hyperviscosity In myeloma, symptoms of this condition are difficult to manage since the cause is not an excess of blood cells which can be managed by venesection but high levels of paraprotein. In acute problems, plasmapheresis may be considered but this is rarely a long-term solution as within a short time more paraprotein is produced by the myeloma unless effective chemotherapy can be given. It is, however, one important reason for maintaining high levels of fluid intake for patients with myeloma.

Anaemia may require blood transfusions to maintain the haemoglobin at a level tolerated by the patient. Many patients with myeloma will become adjusted to chronic anaemia and be maintained at levels of 9–10 g/dl without significant symptoms. Synthetic erythropoietin is now available and there is some evidence that this is effective in myeloma to maintain levels of haemoglobin. It is, however, an expensive drug requiring intermittent subcutaneous administration.

Infections are particularly common in myeloma affecting up to 80 per cent of patients at some time in their course. Active treatment of these should be encouraged with broad-spectrum antibiotics.

Neutropenia (total neutrophil count less than 1.0×10^9/L) is rare unless associated with chemotherapy. Neutropenic sepsis should be treated in the usual way with intravenous broad spectrum cephalosporin or aminoglycoside antibiotics. Care should, however, be taken in myeloma patients with these drugs since they both are affected by impaired renal function. Gentamicin may be the drug of choice in this situation since monitoring of blood levels is freely available and provided prolonged inter-dosing intervals are used can be safely administered.

Key points

- Intensive supportive therapy is essential for the management of myeloma, with attention to fluid replacement, renal function, antibiotics for infection and transfusion for anaemia.
- Chemotherapy with either combination chemotherapy or alkylating agents alone will control the initial phase of the disease and enable a plateau phase to be reached.
- Consolidation with high dose chemotherapy strategies may be considered at plateau phase in younger patients.
- Bisphosphonates will reduce the incidence of hypercalcaemia, pathological fracture and spinal cord compression. They may also be effective in scattered bone pain.
- Radiotherapy should be given for local bone pain and inoperable pathological fracture; hemibody radiotherapy may gain further remission for advanced chemo-resistant disease.
- Recurrence often responds to further chemotherapy using an alternative to that given initially, but long-term survival is rare, the average life expectancy being around 3 years from diagnosis.

Supportive care for patients with haematological malignancies:

◆ Once anti-tumour treatments are discontinued, the terminal phase usually develops quickly.

◆ Patients have had prolonged and close contact with the haematology/oncology teams over the preceding months or years, and often prefer to remain under their direct care.

◆ Options including care at home should be encouraged but success requires good liaison between hospital and community teams.

◆ Often patients have means of central venous access; unless infected these can be useful if further blood products are likely to be administered; in these situations the regular care regimen must be maintained. Otherwise it is preferable to take them out.

◆ Absolute decisions such as 'no further blood products or antibiotics' are best avoided; instead consider the value of such interventions in relation to specific situations and the wishes of the patient.

◆ Subcutaneous infusions may be used in patients with thrombocytopaenia but require close monitoring of the sites for bruising or oozing. Caution is needed with NSAIDS with assessment of benefits versus increased risks of bleeding.

Case History 16.2

Mrs W is a 75-year-old lady with a long history of back problems and several fractures after minor falls. X-rays had shown marked osteoporosis and she was commenced on oral etidronate.

Some months later, she is found to be anaemic. Investigations find a paraprotein and 35 per cent plasma cells in a sample of bone marrow. Ig G myeloma is diagnosed. Oral chemotherapy with melphalan and prednisolone is commenced and the falling immunoglobulin levels show a good response to this. However she has a severe exacerbation of pain in her lower dorsal/upper lumbar spine which radiated around her sides. X-rays show wedging and loss of height of multiple vertebral bodies and there appears to be a new collapse of T10. She is referred to the palliative medicine clinic.

Mrs W is struggling with pain as well as loss of independence. Previously active and sociable, she now spends everyday lying on the settee at home, looked after by an anxiously attentive husband. She feels useless and a burden on her family; she admitted to a persistently low mood for several weeks. Her GP had prescribed control release morphine with some improvement and she was now taking 120 mg daily but did not want to increase because of the side effects (sleepiness and constipation). The haematologist had advised against NSAIDS although she did take regular paracetamol.

After discussion with Mrs W and her husband, the following plan was agreed:

- Radiotherapy to her lower dorsal spine.
- Oral etidronate switched to zoledronate given by short infusions each month.
- Physiotherapy input for trial of TENS and assessment of mobility.
- Switch from morphine to an alternative opioid was discussed but Mrs W wants to keep this in reserve.

Radiotherapy in this case proved very helpful in reducing pain at the site of recent collapse suggesting that myeloma infiltration was a contributory factor as well as a structural weakening due to osteoporosis. She also found relief from the use of TENS. A gentle program to increase activity was drawn up. This made a big difference to her morale and self esteem such that antidepressants were not necessary.

Practice points

- Osteoporosis is a common radiological finding in myeloma.
- NSAIDS should be used with caution and avoided if there is evidence of renal impairment.
- Regular administration of bisphosphonates may reduce the incidence of skeletal events such as fracture and vertebral collapse.

Chapter 17

Skin tumours

Whilst pathologically distinct skin and soft tissue tumours present very similar problems when advanced.

Skin tumours may be classified into two main groups:

- Basal and squamous cell carcinomas

- Melanoma

Primary skin tumours are often related to sun exposure and their incidence is increasing in non-pigmented races. It is seen particularly in Australia and South Africa but is also increasing in incidence in Western Europe due to altered leisure activities.

Basal cell carcinoma (also known as rodent ulcer) is a disease predominantly of the elderly and is rarely a major clinical problem except in a few neglected cases or where there is extensive invasion of local soft tissues and bone. Squamous carcinoma tends to arise in middle aged and elderly patients but is potentially more sinister as it spreads to local and regional nodes and may also develop blood borne metastases with an associated mortality. Both basal and squamous cancers of the skin typically, although not exclusively, develop on sun-exposed areas of the face and limbs.

Melanoma is by far the most sinister of the trio presenting in patients at any age although it is rare in children. It is associated with previous episodes of sunburn, especially as a child. Whilst superficial melanoma may be a relatively straightforward condition dealt with by surgical excision the reputation of this tumour for rapid blood borne dissemination and ultimate death is well earned.

There are other rare tumours arising from adnexal structures such as the hair follicles, sweat and sebaceous glands. Merkel's tumour is a tumour arising from the neuroendocrine tissue which is highly malignant behaving in a fashion like melanoma or small-cell lung cancer.

Key points

- Skin tumours are of three main types: basal cell or squamous cell carcinomas and melanoma.
- Skin cancer is often due to sun damage particularly in Caucasian races.
- Basal cell carcinomas will infiltrate and invade locally but do not metastasize.

- Squamous carcinomas invade locally and spread by lymph node involvement; blood borne metastases are unusual except in advanced cases.
- Melanomas disseminate widely by blood borne spread to liver, lungs bone and CNS.

Basal and squamous cell carcinomas of skin

Natural history and prognosis

Basal cell carcinoma

Basal cell carcinoma is a local condition which grows and invades the surrounding tissues. The majority are small superficial lesions which may be nodular, cystic, diffuse spreading superficially. They subsequently erode and ulcerate, hence their name 'rodent ulcer'. They usually have a long natural history. Their extent may be underestimated because of invasion along tissue planes, and particular areas of concern are around the orbit, auditory meatus and naso-labial region where they are particularly common. Metastases are extremely rare, (<0.01 per cent, usually occurring in bone), but where primary treatment is inadequate then recurrence and progressive local tissue destruction may occur. They may also present in an advanced incurable state due to neglect particularly in the elderly and in sites not readily inspected such as the scalp.

Squamous carcinoma

Squamous carcinoma tends to arise on sun exposed areas in particular around the face, dorsum of hands and lower limbs but can arise in any site. A less common predisposing factor is chronic skin damage and squamous skin cancer is well recognized developing at oprevious sites of traumas such as burns; historically they were associated with exposure to surface carcinogens such as soot, tar and mineral oils. There is an increased incidence in patients who are immunosuppressed, including post-transplant patients. It spreads by lymph node metastasis to adjacent regional lymph nodes and also blood borne spread.

Symptoms

Pain

Pain is rarely a feature of primary skin cancer unless there is extensive local tissue damage, bone or nerve infiltration. Metastatic lymphadenopathy from any of these primary sites may cause local pain in the draining node area, for example the groin from the leg and axilla from the upper limb.

Haemorrhage

Surface bleeding from skin tumours is common and indeed any skin lesion which starts to bleed should immediately be investigated for malignancy. Large lesions such as a neglected basal cell carcinoma can result in considerable surface haemorrhage which may be difficult to control.

Regional node metastases may grow to a large size with fungation and local haemorrhage. Erosion of a major vessel, in particular the carotid with neck nodes or the femoral artery from the groin is a recognized hazard in advanced disease.

Obstruction

Primary skin tumours rarely cause problems with obstruction unless regional lymph nodes cause peripheral swelling of an associated limb.

Other symptoms

Tumours within the skin and soft tissues are at particular risk of ulceration and fungation. This may be painful especially when associated with secondary infection. Surface discharge and malodour may develop. Neglected or locally recurrent basal cell carcinomas can similarly result in extensive tissue damage around the orbit, oral and nasal cavities affecting vision, breathing, speech and food intake.

Key points

- The main symptoms from skin tumours are due to local growth, surface bleeding and fungation.
- Metastatic lymph nodes may cause limb swelling, pain and fungate.
- Skin tumours around the eye, nose or mouth may cause additional problems due to local damage.

Treatment

Surgery

Surgery is the primary modality of treatment for both the skin tumours. Most small basal cell carcinomas will be treated in the dermatology clinic by curettage or simple excision. More advanced tumours may require extensive resection and occasionally repair with a skin flap. Squamous cell carcinomas will be dealt with in a similar fashion but require a wider surgical margin to ensure local control.

In cases presenting with advanced disease, primary surgery may be impossible. Surgery may still have a role with a limited resection of a fungating tumour to achieve local skin cover or following a course of radiotherapy using a skin flap to repair an extensive defect where the area has been sterilized with radiation.

Radiotherapy

Radiotherapy is indicated for certain basal cell carcinomas and squamous cell carcinomas of the skin. Its use as the primary treatment modality depends upon the site and size of the lesion and a consideration of the cosmetic results of treatment. It is of particular value in areas where surgical excision would involve extensive surgical repair and possible functional or cosmetic deficits. These include the lower eyelid, nasolabial region and external pinna. In most other sites, primary surgery is usually to be preferred but in advanced neglected tumours a combination of radiotherapy and surgery may be of value. Certain areas are particularly slow to heal after radiotherapy and in these surgery is to be preferred; they include the lower leg, dorsum of hand and skin over the back. Where surgery is considered unwise due to extreme old age or other concerns, more complex radiotherapy techniques such as surface brachytherapy may be successful.

Radiotherapy also has an important palliative role for locally advanced disease and recurrent squamous or basal cell carcinomas. Relatively small doses of 8–10 Gy in a single fraction or 20–30 Gy over 1–2 weeks can prevent fungation or where this has occurred reduce surface haemorrhage and allow the surface to dry reducing nursing care requirements.

Case History 17.1

A 77-year-old woman with liver metastases from colorectal cancer attends the Day Hospice. One of the nursing staff notices that she has a persistent, scabbed nodule on her lower eyelid, close to her nose. It is about 1.5 cm across and the appearance is typical of a basal cell carcinoma. There is some difference of opinion within the team about what action should be taken. The oncologist is asked for his opinion and she attends for radiotherapy three weeks later.

Practice points

- Radiotherapy is an easy treatment option which will almost always cure a lesion of this type.
- Left for 12–18 months – which may be possible even in a patient with liver disease from bowel cancer – the nodule will become an unpleasant, disfiguring ulcer which would necessitate major surgery or be less likely to be controlled by radiotherapy.

Chemotherapy

In general, chemotherapy has little role in the management of basal cell carcinoma or squamous carcinoma of the skin.

Other treatment

Management of the advanced local skin tumour is that of any fungating wound with regular nursing care and the use of topical antibiotics such as metronidazole, haemostatic dressings where there is local haemorrhage and activated charcoal where there is necrosis and malodour. Patients often also need considerable psychological support and practical help so that a disfiguring or smelly tumour can be hidden successfully to enable them to interact socially as far as possible.

The development of skin cancer in the immunosuppressed patient should lead to a review of their immunosuppression reducing this as far as possible without compromising the success of a transplant; it should also herald a higher level of surveillance for these patients.

Key points

- The most effective treatment for primary skin tumours is local surgical excision.
- Lymph node dissection as the best treatment for involved lymph nodes.
- Radiotherapy is indicated for basal cell and squamous cancer around the eyelids and nose where better cosmesis may be obtained.
- Very large tumours may require both surgery and radiotherapy.

Melanoma

Natural history and prognosis

Melanoma usually arises in a pre-existing 'mole' although amelanotic melanoma is a recognized entity. They may occur on any site of the body, those occurring on the limbs tending to be associated with a better prognosis than those on the trunk, and also, less commonly, from mucosal surfaces and the nail bed (sub-ungual melanoma). They are classified according to their depth of infiltration either anatomically (Clarkes level) or by measurement of the histological specimen after excision (Breslow thickness). Melanoma invading greater than 1.5 mm generally has a poor prognosis and rapid dissemination to regional lymph nodes and through the circulation to liver, lungs, bone and brain is well recognized. Other recognized patterns of metastases from melanoma are with satellite nodules spreading in the skin away from the primary site due to infiltration of subdermal lymphatics and metastases in the bowel particularly small bowel nodules. Long periods of many years between treatment of a primary melanoma and the appearance of metastases are well-recognized.

Symptoms

Pain

Metastasis however, in particular, from melanoma can cause liver pain due to rapid enlargement and massive hepatomegaly. Headache may be a feature because of brain metastases again particularly associated with melanoma, which also disseminates to bone causing metastatic bone pain and the thorax causing chest and pleuritic pain. Metastatic lymphadenopathy may cause local pain in the draining node area, for example the groin from the leg and axilla from the upper limb.

Haemorrhage

Melanoma is considered a particularly haemorrhagic tumour and metastases from this tumour can spontaneously bleed which may result in an intracerebral haemorrhage from brain metastasis, intrapulmonary haemorrhage from pulmonary metastasis, gastrointestinal haemorrhage from any site within the gastrointestinal tract and intrahepatic haemorrhage from hepatic metastasis. This will often present with a rapid deterioration either neurologically in the case of brain metastasis or with increasing local pain and discomfort in the case of lung and liver metastasis. Regional node metastases may grow to a large size with fungation and local haemorrhage.

Obstruction

Melanoma frequently metastasizes to regional lymph nodes which can cause limb swelling often with associated fungation of the node mass. Nasal cavity, sinuses and nasopharynx are rare, but well-recognized sites for melanoma to develop resulting in obstruction of the nasal airway. Rarely melanoma within the gastrointestinal tract may cause sub-acute obstruction.

Local sites of melanoma may ulcerate. Mucosal melanomas within the oral or nasal cavity may cause local pain, discharge and foul taste. Within the head and neck region, melanoma may affect the orbit and eye resulting in disfigurement either from the tumour itself or the need for radical surgery.

Key points

- Melanoma usually arises in a previous mole, heralded by an increase in size, pimentation of shape and itching or bleeding.
- Prognosis is related to depth of invasion; most superficial melanomas <0.75 mm deep are cured, deeper melanomas carry a risk of distant metastases.
- Melanoma may be associated with symptoms due to liver, lung, bone or brain metastases which may appear several years after diagnosis of the primary lesion.
- Mucosal melanomas arising in the head and neck region, bowel and perineum can cause additional local symptoms.

Management

Surgery

The primary site of melanoma is resected widely with a margin of at least 2 cm of normal tissue and in more deeply invading melanomas a wider margin is sometimes recommended. There has been controversy as to whether elective block dissection of regional lymph nodes is of value. Randomized trials have failed to show any overall survival advantage but in the case of involved lymph nodes then surgical dissection is the treatment of choice.

Radiotherapy

Whilst of little value in the primary treatment of melanoma, radiotherapy may be given where excision margins are close and in surgically difficult sites such as the head and neck region where an increased rate of local control will be achieved using post-operative radiotherapy. Radiotherapy is also the treatment of choice for a characteristic melanoma occurring on the face of elderly people termed lentigo maligna. These appear exquisitely sensitive to radiation and this is usually curative.

In the palliative setting radiotherapy has an important role in reducing local symptoms from painful or bleeding skin nodules and in the control of advanced, inoperable regional nodes. Typically larger fractions are delivered in melanoma; single doses of 8–10 Gy are usually sufficient for control of haemorrhage, higher doses up to 30 Gy in 5 fractions may be given for large tumour masses where growth restraint and shrinkage are required for satisfactory palliation.

Case History 17.2

Julie had a mole removed from her calf because it had become larger and itched. This turned out to be a malignant melanoma so a further wide excision of the area was undertaken.

Four years later she has developed extensive metastases involving the subcutaneous tissues, lungs and liver. She has a trial of temozolomide with some response, but the disease progresses within weeks. She decides that she does not want more chemotherapy and is doing well to accept the situation.

She finds the superficial tumours one of the worst features of the illness because they are such an obvious reminder to herself and others. To begin with, she had requested surgical excision as they appeared but they were now too numerous. A radiotherapy opinion was sought.

It was suggested that a single treatment could be given to the most troublesome lesions, and that if these responded it might be worth giving treatment to others in the future. She was most concerned over a 3 cm nodule on her neck that was unsightly and bled from the surface; there was also a larger lump on her back which was uncomfortable when she lay in bed. Palliative radiotherapy, using electrons, was used to treat the sites. The tumours regressed substantially and the bleeding stopped.

Practice points

- Metastatic melanoma may not appear for several years after the initial diagnosis.
- Metastatic disease is often widespread and may respond poorly to chemotherapy.
- Palliative radiotherapy can be a way of dealing with symptomatic superficial tumours.

Radiotherapy is also indicated in the management of brain, bone and occasionally liver metastasis from melanoma, and for the palliation of painful or bleeding skin nodules. There is no evidence that dose fractionation schedules other than the standard palliative schedules are advantagous, i.e. 8 to 10 Gy in a single fraction for a bone metastasis, 12 Gy in 2 fractions or 20 Gy in 5 fractions for brain metastases and 20–30 Gy over 2–3 weeks for liver metastases.

Chemotherapy

Whilst many trials have been performed in melanoma it remains a chemoresistant tumour with few drugs having an influence upon its natural history. In advanced disease attempts may be made to achieve some degree of control using drugs such as vindesine or dacarbazine (DTIC). In general response rates are only of the order of 20–30 per cent and shortlived; for most patients this treatment is not appropriate. A new drug, temozolomide, appears as effective in melanoma as other chemotherapy agents and has the advantage of oral administration and low toxicity.

Other treatment

Melanoma is one of the few tumours which has shown responses with biological agents in particular interferon or interleukin 2. Again however the response rate is relatively modest, of the order of 30 per cent. This treatment is given by subcutaneous injection three times per week on a continuous basis. It may be associated with debilitating general malaise and flu-like symptoms. Significant impacts upon the overall natural history of the disease are relatively rare, although small improvements in survival may be seen if given adjuvantly in high risk cases.

Patients with melanoma who present with a limited number of localized lung metastases should be considered for metastatectomy in which surgical excision of the metastases is attempted. In a small number of selected patients where the lung is the only site of limited relapse this can result in a further long disease-free interval.

Key points

• Melanoma requires a wide margin of excision.
• Metastatic melanoma may respond to chemotherapy such as dacarbazine or temozolamide and is responsive to interferon.

Case History 17.3

A 34-year-old fair-haired man saw his general practitioner about a mole on his back. His wife had noticed that it seemed to be darker and it occasionally bled. He was sent to the local 'Pigmented Lesion Clinic' and the clinical diagnosis of malignant melanoma was confirmed on biopsy.

He underwent a wide excision of the mole and surrounding tissue, using a split skin graft to cover the defect. Histology showed tumour invasion to a depth of 2.1 mm with lymphatic invasion. A chest X-ray was normal and no further treatment was given at this stage.

Twelve months later, at a routine clinic visit, he is found to have a 2 cm enlarged node in the axilla on the same side as his melanoma. A fine needle aspirate confirmed that this contained melanoma and he underwent axillary node dissection. Five of the eighteen nodes removed contained tumour and there was spread beyond the node capsule in some. Radiotherapy was recommended as there was a high risk of recurrence, but he was warned that this might lead to the development of lymphoedema of his arm. He completed a course of treatment and remained well. He did develop mild arm swelling about 9 months later but with no evidence of disease and this was managed with a compression sleeve.

Three years later he developed persistent upper abdominal discomfort and was found to have an enlarged, hard liver. He was reviewed by the oncologist and investigations now showed liver and lung metastases. He was offered palliative chemotherapy and commenced intravenous dacarbazine. This caused nausea and vomiting, despite ondanstron, on the first day of treatment but he coped with this. After 6 weeks he developed severe headaches and a brain scan showed multiple metastases. His condition deteriorated rapidly and in view of this, with a poor response to chemotherapy for his widespread disease, it was decided not to advise cranial irradiation. A few days later he developed sudden severe pain and became comatose.

Practice points

- Deeply invading melanoma has a bad outlook, with a high probability of regional and distant spread.
- Even in poor prognosis disease, aggressive treatment to local and regional disease is important to avoid uncontrolled tumour at these sites.
- Patients with brain metastases who have widespread disease and poor performance status will be unlikely to benefit from radiotherapy.
- A bleed into a secondary tumour is not unusual and can cause severe hepatic pain or an intracerebral haemorrhage.

Chapter 18

Bone and soft tissue tumours

Bone and soft tissue tumours, whilst relatively common solid tumours in children, are rare in adults. They may occur at any age although certain types of tumour follow a recognized pattern, for example osteosarcoma is seen in adolescents and then a second peak of incidence in patients aged 60–70 whilst most soft tissue sarcomas are seen in patients over the age of 50. There are a number of sub-types of primary bone tumour, the classification being related to behaviour, some of these being highly malignant metastatic tumours such as osteosarcoma whilst others are relatively benign tumours with low metastatic potential such as osteoclastoma (see Table 18.1). In contrast, whilst there are many different histological sub-types of soft tissue sarcoma depending upon the normal tissue type they resemble, their behaviour is not greatly influenced by their sub-type. A list of the common sub-types is shown in Table 18.2. The aetiology of bone and soft tissue sarcomas is largely unknown. Whilst patients may relate the diagnosis of a bone tumour to local trauma this is not a recognized aetiological factor but rather a feature in drawing attention to a particular site. Osteosarcoma in elderly patients is typically secondary to underlying Paget's disease of bone. Soft tissue sarcoma may rarely be secondary to previous local irradiation and there are rare familial syndromes for example the LiFraumeni syndrome. In the majority of adult soft tissue sarcomas however there is no recognized underlying cause.

The natural history of these tumours is to grow and infiltrate locally, often extending widely through tissue planes at their site of origin either involving extensively bone or in the case of soft tissue tumours infiltrating entire muscle compartments. This has important implications for the extent of local treatment required and probability of local recurrence. These tumours typically spread distally by blood borne metastasis to the lungs with less commonly liver and bone involvement. Nodal involvement is rare except in a few specific examples, for example synovial sarcoma and alveolar rhabdomyosarcoma of adults.

Key points

- Osteosarcoma is an aggressive tumour invading locally and metastasizing particularly to lungs.
- Other malignant bone tumours include osteoclastoma and chondrosarcoma which are typically localized to the site of origin.
- Soft tissue sarcomas will infiltrate widely at their site of origin and spread by blood borne metastases most commonly to the lungs.

Table 18.1 Common types of primary malignant bone tumour

Osteosarcoma	10–20 years & 60–70 years	Local infiltration
	Femur, tibia, (45%); humerus(10%)	Blood borne mets to lung
Chondrosarcoma	>50 years	Local infiltration
	Pelvic bones most common	Metastases only in high grade
Osteoclastoma	40–60 years	Local growth
	Knee, radius, humerus	Metastases rare
Ewings tumour	5–15 years	Local infiltration
	Any bone	Blood borne mets to lung

Table 18.2 Types of soft tissue sarcoma in adults

Most common	Least common
Fibrosarcoma	Synovial sarcoma
Liposarcoma	Clear cell sarcoma
Leiomyosarcoma	Malignant fibrous histiocytoma
Rhabdomyosarcoma	Angiosarcoma
Neurogenic sarcoma	Lymphangiosarcoma

Common symptoms

Pain

Most of these tumours present as a palpable mass which may be associated with local pain and tenderness, although many are pain free at presentation. Forty-five per cent of osteosarcomas arise around the knee, with a ratio of femur to tibia involvement of 2:1. Local pain, particularly worse on weight bearing, is a typical feature and increasing pain in patients with underlying Paget's disease should alert to the diagnosis of malignant change. Bone tumours may result in pathological fracture and this may be the presenting feature.

Forty per cent of soft tissue sarcomas arise in the lower limb or buttock and 20 per cent in the retro-peritoneal area. In the limb they are often painless whilst in the retroperitoneal area persistent and increasing back pain may be the only symptom. They may grow to a substantial size before diagnosis particularly where they arise in a body cavity such as the abdomen or a large muscle such as the thigh or buttock.

Fungation and haemorrhage

Whilst bone tumours may cause deformity of bone they rarely fungate through the skin. In contrast soft tissue sarcoma left untreated will progress and cause a large fungating mass. Surface haemorrhage may also be a problem in the management of locally advanced diseases.

Other symptoms

Soft tissue masses may result in nerve compression and neuropathic symptoms. Within the retro-peritoneal space progressive enlargement may cause distal venous or lymphatic obstruction with lower limb swelling and ureteric obstruction causing hydronephrosis.

Lung metastasis being a common feature of the natural history may present with typical symptoms (see Chapter 23) including cough, haemoptysis, dyspnoea and pleuritic chest pain.

Key points

• Bone tumours usually present with local swelling and pain which may lead to pathological fracture.

• Soft tissue sarcomas will cause a swelling at their site of origin; in large muscles such as the thigh and buttock, and in the retroperitoneal cavity the primary can reach a large size before detection.

• Low grade tumours may grow slowly but inexorably causing deformity and impairing function whilst the patient remains well.

• Sarcomas may ulcerate and fungate if left untreated.

• High grade tumours may progress rapidly with symptoms from widespread metastases at presentation.

Management

Bone tumours

Surgery

Surgical removal is the mainstay of treatment for bone tumours. For the less malignant types, osteoclastoma or chondrosarcoma, then radical surgical excision is the treatment of choice where technically possible. Similarly for osteosarcoma radical excision of the affected area is important aiming wherever possible at limb conservation and appropriate prosthetic bone replacement. This will be preceded by chemotherapy in osteosarcoma to obtain early control of micrometastatic disease and reduce the extent and viability of the primary tumour mass enabling more complete surgery whilst preserving function.

Radiotherapy

Radiotherapy has a limited role in the management of bone tumours which generally have limited radioresponsiveness. It may be used for local recurrence after extensive surgery and will be used in primary treatment for surgically inoperable bones. Examples will include bone tumours arising in the vertebral column or pelvic girdle bones. These tumours require relatively a high dose of radiotherapy to doses of at least 60 Gy for local control. Such doses cannot be achieved in the spinal column without spinal cord damage and the control of tumours in this region is therefore a major problem. Fortunately it is a relatively rare site for primary bone tumours.

Chemotherapy

Chemotherapy has a major role in the management of osteosarcoma, modern treatment protocols using primary chemotherapy followed by surgical removal of the site of origin. In the past complex drug schedules using high dose methotrexate have been used. It is now more usual to use schedules containing drugs such as cisplatin, ifosfamide and Adriamycin.

A rare tumour in adults is Ewing's sarcoma, typically seen in patients aged between 10 and 20 years. This will also be treated with primary chemotherapy using combinations of vincristine, Adriamycin, actinomycin D and cyclophosphamide followed by local treatment, usually radiotherapy in this relatively radiosensitive tumour.

Case History 18.1

A 62-year-old man presents with pain in right upper chest and elbow. On examination a swelling is discovered in the supraclavicular area. CT scan shows tumour arising from the right first rib. Appearances are those of a primary osteosarcoma, which is confirmed by biopsy. No evidence of distant metastases is found.

He is treated with combination chemotherapy but this achieves only partial regression of tumour. He proceeds to radical surgery but limb preservation is not possible. He undergoes upper lobectomy and forequarter amputation

Eight months later he is complaining of pain in his shoulder and this radiates to his phantom limb. An MR scan is requested which unfortunately shows recurrent tumour around the brachial plexus. He also has multiple nodules on a chest X-ray which appear to be lung metastases.

The plan is to give further chemotherapy but he understands that his disease is incurable. His main problem is pain, which clearly has a neuropathic component. This responds to morphine in combination with gabapentin. At this point the palliative care team are involved to help with on-going support and symptom control.

There is progression of lung and soft tissue disease so chemotherapy is stopped after 2 cycles. Palliative radiotherapy is given to the mass on his upper chest wall. Within a few months he is less well. His lung metastases are causing cough and breathlessness on exertion. A further increase in his morphine helps and he agrees to use a wheelchair outside the home.

The treated area on his upper chest wall breaks down because of tumour infiltration. The terminal event is a massive haemorrhage from the wound.

Practice points

♦ Although commonly arising in a long bone, primary osteosarcoma can arise at other sites and these are associated with a worse prognosis.

♦ If metastases had been detected earlier, radical surgery would not have been attempted.

♦ Some tumours prove to be extremely resistant to chemotherapy or radiotherapy: here failure to control local disease was the cause of death.

Soft tissue sarcoma

Surgery

Surgery is the most important treatment modality in the management of soft tissue sarcoma. It is widely recognized that simple excision of these tumours is inadequate and will inevitably be followed by local recurrence. They require wide radical resection with compartmentectomy, that is removal of all muscle groups in a muscle compartment, within the limbs, and equally radical wide excision in other sites. In the past limb tumours were thought to require amputation but now limb conservation is practised by the use of wide excision and post-operative radiotherapy. There may however, be instances where amputation is the only means of obtaining clearance and control of an extensive soft tissue sarcoma arising proximally in the thigh or upper arm. Retro-peritoneal sarcomas present a more difficult problem often being unresectable or a debulking procedure being all that is technically feasible.

Radiotherapy

Radiotherapy has an important role in the post-operative treatment of soft tissue sarcomas. Following the same principles as surgical treatment wide radiation fields covering the entire muscle compartment and also including any surgical scar within which implantation and local recurrence is a recognized risk, should be used. This can result in very large radiation fields and typically treatments will involve two or three phases over 6–7 weeks to cover an initial large volume and then smaller areas focusing on the original site of origin to increase the dose to that site. Doses of around 60 Gy are required to expect good durable local control rates. Techniques using brachytherapy insertion of afterloading tubes into which radioactive sources can be placed post-operatively have also been described but have not been shown to have any great advantages over modern external beam treatment. Tumours which are inoperable, commonly those in the retro-peritoneal region, will be treated by radiotherapy, but there will be limitations in terms of the total dose that can be safely delivered because of tolerance of surrounding normal tissues in particular small bowel and kidneys.

Radical high dose radiotherapy to the limbs may have long-term side effects. In particular fibrosis and shortening of muscles can result in restriction of movement at joints. A general principle of limb radiotherapy is to attempt to preserve a lymphatic channel by leaving as much of the circumference of a limb out of the high dose volume as possible and unless absolutely essential never covering the entire circumference of a limb. However, this may not always be possible and lymphoedema may occur distal to the site of treatment.

Radiotherapy also has a role in tumours presenting as large fixed inoperable masses. High dose primary radiotherapy may be given and in some circumstances may then allow after a period of regression radical surgery. Locally recurrent tumours may also be treated with radiotherapy to achieve growth delay and prevent local fungation. Tumours which have fungated or have surface bleeding will also be palliated by local radiotherapy often using shorter treatment schedules in larger doses per fraction, for example 30 Gy given in 5 treatments on a weekly or bi-weekly basis.

Chemotherapy

Soft tissue sarcoma is a relatively chemo-resistant tumour. Only limited responses are seen with current drugs the most active of which is Adriamycin. Chemotherapy may considered for selected patients with symptomatic metastatic disease and periods of disease stabilisation or even partial remission may be seen in up to 30 per cent although ultimately progression is to be expected. The 5-year survival of patients presenting with distant metastasis from soft tissue sarcoma is less than 5 per cent.

An exception to this is the rare gastrointestinal stomal tumour which appears particularly sensitive to the new drug Imatinib Mesylate (Glivec). It is therefore important to distinguish this type of bowel sarcoma from the more common leiomyosarcoma; immunohistochemical stains on the biopsy for CD34 and CD117 are characteristic of gastrointestinal stromal tumours.

Key points

- Primary bone tumours are treated by local resection; in osteosarcoma this will be preceded by chemotherapy incorporating cisplatin, adriamycin and ifosphamide.
- Radiotherapy may be used for primary bone tumours in inoperable sites such as the vertebrae or pelvis.
- Soft tissue sarcomas are best managed by wide local resection followed by wide field radiotherapy.
- Metastatic sarcoma responds poorly to palliative chemotherapy.

Case History 18.2

A 58-year-old woman had suffered lower back pain for two years. During this time X-rays of the spine had shown no abnormality and she was treated by her general practitioner with anti-inflammatory drugs and physiotherapy. She had also sought help from a local osteopath.

The general practitioner finally referred her to an orthopaedic surgeon, who arranged a MR scan of the spine. After a delay of several more weeks – during which time her symptoms were getting worse – this was performed. It showed a large soft tissue mass in the retroperitoneal tissues, just below the level of the renal vessels. There was unilateral ureteric obstruction with hydronephrosis. A radiological diagnosis of a liposarcoma was made from the MR tissues characteristics and a needle biopsy confirmed a myxoid liposarcoma.

She was seen urgently by a specialist sarcoma team to assess and plan treatment. A CT scan of her chest showed no evidence of lung metastases. However the primary tumour was considered to be inoperable and therefore the alternative would be radical radiotherapy. It was explained to the patient and her husband that the size and nature of the tumour meant that complete eradication and cure were very unlikely. However as large a dose of radiotherapy as possible (within the limits of tolerance of the surrounding tissues) would be worthwhile to offer the best chance of controlling the tumour for some time. This would also help her pain. They were informed that treatment would inevitably include the ipsilateral kidney and the dose received would destroy its function. While her biochemical profile was normal, an isotope renogram showed that there was in fact little contribution from the obstructed kidney; fortunately that on the other side was working normally.

CT scans were used to plan the radiotherapy treatment which was given over a 6-week period. The detailed plan ensured that the normal kidney was not irradiated. From the start of treatment she was quite nauseated but this improved with regular ondansetron.

In the third week onwards, she developed diarrhoea with occasional colic. Her pain at this stage was controlled by slow release morphine; laxatives were stopped and additional loperamide was given to reduce bowel frequency. This gradually settled within another 3 weeks after her radiotherapy finished.

Her analgesic requirement reduced considerably over the next few months and she was able to resume work and her usual activities. A repeat CT scan 12 months later showed a residual tumour mass but was causing no symptoms. There was evidence of a small amount of subcutaneous fibrosis in her flank.

Unfortunately pulmonary metastases appeared soon after this. Chemotherapy was deferred until these were causing symptoms and she had a transient symptomatic response. Throughout this time she had no further problems from the primary site but died from metastatic disease two and a half years after the radiotherapy.

Case History 18.2 (continued)

Practice points

- Retroperitoneal sarcoma may be hard to diagnose in its early stages.
- They are often inoperable and radiotherapy is important for local control.
- Acute effects of abdominal radiotherapy frequently include nausea and vomiting, attributed to stimulation of gut 5HT receptors. 5HT3 antagonists such as ondansetron or granisetron are very effective.
- Another acute effect is diarrhoea, due to loss of cells from the epithelial lining.It is self limiting and resolves as the mucosal surface repopulates but some individuals may need inpatient care and fluid replacement.
- Lungs are a common site of distant haematogenous spread from sarcomas of all types.

Chapter 19

Malignancy of unknown primary site

Metastatic cancer in which the site of origin of the disease is not immediately obvious, accounts for up to 10 per cent of new diagnoses of malignancy. A classic example is the middle-aged man with back pain and weight loss, who after a succession of diagnoses and consultations is eventually found to have vertebral and liver metastases but there are no clinical or radiological clues as to the source of these. It is a devastating and bewildering diagnosis for the patient and family and one which presents dilemmas to the clinician. What further investigations are indicated, and how far should the search for a primary carcinoma be pursued, if at all? Which patients should be referred to an oncology specialist for a further opinion? And for the oncologist, is systemic treatment such as chemotherapy justified in addition to symptomatic management of the obvious disease? If, after careful consideration, no treatment or minimal local treatment with no further investigation is planned, it is often difficult for patient and family to accept such a strategy; other opinions and alternative therapies may be sought.

There are a number of reasons why the primary site may be difficult to find. These might include a previously missed diagnosis, such as failure to send an appendicectomy specimen or an innocuous skin lesion for histological examination, thus missing a carcinoma of caecum or an atypical melanoma. The surgeon or physician may miss a small primary tumour at endoscopy because it is genuinely occult: a very small lesion or one which is spreading in the sub-mucosal layers with no surface abnormality. A number of these patients have small primary cancers which appear to be biologically aggressive and metastasize widely. Rarely the primary cancer may regress spontaneously. The resolution of even the most advanced radiological imaging is limited to lesions of around 5 mm; a primary tumour however will be a long way through its growth cycle containing at least 10^8 cells by this time, with metastasis occurring long beforehand. The primary cancer is detected in about 20 per cent of patients in their remaining lifetime but is subsequently discovered in 75 per cent who have a post-mortem examination. Post-mortem series show that lung and pancreas are the commonest primary sites.

Aims of management:

- Establish a histological diagnosis if this has not already been done.
- Further investigations as appropriate to help detect primary site or plan management.
- Treatment to local, symptomatic disease.

- Consideration of systemic treatment.
- Provision for future follow-up and care.

Confirmation of malignancy

Every effort should be made to establish a tissue diagnosis, even when there is little doubt that the clinical and radiological picture is of widespread cancer. Multiple pulmonary lesions may be due to carcinomatosis, but the differential diagnosis includes sarcoidosis, allergic alveolitis, pneumonia, and other infections (tuberculosis, fungal). Areas of increased activity on a isotope bone scan have a number of possible causes. These include trauma, inflammatory arthropathies, osteomalacia, and Paget's disease as well as metastatic cancer. Cerebral masses on a CT scan may be tumour, but must be distinguished from non-neoplastic cysts, or abscess.

Definition of tumour type

The majority of patients are found to have adenocarcinoma, often poorly differentiated; less than 10 per cent are of squamous origin and a small number cannot be classified by light microscopy alone. Other techniques including immunocytochemistry and electron microscopy can distinguish between tumour types such as lymphoma, melanoma, or carcinoma and tumours of neuroendocrine or mesenchymal origin. Non-Hodgkin's lymphomas account for at least a third of undifferentiated tumours and this has important implications for treatment. Other specific cell markers can also be detected by immunohistochemistry, for example oestrogen receptors for breast cancer, prostate specific antigen (PSA) for prostate cancer and CD99 for primitive neuroectodermal tumours (PNET).

In addition to detailed histological examination, specific serum markers may be of value in identifying certain primary types for example prostate specific antigen (PSA) for prostate cancer, CA125 in epithelial ovarian cancer, carcinoembryonic antigen (CEA) in colorectal cancer and alphafetoprotein (AFP) for primary hepatocellular cancer. In germ cell tumours AFP, beta-human chorinic gonadotrophin (HCG) and serum lactate dehydrogenase (LDH) are often raised.

Imaging may help to identify a hidden primary site. Patients presenting with a neck node containing squamous carcinoma will usually have a primary site in the head and neck region; MRI is a valuable tool for detecting such tumours. Positron Emission Tomography (PET) scanning is a relatively new tool which, using uptake of a radiolabelled tracer fluorodeoxyglucose (FDG) can identify hypermetabolic sites otherwise undetectable with conventional imaging (Fig. 19.1). Whilst not specific for malignancy, similar changes being seen at sites of infection or acute inflammation, PET scanning will often help to direct a further search for an unknown primary site; it appears more useful for sites in the head and neck region than in the abdomen and pelvis.

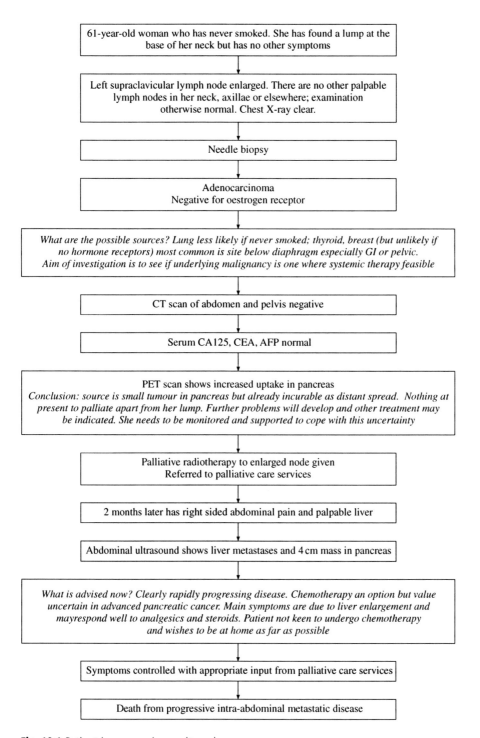

Fig. 19.1 Patient journey: primary site unknown.

Identification of important sub-groups

It is important to identify the following categories of patients who may be offered useful treatment:

- those with an underlying occult head and neck cancer,
- those with other potentially curable cancers – germ cell tumours, lymphoma, choriocarcinoma,
- those who would benefit from hormone treatment: breast, prostate, and endometrial cancer,
- those who might have a useful response to palliative chemotherapy: breast, ovarian, and small cell lung cancer.

Prognosis

As one would expect, patients with widespread malignancy at diagnosis have a poor outlook and for most of these individuals there will be no treatment offered to halt the progression of disease. The median survival for these patients as a whole is 3–4 months and less than 25 per cent are alive after 1 year. Those with multiple sites of involvement, particularly if these include lung, brain or liver, have a life expectancy measured in weeks. However, the prognosis is sometimes better for the patient with a solitary metastasis who seems otherwise well, especially if arising in bone.

The patients with occult head and neck cancer as a group do much better with appropriate management, with up to 20 per cent who survive 5 years from presentation. The other important groups, although representing small numbers of patients, are those with lymphoma or germ cell tumours in whom treatment offers a chance of prolonged remission and long term cure.

> ## Key points: carcinoma of unknown primary site
>
> - Histological confirmation of the diagnosis should be obtained; the aim is to identify treatable tumour types.
> - Specific immunohistochemistry and serum markers such as PSA, CA125, CEA, AFP and HCG may help identify the primary.
> - CT, MR and PET scanning may give additional anatomical localization.

Metastatic lymph nodes in the neck

A *supraclavicular node* is highly likely to be due to a primary tumour arising in lung, or if on the left side, drainage from sites below the diaphragm such as stomach, bowel, pancreas or in women the ovary. The node is commonly found to contain metastatic adenocarcinoma although lymphoma and germ cell tumours must be excluded. If the chest X-ray is normal, CT scanning of the abdomen and pelvis will detect the primary source in around 30 per cent of cases. Unfortunately the common scenarios of primary tumours in the lung, stomach or pancreas are rarely helped by aggressive treatment of the primary but other sites such as breast, colorectal and ovary tumours may well benefit from palliative systemic treatment.

Management of the node itself will typically include local excision for biopsy, or a needle biopsy followed by local radiotherapy for residual or symptomatic disease. In asymptomatic patients a 'wait and see' policy is often adopted.

An enlarged neck node above the supraclavicular fossa requires careful assessment and a planned approach. Fine needle aspiration is preferred to open biopsy and every effort is made to discover the primary source, which can be biopsied to obtain certain histological diagnosis. The investigations will include panendoscopy of the respiratory and upper digestive tracts, MRI scanning and increasingly, where available, PET scanning.

Squamous carcinoma presenting in a lower neck node may be from a cancer of the bronchus, but mid-upper neck nodes are almost certainly from a primary tumour somewhere in the head and neck region. Frequent sites for unsuspected cancers are the base of tongue, tonsil, hypopharynx, and nasopharynx. Thorough examination under an anaesthetic is performed and 'blind biopsies' are often taken in these areas if there is no tumour; these can reveal the occult primary lesion. If so, the management of the involved node is then planned as part of the entire treatment approach. This may mean a block dissection or inclusion in a radiotherapy treatment volume.

If no primary tumour is discovered, the treatment plan may well be a radical node dissection of the involved side of the neck or radical radiotherapy planned to include the common occult sites in the oropharynx and hypopharynx, followed by close and careful ENT follow-up. Appropriate treatment to the primary cancer is given as and when it declares itself. The outlook for patients with occult head and neck squamous cancer is certainly better than others with metastatic disease, justifying a radical approach to the sites of disease. Five year survival rates may reach 20 per cent.

Although squamous carcinoma is the commonest finding, other pathological types of tumour involve local lymph nodes. These include adenocarcinoma, perhaps from thyroid or salivary gland and adenoid cystic carcinomas from salivary gland tissue; as with all head and neck cancer a careful search for the primary site radical treatment where possible is performed. Malignant melanoma which may arise from skin or mucosa should always be considered and has a worse prognosis especially if regional nodes are already involved.

Metastatic lymph nodes at other sites

Fine needle aspiration for cytology or excision biopsy is easily carried out where there is an enlarged superficial node and the histology established as precisely as is possible.

As before, it is very important to diagnose accurately lymphoma and then proceed to staging investigations in these patients. Men with retroperitoneal or mediastinal disease may have germ cell tumours and even if this is difficult to establish, may respond to platinum-based chemotherapy regimens.

An enlarged *axillary node* in a woman, if found to be adenocarcinoma, is highly likely to be associated with a cancer in the ipsilateral breast. This must be pursued further, including mammography, to plan the best management of local disease and also because a firm diagnosis of breast cancer means that useful systemic treatment can be used to control widespread cancer.

Nodes in the *groin* have more diverse origins. Cancers of the lower limb skin, vulva, and anus are possible primary sites and CT scanning may reveal a source within the pelvis in a third of these patients. If melanoma is found, there would be a careful search for the primary in the adjacent limb or quadrant, not forgetting the soles of feet, nail beds, and inspection of vulva and anus. Patients should be questioned about removal of a mole or other skin lesions in the past.

In the absence of a documented primary cancer or if there is no useful systemic therapy, most patients will undergo surgical node dissection to achieve local control and are then carefully watched on follow-up. If the nodes are fixed, or the patient is in poor condition or with untreatable disease elsewhere, a short course of palliative radiotherapy may be given to prevent ulceration of the surrounding skin or swelling of a limb, and to relieve local pain.

Key points: metastatic lymph nodes

◆ Nodes above supraclavicular fossa are usually due to an occult head and neck primary and should be treated radically with a 20 per cent long-term cure rate.

◆ Left supraclavicular nodes are usually due to an intra-abdominal or pelvic primary.

◆ Groin nodes may be due to lower limb, anal or vulval tumours but 30 per cent will be due to intrapelvic tumour.

◆ Always consider an occult or undiscovered malignant melanoma.

Metastatic disease involving other tissues

Up to 60 per cent of patients with occult primary malignancy have widespread dissemination at diagnosis. This is often found to be adenocarcinoma and cancer in the lung, pancreas, or other gastrointestinal sites are usually responsible. In 50 per cent of women who have extensive intraperitoneal spread, pathological findings point to an ovarian cancer and they may have a worthwhile response to treatment. This also applies to a few who have underlying breast cancer but most patients with disease originating in bowel and other gastrointestinal sites will have no treatment apart from palliative surgery to relieve obstruction.

Common presentations of advanced malignancy are with jaundice or liver enlargement; pleural effusions or ascites and painful secondary deposits in bone. The management of patients with metastases in specific sites is discussed elsewhere.

The absence of an obvious primary source may cause additional anxiety for the patient, but in the majority of cases will not significantly alter the dismal prognosis, the median survival of patients presenting with bone or liver metastases being between 4 and 6 months. Invasive tests which are unlikely to benefit management should be avoided, especially as many patients are elderly and already quite ill. Empirical treatment with tamoxifen or megestrol acetate is well tolerated and may benefit a few. However, some patients with adenocarcinoma from an indeterminate site may be relatively well at diagnosis and desperate for something to be tried. In these situations, chemotherapy, using a drug combination which may include adriamycin and cisplatin, is sometimes given. The disease often shows a short-term response in 30–40 per cent which can help symptoms and undoubtedly improves psychological well-being. Sadly this is unlikely to make the patient live much longer and published results show a median survival for treated patients of still only 4–5 months.

Key points: distant metastases of unknown primary

- Liver metastases are usually due to colorectal, breast, pancreatic or stomach primaries.
- The diagnosis of myeloma should be considered in patients with multiple lytic bone lesions.
- Sclerotic bone metastases are likely to be from prostate cancer in a man and breast cancer in a woman.
- Worthwhile responses from systemic treatment may be obtained particularly in prostate and breast cancer but the mean survival is poor at around 4 to 6 months.

Case History 19.1

A 46-year-old man has smoked heavily for thirty years. He works in the construction industry and sees his GP about a pain in his hip on several occasions. He is reassured and anti-inflammatory painkillers are prescribed. One evening the pain is unbearable and he takes himself to the accident and emergency department of his local hospital. An X-ray of his pelvis shows a lytic tumour in the right ilium and he

Case History 19.1 (continued)

has multiple small metastases in both lungs. A needle biopsy demonstrates squamous carcinoma and a lung primary seems likely.

Not surprisingly, he and his family are devastated by this news and are extremely angry. Most of this is directed at the GP for failing to refer him for tests, but their bitterness leads to a distrust of all professionals who encounter them. They are told that he will be seen by a cancer specialist, who will arrange treatment. There follows a difficult consultation period during which the oncologist has to explain the poor outlook and recommends palliative radiotherapy, in a single session to be arranged as soon as possible. Suggestions of referral to a Macmillan nurse are rejected. He attends the radiotherapy department about two weeks later, this time with the information about the treatments downloaded from the internet. The oncologist is accused of giving him inadequate treatment and not offering him any chance at all. As well as the outburst of anger, it is clear that this man is in considerable pain and distress, made worse because he refuses to have anything to do with his GP.

The oncologist negotiates admission to the ward to assess the situation and to get the symptoms under control and the palliative team become involved to help with this. With regular analgesics his pain improves and he can now lie in position for his radiotherapy, but he remains desperate to have further treatment for his cancer beyond this. The value of chemotherapy is discussed; this might delay symptoms from his lung metastases but any gain in survival was likely to be small and uncertain. However the patient found that the thought of having no treatment was extremely hard to accept and was anxious to try something while still well enough to do so.

It was agreed to give him 2–3 courses of chemotherapy (MVP) initially, with clear understanding that the treatment would be discontinued if his cancer was not responding. Fortunately there was some regression of his lung metastases on repeat chest X-ray and he continued with a further 2 cycles. Despite professional reservations, he tolerated chemotherapy extremely well, and having some treatment 'to fight it' did enable this man and his wife to come to terms with the situation and also prepare their children.

The hospital team provided support to both of them while another partner in the practice negotiated to take over care at home. He developed headaches and left sided weakness from cerebral metastases about a year after the initial diagnosis. This time he had a short course of cranial radiotherapy which controlled his symptoms for a few weeks more, but he did not seek further treatment. He was deteriorating generally but remained at home (where he could smoke without restriction!) until he died.

Practice points

- Situations where presentation of cancer by commonly-encountered musculo-skeletal symptoms are a source of delayed diagnosis, anger and often loss of confidence in healthcare professionals.

- It is important to recognise that people often have high – and sometimes unrealistic – expectations of cancer treatment, regardless of stage of disease.

- Active treatment should not be offered to avoid recognition of a poor outlook and unproven treatments should be used in the context of a clinical trial.

- However some individuals can appreciate that benefit for them might be small and uncertain, but would still choose treatment when discussed. In these situations, honest information and a plan to reassess with clear objectives is essential.

Chapter 20

Malignancy associated with HIV infection

Cancer is only one of the spectrum of problems associated with HIV infection. Some form of malignancy develops in around 40 per cent of infected people and with the steady prolongation of life expectancy for these patients, numbers are bound to increase. Kaposi's sarcoma has long been perceived as a diagnostic marker of AIDS and the description of lymphoma occurring in immunosuppressed homosexual men heralded the recognition of the HIV-associated syndrome in the mid 1980s.

The tragedy of AIDS and the unusual and atypically behaved cancer linked with it has brought new understanding of the biology of malignancy itself. It has also produced new challenges for palliation when potential toxicity may outweigh benefit and the objectives of any treatment must be considered in the context of a universally fatal illness.

The following are recognized to be AIDS-defining malignancies occurring with HIV infection:

◆ Kaposi's sarcoma

◆ high grade non-Hodgkin's lymphoma

◆ squamous carcinoma of cervix and anus

There are also other cancers that may be increased in people infected with HIV including:

◆ Hodgkin's disease

◆ head and neck cancer

◆ lung cancer

◆ testicular cancer

◆ myeloma

Immunosuppression is well known as a factor in carcinogenesis; there is an increased number of lymphomas and skin cancers in transplant recipients. It may be this rather than the HIV virus itself that enables other transmissible factors (often carcinogenic viruses) to induce malignant transformation of infected cells. Examples include EB virus and lymphoma; papilloma virus and anal/cervical cancers; and more recently, the identification of herpes virus with Kaposi's sarcoma.

In some patients with HIV-associated malignancy, and up to a third of those with lymphoma, the cancer is the presenting pathology and evidence of infection is discovered concurrently or afterwards. Among those with established AIDS, the diagnosis of malignancy may itself present problems. Lymphadenopathy is common in this group of patients as are systemic symptoms such as sweats or weight loss, which may delay the diagnosis of lymphoma; enlarging nods, particularly when in isolated sites require biopsy. Intracerebral lymphoma has to be distinguished from other pathologies such as intracerebral toxoplasmosis. MRI and gadolinium scanning may be helpful; also lymphoma tends to be a solitary lesion and toxoplasmosis usually multiple. The pigmented cutaneous and oral lesions of Kaposi's are pathognomonic, those arising in the lungs produce non-specific abnormalities on a chest X-ray. Soft tissue and visceral lesions may be biopsied but with a risk of bleeding. In other patients, it may be the diagnosis of an unusual malignancy in a young adult that leads to the discovery of the HIV infection.

The overall prognosis is frequently dominated by the underlying immunosuppression rather than the cancer. Treatment has to be carefully tailored to the individual situation and the symptomatic problems. These patients are especially vulnerable to any additional risk of opportunistic infection and also the tolerance of normal tissues to radiotherapy is lowered, leading to troublesome acute effects which limit useful treatment. A further coexisting problem may be that of continued drug abuse and opioid dependency.

The introduction of effective systemic antiviral treatment (Highly Active Antiretroviral Therapy: HAART) has modified the natural history of HIV infection in the developed countries where it is now readily available with many patients having a prolonged period of remission with improved immune function and reduced viral load. This is now an important component of the management of malignancy in patients with HIV infection. However, the side effects of anti-viral drugs are often troublesome for patients and add to the toxicity of chemotherapy regimens, sometimes with a synergistic effect:

- anaemia and neutropaenia: zidovudine (AZT)
- peripheral neuropathy: stavudine, lamivudine, zalcitabine
- CNS effects (nightmares, acute psychosis): efavirenz
- stomatitis: zalcitabine

Key points

- Malignancy is seen in at least 40 per cent of HIV infected patients.
- AIDS defining malignancies are Kaposi's sarcoma, non-Hodgkin's lymphoma, anal and cervical cancer.

Kaposi's sarcoma

This was, prior to HIV infection, a rare malignancy of mesenchymal tissue; the cell of origin may be endothelial or possibly smooth muscle. It is characterized by angiogenesis: new blood vessel proliferation that appears to be influenced by cytokines such as growth factors. In 1994, an association between Kaposi's sarcoma and the human herpes virus 8 was demonstrated. This sexually transmitted virus is now thought to be the carcinogenic agent in all cases, including the endemic or African forms and Kaposi's arising in transplant recipients.

Typical lesions are purple macules of up to 2 cm, commonly arising on the lower extremities but can affect all areas of skin. They also arise in mucosal surfaces, especially the junction of soft and hard palate in the mouth. These lesions progress to nodules and confluent plaques, sometimes with haemorrhage into the surrounding tissue; this leaves permanent pigmentation. There may be associated lymphadenopathy which, together with extensive skin infiltration, produces lymphoedema. Kaposi's sarcoma was once regarded as disfiguring but an otherwise incidental complication of AIDS.

It is now clear that patients who survive longer through control of infections develop more aggressive and generalized involvement of other systems. This produces many symptoms and may itself be life-threatening. Multiple lesions are present in the mouth and throughout the gastrointestinal tract in 50 per cent of patients with cutaneous disease. These may cause pain and difficulties with swallowing and speech; bleeding and abdominal colic can occur. Diffuse gastric infiltration has also been described. Involvement of the respiratory tract and lungs develops in up to a third of patients. These may experience hoarseness and stridor from laryngeal deposits, haemoptysis, dyspnoea, and wheeze. The chest X-ray often shows nodular or reticular shadowing, sometimes with pleural effusion. The diagnosis is confirmed by bronchoscopy which may identify typical endobronchial lesions. Pulmonary involvement by Kaposi's sarcoma shortens the prognosis and is associated with a median survival of 6 months.

Management

Indications for treatment include:

- cosmetic: disfiguring or obvious lesions on exposed sites, especially the face
- lymphoedema: periorbital, limb, lower trunk
- bleeding from localized lesions
- painful or uncomfortable lesions (e.g. in oropharynx, soles of feet)
- laryngeal deposits causing stridor
- dyspnoea due to pulmonary infiltration

Although localized radiotherapy can effectively treat localized areas of Kaposi's sarcoma it was soon found that the doses usually well tolerated in palliation produced severe mucosal reactions in these patients. This is probably due to the vulnerability to infection following acute radiation damage to the epithelial lining.

Local radiotherapy can achieve good palliation of sites that are bleeding, painful, obstructing or cosmetically unacceptable by using single doses of no more than 8 Gy or a dose per fraction of no more than 1 Gy when the mucosal surfaces are treated. Disfiguring skin deposits are well worth treating, but respond slowly and pigmentation secondary to haemosiderin deposition will persist; local recurrence is reported in up to 10 per cent. Larger fields are used if indicated: parallel opposed beams are directed at confluent skin nodules and nodes in part of a limb or trunk to treat swelling due to lymphatic obstruction. Occasionally, whole body electron treatment is used for extensive skin infiltration. This causes loss of hair and nails unless the scalp and nail beds are shielded.

Kaposi's sarcoma responds to chemotherapy but benefit has to be balanced against the increased susceptibility to infection associated with further suppression of the immune system and bone marrow. The T-helper lymphocyte (CD4) counts correlate with the existing level of immunosuppression and can be used as a guide to whether the patient can tolerate chemotherapy; a CD4 count of $<200 \times 10^9$/L is associated with poor prognosis.

Unfortunately it is the more immunocompromised patients who are more ill and also the most likely to have significant symptoms from their Kaposi's sarcoma. Side effects such as alopecia and nausea and vomiting are also unacceptable in patients who are also coping with other symptoms and reduced life expectancy. In spite of these constraints, examples of effective and tolerated regimens are intravenous vincristine and bleomycin; weekly epirubicin and low dose oral etoposide. Adriamycin (doxorubicin) encapsulated in liposomes is selectively taken up by the tumour and is less toxic than the drug in solution. Chemotherapy can be used to palliate symptoms related to widespread disease, particularly if there is pulmonary involvement. Marrow suppression caused by cytotoxic drugs can be counteracted by the use of colony stimulating factors. Responses to chemotherapy are obtained in 40–60 per cent, but there is usually prompt relapse or progression on stopping treatment.

High doses of alpha-interferon (e.g. 10–18 megaunits daily) are also used and will be of benefit in 40 per cent but at the price of flu-like symptoms which may not be well tolerated. Intralesional injections of interferon or vinblastine are also tried, but may be painful.

Although in some patients the disease may remain asymptomatic for a long time, the median survival of AIDS patients with Kaposi's sarcoma is only 18–24 months. Poor prognostic features include gastrointestinal or other visceral involvement, opportunist infections, B symptoms (fever, night sweats, >10 per cent weight loss or diarrhoea for >2 weeks) and CD4 count $<220 \times 10^9$/L.

Key points

- Kaposi's sarcoma is characterized by a highly vascular tumour, typically arising in skin, but may also involve gastrointestinal tract, oral cavity and pharynx, lung and other viscera.

- Local symptoms may be successfully palliated by low dose radiotherapy, e.g. single fractions of 8 Gy but residual pigmentation is common in skin lesions.

- Visceral and widespread cutaneous disease may respond to systemic chemotherapy; liposomal daunorubicin is well tolerated and as effective as more toxic combination chemotherapy.

- Visceral disease, opportunist infections, B symptoms and a CD4 count $<220\times10^9$/L are poor prognostic features.

Non-Hodgkin's lymphoma in association with HIV

Lymphoma is diagnosed in up to 10 per cent of HIV-infected patients and is nearly always of high grade, B cell type. This includes primary intracerebral lymphoma which is extremely rare outside this group. The lymphoma may be the presenting feature of the HIV infection and those patients who are identified while relatively well can at least be offered more intensive and effective treatment for their malignancy.

These types of non-Hodgkin's lymphoma are rarely confined to the lymph nodes alone and behave in an aggressive fashion. Involvement of the bone marrow and central nervous system is not uncommon and confers a worse prognosis.

Primary CNS lymphoma is a recognized feature of HIV infection and rare as a sporadic form of lymphoma. Another rare form of lymphoma recognized in this group of patients is the unusual primary effusion lymphoma, presenting as serous effusions in the thoracic or abdominal cavities, typically comprising lymphoma of anaplastic large cell or immunoblastic type. Plasmablastic lymphoma of the oral cavity is another rare entity associated with this group of patients.

The principles of treatment follow the same lines as for NHL in immune competent patients, however the tolerance of this group of patients to intensive chemotherapy schedules such as CHOP or M-BACOD is poor. Reduced doses and increased use of granulocyte stimulating factors (GCSF) and prophylactic antibiotics alongside HAART may increase the chances of delivering effective chemotherapy and improve the success of treatment. Weekly schedules may prove easier in terms of close patient monitoring and individual tailoring of drugs than 3 or 4 weekly chemotherapy.

Primary cerebral lymphoma has an extremely poor outlook. Systemic treatment may be of value but often palliative treatment is confined to a short course of cranial radiotherapy. Median survival following this is only 2.5 months. Similarly localized lymphoma in other sites may also respond to local radiotherapy but tolerance to radiation is also reduced and severe mucositis may complicate even modest doses to the head and neck region or mediastinum.

Untreated patients will succumb within weeks of diagnosis; chemotherapy offers a chance of remission and short-term control although less than 5 per cent survive beyond 2 years; patients with a low CD4 count and a pre-existing AIDS diagnosis have a particularly poor outlook with a median survival of only 3 months.

Key points

- Non-Hodgkin's lymphoma in HIV infection is usually the common diffuse large B-cell type of high grade lymphoma.
- Other characteristic types include primary CNS lymphoma, primary effusion lymphoma and plasmablastic lymphoma of the oral cavity.
- Treatment follows the same guidelines as in non-AIDS patients but tolerance of combination chemotherapy and radiotherapy is relatively poor in this group of patients.
- The overall median survival is around 12 months but is worse in patients with a previous AIDS diagnosis, low CD4 count and primary CNS disease.

Cervical cancer

Invasive cancer of the cervix in the presence of HIV infection is typically an end result of progressive high grade cervical intraepithelial neoplasia (CIN) due to human papilloma virus infection of the female genital tract. The risk of developing CIN and of progression to invasive cancer is related to the CD4 count and as with other AIDS related malignancy a poor outlook with rapid progression through CIN to invasive cancer is most likely with a CD4 count of $<200 \times 10^9$/L. This is group of patients in whom regular frequent screening with cervical smears is important and current recommendations are that this is performed annually with many recommending 6 monthly smears in HIV positive sexually active women, particularly where previous dysplasia has been encountered.

Management of CIN and cervical cancer in HIV positive women is the same as for uninfected women. Radical surgery should not be denied those presenting with an early invasive cancer in the absence of other poor prognostic features of AIDS.

Other cancers

Epithelial tumours of the anal canal, head and neck region and lung are all more common in the presence of HIV infection. No specific features distinct from other populations has been identified and in general their management will follow standard guidelines modified where necessary in the light of other complications from AIDS and in the knowledge that systemic chemotherapy and radiotherapy will be less well tolerated.

An increase in testicular germ cell tumours has also been recognized, both seminoma and teratoma are seen in similar proportions to the general population. Again treatment should follow standard guidelines.

Key points

- Human papilloma virus infection causing CIN and invasive cervical cancer is a recognized risk for HIV positive women.
- Regular cervical smear screening 6–12 monthly is important in this patient group.
- Management of epithelial malignancies of the cervix, anal canal, and head and neck region should follow standard guidelines for the general population.
- An increased incidence of testicular germ cell tumours is also seen which are managed in the same way as patients not infected with HIV.

Chapter 21

Bone metastases

Bone metastases may arise in any bone in the skeleton but are most commonly found in those of the vertebrae, pelvis, and ribs, the next most common site being long bones, in particular the femur and humerus. Metastases in bones of the lower leg, hands, and feet although recognized are rare. Tumours may invade bone directly if they arise from adjacent sites as can be seen in the head and neck region or where there are paravertebral masses but most commonly bone metastases reflect blood-borne dissemination.

Whilst almost any primary site can be associated with bone metastases they are most commonly seen in association with primary tumours of the breast, prostate, and lung and are also common in the rarer tumours of kidney and thyroid. Details of their incidence are shown in Table 21.1.

The arrival of a tumour cell on the surface of a bone stimulates an osteoclastic response. This is mediated by the release of various chemical factors termed osteoclast activating factors (OAFs) which include prostaglandin, parathyroid hormone, and other related peptides. The osteoclastic activity results in bone reabsorption and allows tumour cells to penetrate into the marrow cavity of the bone and establish a tumour colony which becomes the clinically apparent bone metastasis. In response to this activity the bone mounts an oesteoblastic reaction attempting to lay down new bone to repair the areas of reabsorption. Virtually all metastases have a combination of this osteoclastic and osteoblastic activity happening within them. It is the osteoblastic reaction that results in uptake of radioisotopes which provide the basis of a diagnostic bone scan and also potential for therapy. The balance between the two processes results in different clinical scenarios even in the same patient, extremes of which are shown in Fig. 21.1. Where the osteoclastic response predominates then lytic lesions are seen characterized by renal metastasis and myeloma. Where osteoblastic reaction predominates then sclerotic metastases are seen characterized by those of breast and prostate cancer.

The prognosis for a patient presenting with bone metastases is generally poor. Whilst bone metastases in themselves are not life-threatening they represent blood-borne metastatic spread of the primary tumour and are therefore very often associated with soft tissue metastases. Even where this is not the case the complications of bone metastases such as spinal cord compression, pathological fracture, hypercalcaemia, or chronic musculoskeletal pain may all contribute to the patient's decline. Despite this, however, some patients will survive for many months and even several years with bone metastases, particularly those whose tumours are amenable to systemic treatment such as

Table 21.1 Incidence of bone metastases in different primary tumours

Primary site (%)	Incidence of bone metastases
Breast	73
Prostate	68
Thyroid	42
Kidney	35
Bronchus	35
Colorectal	11

primary cancers of the breast and prostate. Occasionally, bone metastases may be solitary and this is a well-recognized occurrence in renal cell carcinoma where radical treatment of a solitary bone metastasis may be associated with a long disease-free interval of several years. These events tend to be exceptional, however.

Clinical presentation

Many bone metastases are asymptomatic and may on occasion be found incidentally because of an X-ray or scan taken for other reasons. Ultimately, however, symptoms arise and these may include local pain, fracture, neurological complications, or hypercalcaemia.

Pain associated with bone metastases is typically persistent and associated with local tenderness. It is often related to movement or weight bearing. Bone pain may be disproportionate to the appearances on X-ray or bone scan. Despite multiple metastases

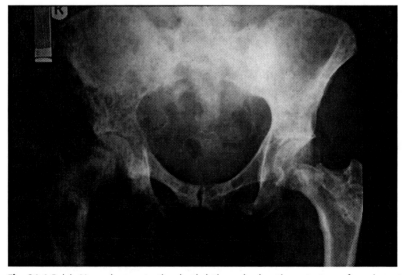

Fig. 21.1 Pelvic X-ray demonstrating both lytic and sclerotic metastases from breast cancer.

some patients may have only one site of pain whilst others may have multiple sites of pain despite relatively normal radiological examinations. Neuropathic pain may be arise because of nerve root involvement particularly where there is vertebral collapse or a large soft tissue component to the metastases.

Pathological fracture may occur spontaneously or after only minor trauma. The most common site for pathological fracture is the upper femur but other long bones may be affected. Vertebral collapse is also a common observation in patients with bone metastases. Pathological fracture may present with increasing pain or inability to bear weight. There will be obvious localized tenderness and frequent deformity of the limb. In some circumstances, however, pathological fracture may not be clinically apparent and persistent pain, particularly of the hip, in patients with bone metastases should always be investigated with an X-ray to exclude underlying fracture which would benefit from active intervention.

Neurological symptoms may arise either because of spinal cord or cauda equina compression due to encroachment of tumour or collapsed bone into the spinal canal, or because of involvement of a peripheral nerve root in the spinal root canal.

Hypercalcaemia is commonly associated with bone metastases but is often not directly due to bone damage. The usual cause for malignant hypercalcaemia is the production by the primary tumour of parathyroid hormone-like peptides affecting calcium metabolism both in bone and at the kidney. Patients with hypercalcaemia, however, often have an exacerbation of bone pain and bone metastases are frequently found in association with this. Treatment of the hypercalcaemia may result in dramatic resolution of the bone pain.

Key points: bone metastases

- The common primary sites are breast, prostate and lung.
- All bone metastases have both an osteoblastic and osteoclastic component; in some the osteoclastic response may predominate giving lytic lesions and in others the osteoblastic response predominates giving sclerotic metastases.
- Overall survival is on average a few months with multiple bone metastases.
- In addition to pain complications include neurological effects, fracture and hypercalcaemia.

Bone pain

Pharmacological approach

In most patients initial management will entail the use of simple analgesics and non-steroidal anti-inflammatory drugs, titrating through the analgesic ladder to stronger opioid drugs as indicated by their pain response. Sometimes trying different non-steroidal anti-inflammatory drugs may be of value, no particular drug having been shown to be superior in this setting. The COX-2 inhibitor drugs are other alternatives to try if standard NSAIDs do not work.

Bisphosphonates have an expanding role in the management of bone metastases. In both breast cancer and myeloma they have been shown to reduce the clinical impact of metastatic bone disease when given in a prophylactic setting to patients with asymptomatic disease. In particular they reduce the number of vertebral fractures and the need for radiotherapy, suggesting they supplement pain control. For established bone pain there is increasing evidence that intravenous infusions of bisphosphonates such as pamidronate or clodronate can be effective. Their relative efficacy compared to radiotherapy is uncertain; direct comparison of response rates suggests that they may be only effective in approximately half the number of patients (i.e. the response rates are around 40 per cent compared to 80 per cent with radiotherapy), but this may reflect different patient populations and methodology. They should be regarded as a valuable addition to the therapeutic armamentarium available for metastatic bone disease used alongside radiotherapy and analgesics. Oral formulations of clodronate are available but their absorption is variable and the intravenous route is generally best to establish the efficacy bisphosphonate therapy in this setting with an infusion delivering 1500 mg of clodronate or 30–60 mg of pamidronate over 4 h. In patients who benefit then a maintenance programme with 3 to 6 weekly infusions may be valuable. Zolendranate and ibandranate are two newer more potent bisphosphonates which may well replace these older drugs in the near future and be available not only as intravenous infusions but also more potent oral formulations.

Dexamethasone in doses of 4–8 mg daily may also be helpful in bone pain. Where there is a neuropathic component then appropriate adjuvant analgesics such as amitriptyline or gabapentin should be considered. Muscle spasm may accompany bone pain and again adjuvant drugs such as diazepam and baclofen may be indicated in selected patients.

Localized bone pain

Despite widespread bone metastases pain is often localized to one particular site. Commonly, this affects the ribs, spinal column, or pelvis. There is no value in treating asymptomatic bone metastases unless there is considered to be a high risk of pathological fracture, as in the case of a large lytic deposit in a long bone, or a risk of spinal cord compression where there is documented encroachment into the spinal canal, a feature increasingly seen with spinal MRI scans. Definitive treatment with local radiotherapy will be indicated where optimal medication is ineffective at achieving pain control.

Single doses of radiation delivering 8–10 Gy are usually sufficient and as effective as more prolonged courses of treatment. Simple treatment techniques using single direct beams or two opposed beams (parallel opposed pair) which minimize planning requirements are used to cover the painful area with a margin of 2–3 cm. The treated volume is usually based on the appearances on plain X-rays which are then reproduced on the treatment simulator. However, approximately 50 per cent of the bone in the affected area has to be destroyed before this is seen on plain X-ray and increasingly the more sensitive changes on isotope bone scan and magnetic resonance scan are used to complement basic X-rays. It is particularly important to define accurately the site of origin of metastatic pain when delivering radiotherapy, a common difficulty being to establish whether local metastases are responsible or spinal deposits causing referred nerve root pain are also contributing which will obviously considerably modify the site to be treated.

Pain relief is rarely immediate after local radiotherapy. Around 50 per cent of patients will experience less pain within 2 weeks and 85 per cent within 4–8 weeks. In around 5 per cent a 'pain flare' is described with the pain worsening in the first few days after treatment before settling; it is always wise to warn patients of this possibility.

The duration of relief varies. For many patients there will be pain relief for several months which will cover their remaining lifespan. For some, however, pain may recur after several weeks. In these patients further response can be expected by re-treatment with radiotherapy and this should always be considered. Difficulties may arise in the vertebral column where the underlying spinal cord may be damaged by relatively low radiation doses but in most cases a second treatment on top of a previous palliative dose is within tolerance (e.g. after a single dose of 8 Gy or 20 Gy in 5 fractions a further single dose of 6–8 Gy can be given). Additional doses beyond this, however, may cause cord damage and will usually be avoided unless the patient is in severe pain with only a few weeks of life remaining, when the need for effective palliation will outweigh the remote chance of cord damage which is not, in any case, expressed for several months after exposure.

Complications from simple single dose radiotherapy to a painful bone are usually minor and self-limiting. Treatment to the lower thoracic and lumbosacral spine may cause nausea but rarely any more serious bowel upset. Similarly, doses to the pelvis may have this effect with associated diarrhoea when large volumes of bowel are included. Often a single dose of dexamethasone 8 mg prior to the radiation exposure is given to prevent side effects and prophylactic anti-emetics can be considered. Treatment to the ribs and limbs is rarely associated with acute morbidity other than some mild skin erythema in the treated area.

Patients who fail to respond to radiotherapy comprise 15–20 per cent of those treated and these present a difficult pain problem. Occasionally second treatments with radiation are effective when the first has failed and this may be considered. There is, however, little evidence to support the common practice of giving a larger dose when a single fraction fails. Resistant pain requires careful analysis to ensure that the underlying pathology has been accurately defined. In particular, it is important to distinguish local pain from referred nerve root pain whose origin may be some distance from the site of pain. It is not uncommon for pain to have more than one component and this can be a particular problem for pain around the hip and upper thigh or buttocks where the origin may be from bone metastases in the pelvis or femur, nerve root pain from the lumbosacral spine, or soft tissue infiltration from within the pelvis.

Scattered bone pain

Many patients with bone metastases at some point in their natural history experience more than one site of bone pain with pain often moving from site to site. This is a more difficult situation and local radiotherapy rarely resolves the situation, as other sites of pain seem to become more prominent after treatment of one area. The drug manoeuvres discussed above should always be considered alongside definitive treatment with radiotherapy or chemotherapy.

Hemibody radiotherapy offers a means of delivering wide field irradiation to cover several sites of bone pain. Typically, this involves the upper or lower half of the body but mid hemibody irradiation can be used if the principal sites of pain are the ribs and dorsolumbar spine for example. In the upper half body, unless the skull is involved and symptomatic this will usually be excluded to avoid hair loss and ocular complications. A single exposure is typically used delivering 6 Gy to the upper half body and 8 Gy to the lower half body. The upper half body dose is reduced because of the increased sensitivity of lung to this large volume irradiation.

Response to hemibody irradiation is similar to local radiotherapy with over 80 per cent of patients reporting pain relief after treatment. The pattern of pain relief, however, is somewhat different with many patients reporting pain relief within the first 24–48 h. In 70–80 per cent pain relief will be maintained over a period of several months until their death.

A major drawback of this type of treatment is the increased associated toxicity which usually takes the form of self-limiting gastrointestinal upset including nausea, vomiting and diarrhoea, and bone marrow depression. Pre-medication with steroids and intravenous fluid is often advocated together with prophylactic anti-emetics and an overnight stay in hospital is usually required. Within a day or two acute toxicity will pass and then transient falls in white cell and platelet count can be observed over the next 4–6 weeks with spontaneous recovery and rarely any clinical sequelae. One major toxicity encountered only rarely but with often fatal results is that of pneumonitis. Provided the lung dose after correction for the reduced density of lung to the X-ray beam is kept to 6 Gy mid-plane dose or lower then the likelihood of this is less than 1 per cent. If pneumonitis does develop, heralded by a dry cough and associated dyspnoea, and confirmed by typical widespread changes on chest X-ray, treatment involves steroids and antibiotics for secondary infection. Unfortunately, because the entire lung volume is usually involved respiratory failure may well ensue.

Bone marrow toxicity is the major limiting factor for repeating hemibody irradiation. Sequential upper and lower hemibody irradiation however, can readily be given provided a gap of 4–6 weeks is left for the bone marrow in the first irradiation area to recover.

Radioisotope therapy is of considerable value in these situations and is associated with less toxicity than hemibody irradiation. This treatment relies on the systemic administration of a radioactive isotope which is selectively taken up at sites of bone metastases to deliver a local dose of radiation. The radiation is typically beta particle emission which has a range of only a few millimetres and is therefore concentrated around the site of uptake in the bone marrow. Some isotopes also emit low energy which enable them to be imaged on a gamma camera and produce pictures similar to diagnostic bone scans.

Tumour specific isotopes are recognized but are only associated with relatively rare tumours. In particular radioactive iodine [^{131}I] is taken up by functioning differentiated thyroid cancer and bone metastases from this tumour can be treated with systemic doses of [^{131}I]. This is taken by mouth but because high doses are required which are cleared relatively slowly it is given as an inpatient procedure often requiring the patient to remain for 5–7 days within a single protected room for the radiation levels to reach safe levels for discharge from the hospital. The other example in this group is *m*IBG (*meta*-iodo-benzyl guanidine) which is a metabolite of the catecholamine pathway and is concentrated in the rare functioning tumours affecting cells with this biochemical function. This includes metastatic neuroblastoma and phaeochromocytoma.

The bone-specific isotopes will be taken up by sites of bone damage where there is active osteoblastic activity independent of the primary tumour type. Osteoblastic activity, as discussed earlier is present in virtually all metastases. Any patient therefore who has a positive diagnostic bone scan with technetium can expect to concentrate a bone specific isotope. These have been used most frequently in patients with multifocal bone pain from prostate and breast cancer. Unfortunately the high cost – at around £1000 per injection – limits their use until sequential, single site external beam treatments are no longer adequate.

The use and administration of radioactive isotopes is under careful regulatory control and should not be performed with a platelet count less than 60×10^9/L or total white cell count less than 2.5×10^9/L. Radioisotopes may not be an option for patients with evidence of progressive marrow failure.

The effect of strontium ^{89}Sr has been studied principally in metastatic prostate cancer. ^{89}Sr has a half-life of 50.5 days and emits beta particles but no gamma rays (thus uptake is not detectable by scanning). It is excreted in the urine and to a lesser extent in the faeces; 25 per cent of the given dose is excreted in the first 24 h after injection. Urinary incontinence is therefore a contraindication. Pain relief is seen within 10–14 days of administration in around 80 per cent of patients which can be maintained for many months. Repeat administrations of ^{89}Sr have been described at 3-monthly intervals in selected patients, although persistent sites of local pain may be better treated with local external beam irradiation. Bisphosphonates may be helpful for diffuse pain.

An alternative isotope to strontium is samarium [^{153}Sm] which is targetted to bone by chelation with a phosphonate compound EDTMP to form a complex Sm-EDTMP. This is now licensed to treat bone pain from osteoblastic disease of any type. Overall results with samarium are equivalent to strontium, with the same predictable mild effects on peripheral blood counts. Samarium has a much shorter half-life of only 48 h which allows for a higher activity to be administered which will decay more quickly, and produces gamma rays in addition to its main beta irradiation enabling imaging of isotope distribution using a gamma camera in the same way as an isotope bone scan.

Case History 21.1

A 56-year-old lady presented with a locally advanced breast cancer. She had three courses of chemotherapy with a partial response, followed by radiotherapy to her breast and regional lymph node areas. She now has recurrent cervical and supra-clavicular nodes and has multiple bone metastases.

She is complaining of difficulty in swallowing and initially this is attributed to the bulky nodes in her neck. However she is also complaining of headaches and so a CT brain scan is requested.

By the time she returns to clinic, her swallowing is much worse and she finds that sometimes fluids come down her nose. Her speech has altered and the headaches persist. However there are no brain metastases on the scan.

When she is examined, she is found to have deviation of her tongue to the left and no palatal movement on that side. Her scans are discussed with a radiologist, who points out that her previous bone scan showed increase uptake in the base of her skull. Metastases at this site appeared to be affecting the lower cranial nerves as they passed through the skull.

She is admitted to hospital and a fine bore nasogastric feeding tube is passed. Her headaches and neurological problems improve with commencement of high dose dexamethasone. She has a course of palliative radiotherapy over two weeks which is directed to a small field – 8 × 6 cm – to treat the skull base. This is well tolerated and causes a small area of temporary hair loss, easily disguised. The steroids are quickly tailed off. Subsequently her neurological problems improve enough to permit normal feeding and she later re-commences chemotherapy.

Case History 21.2

A 75-year-old man was listed to attend for a strontium injection. Meanwhile, he was admitted to the local hospice for respite care and symptom control. Staff were asked to check his blood count, (which showed only mild anaemia), and to catheterize him prior to treatment if urinary incontinence was likely to be a problem. This was not felt to be necessary. Simple precautions were recommended: that for 3 days he should use a toilet designated for his use only rather than a urinal, always flush this twice and wash hands afterwards.

Unfortunately the following morning he was febrile and unwell, due to a chest infection. He required nursing in bed. The staff were advised to be particularly careful for the first 72 h after his strontium administration. In particular they should

♦ Always wear gloves when handling bedpans and urinals.

♦ Take great care to avoid spillages and clean up immediately if they occur.

♦ Domestic staff to wear gloves and clean as for infected material.

♦ Within 72 h, contaminated bedding or clothes should be sealed in plastic bags and after this period may be washed normally but separately from the main laundry.

Despite antibiotics he continued to deteriorate and died 6 days after the injection. The undertakers were made aware that his body contained radioactive material, and precautions to avoid contamination by seepages were taken. The Radioisotope Department at the hospital was contacted for advice, who involved the Radiation Protection Advisor.

If the intended means of disposal was cremation, further precautions would be advised based on the estimated residual activity. This is because of the exposure to the crematorium workers who deal with the bone residue; there is also a small contamination of the environment by ash particles via the chimney. However the family planned for a burial which went ahead without any difficulty.

Key points: radiotherapy

♦ Low dose single fraction treatment is adequate for most situations.

♦ Response may take 4–8 weeks, and an initial pain flare is seen in 5 per cent.

♦ Re-treatment is useful if pain returns.

♦ For multiple sites of pain wide field hemibody radiotherapy is effective but asscoiated with bone marrow and gastrointestinal toxicities.

♦ Isotope therapy with a single intravenous injection of strontium or samarium-EDTMP is as effective in scattered bone pain but has less toxicity.

Chemotherapy

May be considered for selected tumours presenting with scattered bone pain and in these situations may be preferable to the radiotherapy techniques described above. It is important to realize that local radiotherapy may still be given alongside chemotherapy for persistent sites of pain. Chemotherapy should be considered in particular in the following cases:

Multiple myeloma is a tumour commonly affecting bones giving the typical picture of widespread lytic lesions throughout the skeleton. Bone pain is an accompaniment in over 70 per cent of patients presenting with myeloma. Chemotherapy for multiple myeloma is highly effective in previously untreated patients and can be relatively simple consisting of either oral melphalan given for 4–7 days every 4 weeks on an outpatient basis or more complex four-drug combination chemotherapy, for example, ABCM which comprises 6-weekly administration of oral cyclophosphamide and methotrexate alternating with 6-weekly administration of intravenous BCNU and adriamycin. The oral and intravenous drugs are therefore given at 3-weekly intervals on an alternating basis. In patients who have been previously treated with these types of chemotherapy then high dose dexamethasone (40 mg/m^2) is an effective salvage form of chemotherapy given daily for 4 days every 28 days. In selected young patients more intensive chemotherapy may be sought.

Small cell lung cancer may present with multiple bone metastases often in the setting of widespread systemic disease affecting lung, liver, and other sites. It is, however, highly sensitive if previously untreated and relatively simple chemotherapy schedules such as oral etoposide in combination with vincristine, cyclophosphamide, or methotrexate, will produce responses in 80 per cent of patients. Whilst relapse often occurs some months later there is also evidence that further chemotherapy with drugs not previously used in the initial treatment is associated with better symptom control and quality of life than in patients denied this opportunity.

Breast cancer is a common cancer in which symptomatic bone metastases are a common problem. In pre- and post-menopausal women who relapse on tamoxifen, combination chemotherapy offers the greatest chance of further response. There is no clear advantage for any particular drug schedule in these circumstances: CMF (cyclophosphamide, methotrexate, and 5-FU), MMM (mitozantrone, methotrexate, and mitomycin C), and FEC (5-FU, epirubicin, and cyclophosphamide) are common drug combinations currently in use. Response of bone metastases to chemotherapy is often relatively slow and several cycles at 3–4 weekly intervals may need to be given before benefit can be determined.

Lymphoma and germ cell tumours are highly chemosensitive types of malignancy although bone involvement is relatively rare in their natural history. Those patients who do have bone pain from these primary tumour types however should always be considered for active chemotherapy even in relapse.

Other solid tumours which may present with metastatic bone pain where chemotherapy can be of value include bladder cancer, non-small cell lung cancer, typically used in combination with local radiotherapy to the site of presenting pain.

Hormone therapy

May also be of benefit in the management of symptomatic widespread bone metastases.

Prostate cancer is the best example of this approach with androgen blockade resulting in dramatic symptom relief in over 80 per cent of men presenting with metastatic bone pain. The median duration of response in this setting is around 18 months after which further hormone manoeuvres are generally unsuccessful.

Breast cancer is the other common tumour in which hormone responses are seen. Symptomatic bone metastases in a post-menopausal woman will usually be managed in the first instance by a hormone treatment, either tamoxifen, or if this has been previously used, an aromatase inhibitor such as anastrazole. Around 60 per cent of women will respond to first-line hormones and in those responding, 40 per cent to a second-line hormone. Hormone therapy is less successful in pre-menopausal women but should nevertheless be considered for symptomatic metastatic disease particularly relapsing after chemotherapy. In women still menstruating, ovarian ablation should be considered alongside tamoxifen and the second-line hormones described above. Up to 40 per cent of women may have symptomatic response to these measures.

Endometrial cancer can respond to progestogens such as megestrol and symptomatic bone metastases would be an indication for this to be introduced although overall response rates are no greater than 30 per cent.

Key points: systemic treatment for bone metastases

- Chemotherapy is of value in myeloma, lung cancer and breast cancer.
- Hormone therapy is effective in prostate, breast and endometrial cancers.

Fracture

Tumour-bearing bone may fracture after relatively little trauma or indeed spontaneously. High risk lesions can be identified defined by the following criteria:

- More than 50 per cent of cortical bone destruction
- Painful lesions greater than 2.5 cm in diameter
- Diffuse lytic involvement of a weight-bearing bone

Bone metastases that fulfil these criteria should be considered for prophylactic internal fixation to prevent later fracture, as shown in Fig. 21.2. Fracture may be preceded by pain but may also occur in an entirely asymptomatic site of metastases. Treatment will depend upon the bone involved and the general condition of the patient.

Femur or humerus

Surgical internal fixation is undoubtedly the most effective means of obtaining rapid pain relief and return of function if the femur or humerus is involved in a pathological

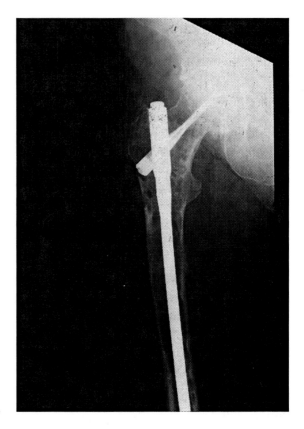

Fig. 21.2 X-ray showing extensive lytic bone disease from multiple myeloma having undergone prophylactic internal fixation.

fracture. In patients who have an expected life expectancy of more than a few weeks then post-operative radiotherapy should be given to prevent further tumour progression within the bone and enable bone healing to occur. In some situations, when fracture occurs at the end rather than shaft of a bone, simple fixation is not possible and an arthroplasty may be the only option.

Other bones

Pathological fracture may occur at other sites, many of which will not be amenable to internal fixation, for example a rib or pelvic bone. In this setting local radiotherapy is of value in relieving pain and facilitating healing of the bone. Doses of 20–30 Gy over 1–2 weeks are usually delivered.

Vertebral fracture

Vertebral fracture is usually seen as collapse of the vertebral body. More extensive destruction of the vertebral arch may result in instability and vertebral displacement. In this setting spinal surgery may be required to ensure spinal stability and avoid neurological complications. In stable vertebral collapse then local radiotherapy may be of value in reducing local pain but the vertebral body is unlikely to re-establish its original contour following treatment, despite local radiotherapy. Persisting discomfort principally due to mechanical pain rather than metastatic pain is common in this situation and may require continuous analgesics and non-steroidal anti-inflammatory drugs.

Poor performance status

Patients who are not ambulant and who have a very limited life expectancy will not be considered for surgical fixation. Simple measures such as limb immobilization or traction may be of value to relieve pain as may single dose radiotherapy.

Case History 21.3

An elderly man is admitted for investigation of back pain and mild iron deficiency. He is found to have liver metastases and sclerotic bone metastases in his dorsal spine. GI tests come up with nothing and prostate cancer is excluded. He is given a single treatment with palliative radiotherapy to his spine. His wife is also unwell so the plan is for intermediate care in a hospice. The day before transfer, he sustains a pathological fracture through the head of his right humerus. It cannot be pinned and so the transfer goes ahead.

The assumption made was that his prognosis would be very short. However, he appears to improve over the course of another 2–3 weeks! By far the biggest problem is the ununited fracture of his shoulder. This makes any attempt to mobilize very painful despite the best efforts to support his arm.

An orthopaedic surgeon is asked to see him and he agrees to perform an arthroplasty. This proves to be straightforward with an uneventful post-operative period. He is able to return home and has several months of pain-free, active time before he becomes less well.

Practice points

♦ While prognosis is usually over-estimated, sometimes people do better than we expect.

♦ Surgical interventions can have a rapid, positive benefit on quality of life and independence in carefully-selected situations.

Neurological symptoms

Bone metastases may affect the neurological system through a number of mechanisms:

♦ Spinal canal compression
♦ Nerve root compression

◆ Skull base infiltration

◆ Skull vault metastases

Spinal canal compression

Encroachment into the spinal canal by tumour arising in the vertebra is a common cause of spinal cord compression or cauda equina compression. Early diagnosis is vital in this condition and any patient presenting with neurological symptoms in the limbs or disturbance of bladder function should be carefully examined for neurological abnormalities as outlined in Table 21.2. Where there are known vertebral metastases and particularly if associated with back pain there is a high likelihood of spinal cord compression, and urgent investigation should ensue. Plain X-rays may be of value to demonstrate bone metastases but the essential investigation is a magnetic resonance scan (MRI) which will give a highly detailed view of the vertebral column and spinal canal. This has largely replaced myelography to image the spinal canal but if MRI is not available then conventional contrast studies are indicated to define a site of compression.

Table 21.2 Neurological signs and symptoms in spinal canal compression

Symptom	Neurological signs and site
Weak shoulders/upper limbs or hands/fingers	*Cervical cord lesion*: may be associated with symptoms/signs in legs or urinary dysfunction
Neck pain or pain radiating from shoulders to arm to fingers	Weakness/sensory signs in upper limbs. Increased tone in legs. Extensor plantar responses
Difficulty walking Stumbling over kerbs or steps	*Thoracic cord lesion*: may be associated with hesitancy of urine or retention and constipation
Unable to climb stairs Difficulty walking	Upper motor neurone weakness in legs (increased tone flexors weaker than extensors) with increased knee and ankle jerks, and extensor plantars
Paraesthesia in lower limbs or buttocks	
Thoracic back pain	'Sensory level' with reduced sensation below level of compression: as a guide level, umbilicus is T10[a]
Loss of bladder/bowel sensation[b]	*Cauda equina compression*
Urinary retention often painless	Reduced tone in lower limbs, global weakness
Leg weakness	Reduced/absent knee and ankle jerks
Paraesthesia/nerve pain in legs or buttocks	Flexor plantar responses
Low back pain	Sensory loss in lumbosacral dermatomes (i.e. groins/legs and buttocks)

[a] Sensory level reflects neurological segment which is usually higher than the actual vertebral level.

[b] This may also be associated with higher cord lesions.

When spinal canal compression has been diagnosed, management should be instigated immediately. In all cases high dose steroids giving dexamethasone 4 mg, 6-hourly should be started.

- Where there is spinal instability then urgent neurosurgical referral is required with a view to spinal stabilization.
- In other cases local radiotherapy is as effective as surgery and may be less traumatic. Doses of 20–30 Gy over 1–2 weeks are generally delivered although in some cases, particularly in those patients with poor performance status or who have established neurological deficits which are unlikely to recover, single doses of 8–10 Gy may be given.
- Progression during radiotherapy or recurrence in a previously irradiated area of spine is another indication for surgery.
- Active physiotherapy and rehabilitation is an essential part of the management of spinal canal compression. Recovery, however, is principally related to performance status at presentation with very few patients who present with established paraplegia ever regaining useful function.

Nerve root compression

This may arise from bone metastases or soft tissue encroaching upon the spinal canal. This can result in pain with neuropathic features which can be very difficult to control. In the first instance, analgesics, steroids, and other drugs specific for neuropathic pain such as antidepressants or anticonvulsants may have a role. Local radiotherapy is often given for this type of pain delivering 20–30 Gy over 1–2 weeks although its efficacy in this particular setting has not been fully evaluated. In difficult cases alternative local treatments include transcutaneous electrical nerve stimulation (TENS), epidural or intrathecal infusions, acupuncture, or specific nerve blocks.

Skull base infiltration

Skull base metastases can result in major disability when cranial nerve palsies develop. Typically this involves the lower cranial nerves as they pass through the foramina of the skull base resulting in bulbar palsy but higher cranial nerves can also be affected. Initial treatment with dexamethasone 4 mg 6-hourly can provide temporary relief and local radiotherapy to the skull base delivering 20–30 Gy over 1–2 weeks will improve symptoms in 80 per cent of cases.

Skull vault metastases

These may result in neurological problems because of pressure on the underlying cerebral cortex causing local epilepsy or hemiparesis. Treatment with dexamethasone 4 mg, 6-hourly may help in reducing underlying oedema and should be followed by local radiotherapy to the site of metastases. This is often best delivered by direct electron beam treating the skull vault to a known depth avoiding radiation beams passing through the brain. Alopecia within the area to be treated is unfortunately inevitable but otherwise there is little associated morbidity and for most patients symptoms will be improved and neurological deterioration avoided. It is particularly important to distinguish extrinsic pressure from a skull metastasis from intrinsic cerebral metastases as a cause of epilepsy or focal neurological deficits since the prognosis for bone metastases in the skull is very much better than that for brain metastases and active treatment should not be denied in these patients.

Key points: complications of bone metastases

- Long bone fractures are best treated with surgical fixation after which postoperative radiotherapy may be of value. Radiotherapy is indicated for fractures of ribs, vertebrae, pelvis, and shoulder girdle.
- Neurological symptoms should always be very carefully evaluated particularly where there are known bone metastases to detect spinal canal or nerve root compression.
- Emergency treatment is required when cord or cauda equina compression is diagnosed with steroids and radiotherapy.
- Cranial nerve palsies and peripheral nerve symptoms from bone metastases benefit from local radiotherapy.

Management of spinal cord compression: practice points

- The key to diagnosis is to look for it – and the key to best results is to refer immediately.
- Among patients with the same neurological impairment, surgery and radiotherapy appear to achieve similar results.
- Patients with chemosensitive tumours and early signs of compression may respond to initial chemotherapy, reserving radiotherapy for progression or relapse.
- Recognition of spinal instability is important: if severe pain on movement or associated deterioration in neurological signs, nurse flat, log roll, use collar if cervical involvement and refer surgery.
- Spinal stabilisation best achieved by anterior approach and usually resolves pain on movement.
- In less fit patients, simple posterior decompression may be the limited option but risk of spinal instability remains.

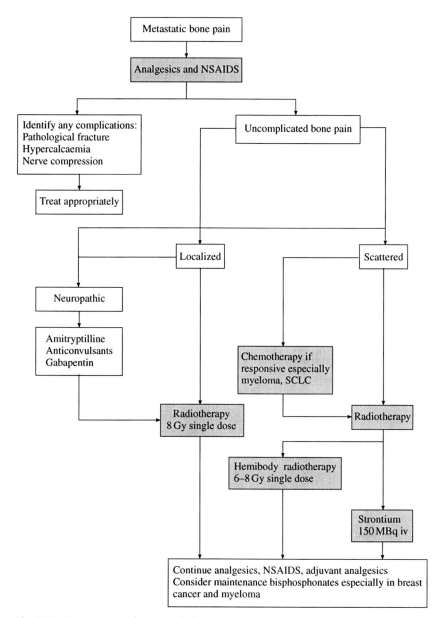

Fig. 21.3 Management of metastatic bone pain: patient pathway.

Case History 21.4

Tom, a 54-year-old engineer, has prostate cancer with bone metastases. His bone pain responded well to hormone therapy but in recent weeks he has been complaining of pain across his shoulders. He also suffers from agoraphobia and has become increasingly reluctant to go out.

He has become increasingly unsteady on his legs and has had several falls, which were associated with panic attacks. Tom was convinced that his difficulty in walking was part of his psychological problems.

The GP asked for the advice of a psychiatrist, who suggested respite stay in a hospice. On admission Tom was found to have a quadriparesis with increased tone in his limbs but intact bladder function.

He was commenced on dexamethasone 16 mg and the cancer centre was contacted immediately. Later the same day, he had an MR scan which showed cord compression at both lower cervical and lower dorsal levels. Immediate radiotherapy was given to both sites. He returned to the hospice for rehabilitation, where he regained full mobility and was discharged home.

Practice points

- To pick up spinal cord compression promptly, a high index of suspicion plus thorough and repeated clinical examination are essential.
- Tumour at more than one level of the spinal canal is not uncommon, and demonstrates the value of MR imaging. If only one level had been treated, the outcome would not have been successful.
- Symptoms and signs of cord compression can evolve slowly. Rapid development may be associated with vascular compromise and recovery is less likely.

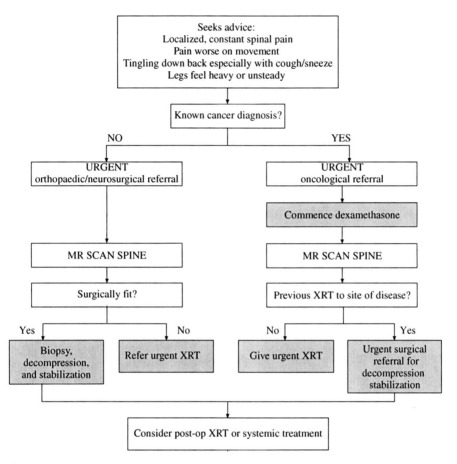

Fig. 21.4 Spinal cord compression: Patient pathway.

Chapter 22

Liver metastases

Up to 50 per cent of patients dying with cancer have liver metastases: it is the organ most commonly involved by secondary spread. This development carries a grave prognosis, as symptomatic liver disease is usually associated with steady physical decline and increasing cachexia to death within weeks or months. For the majority of patients, active treatment may help symptoms but will make little difference to survival. However, within this gloomy picture there is a spectrum which depends upon the extent of metastases and the underlying malignancy. The prognosis is considerably better for the small proportion of patients who have chemosensitive tumours or resectable lesions confined to the liver.

Pathology

The most frequent primary sites associated with liver secondaries are lung, breast, and colon. In colorectal cancer, 28 per cent have documented liver metastases at diagnosis and a further 25 per cent will develop them after resection of the primary disease. They are present in two-thirds of patients dying from breast cancer and in most patients with disseminated malignant melanoma.

The main cause of liver metastases is haematogenous spread. This may be part of widespread tumour dissemination as in breast cancer, when the liver is reached via the hepatic artery. Drainage into the portal venous system from the gastrointestinal tract is another important route of invasion from cancers arising in stomach, pancreas, and bowel. This explains why cancers of the colon and upper rectum may produce metastases apparently confined to the liver as the first and only site of spread which may justify aggressive local treatment in the absence of demonstrable disease elsewhere. Blood borne metastases may occur less commonly in patients with hepatic cirrhosis.

There may also be direct invasion of the liver from cancers arising from adjacent organs such as within the pancreas and biliary tree, or from tumour involving lymph nodes, sometimes with retrograde lymphatic and venous invasion. Superficial deposits can occur as a result of transperitoneal spread: in ovarian cancer, extensive invasion of the liver parenchyma is less common than subcapsular deposits which typically cause local pain.

The rare neuroendocrine tumours (APUDomas), which most commonly arise in lung and small bowel, may spread to the liver. In patients with carcinoid tumours, 95 per cent of those who develop the typical syndrome of flushing, wheeze, and diarrhoea have liver metastases. These patients can live several years with slowly growing tumours and develop massive liver enlargement.

Clinical presentation

Liver metastases may be suspected because of the discomfort of visceral enlargement or pain due to irritation of the stretched capsule. Less often acute pain may arise due to haemorrhage into a metastasis causing a rapid increase in pressure; large subcapsular metastasis can rupture into the abdominal cavity producing a haemoperitoneum and acute abdominal pain with guarding and hypotension.

As the liver enlarges there may be associated nausea, impaired gastric emptying, and oesophageal reflux. Massive enlargement causes dull, aching pain, attributed to drag on the supporting ligaments, and shortness of breath. There may be compression, sometimes with thrombosis, of the inferior vena cava, causing peripheral oedema. Ascitic fluid may develop due to a combination of venous compression causing portal hypertension, obstruction to lymphatic flow across the diaphragm or falling albumin levels. Jaundice due to liver failure is usually a late development, when 75 per cent or more of the liver tissue has been replaced by tumour. The size of the organ is not significant as some patients seem to live with massive hepatomegaly but have adequate liver function and do not become jaundiced. Bruising and bleeding results from impaired production of clotting factors, particularly prothrombin, and hypoglycaemia may occur; encephalopathy will ensue as liver failure advances but acute hepatic failure is an unusual presentation of underlying metastatic cancer. Other causes of jaundice should also be considered such as obstructive jaundice due to intra- or extra-hepatic tumour or sclerosing cholangitis in association with malignant infiltration. Further causes are detailed in Table 22.1.

Key points

- Liver metastases occur due to blood borne spread either via the portal system (e.g. bowel and pancreas) or systemic circulation (e.g. breast and lung).
- The development of liver metastases is associated with a poor prognosis except for rare chemosensitive tumours such as germ cell tumours.
- Small deposits are usually asymptomatic and may be discovered incidentally on routine ultrasound or CT scans.
- Symptoms include vague upper abdominal discomfort, local pain from the liver capsule, anorexia, nausea and gastric reflux.

Investigations

Staging investigations, which are necessary to plan appropriate treatment in apparently early cancer, may detect asymptomatic liver metastases. This is important where radical surgery is envisaged (e.g. amputation for osteosarcoma). The discovery of multiple liver deposits usually indicates incurable disease and in most situations, radical

Table 22.1 Causes of jaundice in patients with cancer

Pre-hepatic

Autoimmune haemolysis (warm or cold antibodies, in lymphoma and leukaemia)

Microangiopathic haemolysis (uraemia, disseminated intravascular wagulation (DIC), septicaemia)

Unrelated causes (e.g. haemoglobinopathies)

Hepatic

Gross parenchymal infiltration by primary or secondary cancer

Intrahepatic biliary occlusion by tumour

Acute viral infections

Drug-induced hepatitis (MAOIs, valproate, methotrexate, 6-mercaptopurine)

Drug-induced cholestasis (erythromycin, chlorpromazine, anabolic or androgenic steroids)

Extrahepatic biliary obstruction

Primary tumours of pancreas, gall bladder and biliary tract

Hepatic portal lymphadenopathy

Gallstones

Biliary stricture post-surgery

Blockage of previously placed biliary stent

---

aggressive local treatment would be abandoned. However, the incidence of positive findings in patients with small primary tumours is often too small to justify routine screening for distant spread at presentation, for example in early breast cancer, only 2 per cent of those who appear to be in stage I and II have any evidence of skeletal metastases and the chances of liver involvement are even smaller.

Biochemical tests

Abnormalities in liver enzymes (aminotransferases (AST), gamma glutamyl transferase (GGT), and alkaline phosphatase (ALP)) are not specific for malignancy, and of course, can still be normal in the presence of liver metastases. Elevated levels have a sensitivity of about 60 per cent in liver metastases, typically causing a rise in GGT, followed by a lesser increase in ALP and AST. In documented liver involvement, a falling serum albumin, rising bilirubin, and a prolonged prothrombin time indicate deteriorating function and a poor outlook.

A rising level of *carcinoembryonic antigen (CEA)* after resection of the bowel tumour correlates with the development and extent of liver metastases in colorectal cancer. CEA levels may also be raised in association with other gastrointestinal malignancies and also with liver metastases from breast, ovarian, and prostate cancer although not with lymphoma, melanoma, or carcinoid tumours. *Alpha-fetoprotein* levels show poor correlation with liver secondary tumours unless due to germ cell tumours, but are raised in 50–75 per cent of cases with primary hepatocellular cancer.

Imaging

Detection of liver metastases is usually by ultrasound, CT, or MRI scanning, confirmed if appropriate by needle biopsy. Isotope scans are rarely used in modern oncology, but there is increasing interest in the role of positron emission tomograpy (PET), using uptake of labelled glucose (FDG) which may increase the sensitivity of detection.

Ultrasound scanning is easily accessible and sensitive; distinguishing between solid lesions and those which may be cysts or abscesses, with resolution of lesions down to 1 cm in size. It is also valuable to assess free ascitic fluid and to define the portal veins and biliary tree. Intra-operative ultrasound can be used to detect tumours deep within the liver prior to surgery.

CT scanning with contrast enhancement can also distinguish between solid and cystic areas; it may be less sensitive than ultrasound in detection of lesions under 2 cm, but is unaffected by excessive overlying fat or gas in the bowel. It is also better than MRI or ultrasound imaging in detection of extrahepatic disease. CT scans can also be used to estimate the proportion of liver invaded by tumour as a prognostic guide and a baseline for assessing response to treatment.

Arteriography may be performed to assess portal perfusion and can more accurately distinguish between benign hyperplastic lesions from malignancy. Its main value is in the assessment of the site of lesions in relation to the vascular anatomy prior to surgical resection. Arteriography has shown that metastases are relatively avascular compared with primary hepatocellular and endocrine tumours. Modern MR techniques can replace arteriography in many situations.

A biopsy is unnecessary where the primary pathology is known and the radiological findings are typical of multiple metastases. Those patients who are found to have one or more lesions in the liver and the underlying pathology is unknown, should have a needle biopsy to establish a tissue diagnosis unless the clinical picture is of advanced carcinomatosis in an extremely ill patient. Biopsy under ultrasound or CT guidance is preferred to ensure that the appropriate tissue is sampled.

Key points

- Ultrasound is the most sensitive investigation for liver metastases.
- CT and MR will give additional diagnostic information.
- Changes in liver function tests occur with metastases; typically the gamma glutamyl transferase is the most sensitive enzyme and first to change followed by transaminases and alkaline phosphatase; bilirubin will rise at a much later stage.
- Ultrasound or CT guided biopsy is required for a tissue diagnosis where there is no previously known malignancy.

Active treatment for liver metastases: when should it be considered?

Active treatment may offer the following:

- palliation of symptoms by reducing the tumour volume in an enlarged liver or relief of jaundice
- possible prolongation of survival compared with supportive care
- possibility of cure in a small minority

A small sub-group of patients with colorectal cancer and metastatic disease confined to one lobe of the liver may be suitable for surgical resection but in most types of cancer there are multiple sites of secondary spread and this would not be an option. Some tumours may be particularly responsive to chemotherapy such as lymphoma, choriocarcinoma, or small cell lung cancer and intensive chemotherapy can achieve prolonged control of the disease. For the majority, however, the aims of reducing symptoms and prolonging life must be balanced against the side-effects and chances of a worthwhile response. The value of various treatment approaches are discussed below. While it is important to be aware of these, most patients will be helped best by direct management of symptoms. This is especially true of those with poor general condition, multiple sites of disease, ascites, or jaundice due to failing liver function.

Surgical resection of liver metastases

Partial hepatectomy should be considered in some patients with liver metastases from colorectal cancer and neuroendocrine tumours. In colorectal cancer, 25 per cent of relapses are confined to metastases within the liver. Of these, 5 per cent have a solitary deposit or metastases confined to one lobe alone: these patients are potentially salvageable by surgery. There is good evidence that this can prolong median survival from 10.6 months for the group as a whole to 22 months. Series of over 200 patients have demonstrated that up to 30 per cent survival at 5 years can be achieved with a 15 per cent long-term survival rate at 20 years. Mortality rates from the procedure in experienced units are less than 2 per cent.

The best candidates will be those with a resectable or resected primary tumour in whom the liver is the only site of spread and where this is either a solitary deposit or unilobar liver involvement. Those with multiple tumours (>4), poorly differentiated cancers, or with lymphatic spread are unlikely to do well. One-third of patients who relapse following liver resection have widespread disease at other sites, but repeat hepatic resections have been performed where the liver is the only site of relapse. The role of chemotherapy given before or following the initial hepatic resection remains uncertain, but will be offered to many patients in the adjuvant setting.

Case History 22.1

Jim is a 54-year-old business man who confesses, at his private insurance medical, that he has been passing blood and mucous from his back passage. Sigmoidoscopy leads to a discovery of a bowel cancer which is arising in the sigmoid colon. Initial investigations show no evidence of spread and he proceeds to have surgery. A complete resection of his bowel tumour is performed but at operation he is found to have three small liver metastases. He is referred to another specialist unit and undergoes a partial hepatectomy; this is followed by six months of adjuvant chemotherapy with 5-fluorouracil. Jim is a philosophical character. He decides to take early retirement on medical grounds and make the most of life. Ten years later he remains well with no recurrence of his cancer.

Practice points

- The liver may be the only site of disease in over 30 per cent of patients with metastatic colorectal cancer.
- Resection of liver metastases may cure some patients.

Techniques for local ablation of liver metastases

Cryosurgery

This has been used to destroy inoperable multiple tumours by injection of liquid nitrogen into the mass. It has been performed for lesions in cirrhotic livers, where resection is indicated but would be hazardous, and also in the management of symptomatic neuro-endocrine tumours.

Embolization

Embolization of the tumour blood supply can be used to treat symptomatic deposits, if painful or in the case of neuroendocrine tumours when causing symptoms due to peptides production. It may also have a role prior to resection of a highly vascular tumour. Contrast media are used to demonstrate vessels which are then occluded by the injection of a variety of materials: gelatin sponge, steel coils, and Lipidiol (iodized oil), among others. The process is carried out under local anaesthetic and is possible because the healthy liver is supplied by the portal vein whereas the tumour relies on hepatic arterial perfusion. The aim is to produce ischaemia and necrosis of the tumour itself. This results in the release of products of tumour breakdown causing local pain and fever. It is contraindicated if there is cirrhosis, portal vein, or biliary obstruction. Embolization has been combined with local perfusion of cytotoxic agents with the aim of improving the local response rates but current evidence suggests that equivalent results can be obtained with intravenous systemic therapy.

Percutaneous alcohol injection

Injection of alcohol under ultrasound guidance can be used to necrose tumours less than 5 cm in size. The technique has been used for primary hepatocellular cancer as well as metastases.

Radiotherapy

The liver is relatively sensitive to radiation; a dose not exceeding 30 Gy in 15 fractions over 3 weeks is tolerated but above 35 Gy radiation, hepatitis will develop. Therefore, the therapeutic dose that can be given to the whole organ is not sufficient to eradicate metastases due to adenocarcinoma but would be effective for infiltration by lymphoma, which is more radiosensitive. Radiotherapy is sometimes given to ease the pain of a tender liver in other primaries such as colorectal or breast cancer if chemotherapy is not appropriate using single doses of 8 Gy. Side effects from hepatic irradiation include anorexia and nausea which are related to the volume of normal liver included in the irradiated volume. It is possible that improved three-dimensional planning (conformational therapy) will enable higher doses to part of the organ while sparing as much normal tissue as possible which may be advantageous where there are localized symptomatic areas of tumour and for tumours of the gall bladder and biliary ducts.

Systemic therapy for liver metastases

Systemic chemotherapy

For widespread metastases resulting from blood borne dissemination systemic chemotherapy is often the only treatment modality which can address the clinical picture of scattered deposits causing multiple symptoms. The decision to offer chemotherapy is therefore not necessarily based solely upon liver involvement alone but on the overall clinical picture of disseminated malignancy. The results of treatment will depend upon the sensitivity of the tumour to chemotherapy; thus good responses with often rapid symptom relief will be seen with small cell lung cancer, germ cell tumour and lymphoma and more modest responses with breast cancer, colorectal cancer, ovary cancer, bladder cancer and non-small cell lung cancer. Other primary types such as renal cell tumours, melanoma and soft tissue sarcoma have only low response rates and the value of palliative treatment is often much less apparent. The drugs chosen are those specific to the primary tumour type, for example anthracycline based scheduled for breast cancer, 5-FU based schedules for colorectal and gastric primaries, cisplatin based for ovary, non-small cell lung cancer and bladder. In most of these scenarios response rates of the order of 30–40 per cent will be achieved with objective tumour reduction and improved quality of life. Often however this will be short-lived with recurrence of symptoms and tumour regrowth with a few months

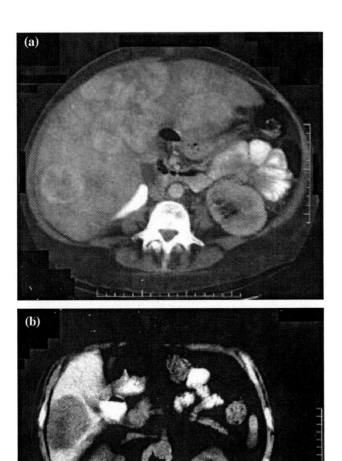

Fig. 22.1 CT scans showing liver metastases from (a) renal cancer and (b) lymphoma.

of the end of chemotherapy. Anthracycline drugs (Adriamycin, epirubicin and mitozantrone) are excreted in the bile and it is important to reduce their dose in patients with a raised bilirubin. The importance of a histological diagnosis when considering chemotherapy is illustrated in Fig. 22.1 showing two cases of liver metastases; the first (a) is from renal cancer, had no response to interferon and resulted in the patients death over a few months, the second (b) is a high grade non-Hodgkin's lymphoma which responded rapidly to systemic chemotherapy and the patient remains alive, well and free from disease.

Regional perfusion

Drugs can be infused directly into the liver by means of a catheter which is inserted in the hepatic artery. This can double the amount of cytotoxic agent reaching the metastatic tumour with less generalized toxicity and fewer side effects. This approach has been used for carcinoid and islet cell tumours, using a perfusion of 5-FU and streptozotocin. It is also used to intensify treatment for colorectal cancer with metastases confined to the liver. Response rates are certainly increased, to around 50 per cent, but randomized trials have failed to show any survival advantage over systemic therapy with the added risk of hepatobiliary toxicity.

Hormone therapy

In common with other metastatic situations, where the primary tumour is hormone sensitive then systemic hormone therapy has a role in the management of liver metastases. This will apply particularly to breast cancer, liver metastases being rare in endometrial cancer and extremely rare in prostate cancer. Previous hormone therapy will be taken into account in deciding upon the best option; tamoxifen, an aromatase inhibitor such as arimidex or a progestogen will be the drugs of choice. Whilst of value in relatively asymptomatic disease, the time course of response is relatively slow typically over a few months and for the patient presenting with jaundice or a rapidly expanding liver, systemic chemotherapy is more likely to provide palliation within a useful time frame. Patients with liver metastases from endometrial cancer may benefit from progestogens or an LHRH antagonist and in the rare event of liver metastases from prostate cancer, antiandrogen therapy is effective.

Biological therapy

In renal cancer short-term palliation may be achieved using interferon, although the toxicity of treatment may be not insignificant. Trials are underway to evaluate any added benefit from the addition of 5-FU-based chemotherapy to an interferon/interleukin regimen. In breast cancer, patients who have tumours positive for the c-erb B2 receptor may have responses to the monoclonal antibody herceptin.

Hepatic transplantation?

A liver transplant is now an accepted option for primary liver cancers. This approach is much more contentious in metastatic cancer but has been tried in a very small number of patients. Experience suggests that the obligatory immunosuppression does not enhance tumour growth, but the fundamental problem is that of the re-seeding of the transplanted organ by circulating tumour cells and of relapse at other sites. It is therefore unlikely to have a major role in the management of metastatic disease until systemic treatment can be effective in mopping up residual circulating cells and micrometastases.

Key points

- A small number of patients may have true solitary or localized liver metastases as the only site of relapse for whom radical resection should be undertaken with a 30 per cent five year survival.
- Other surgical techniques may be used to reduce the size of liver metastases including cryotherapy, embolisation and alcohol injection.
- Radiotherapy has a role in palliation of the symptoms of hepatomegaly but is limited by the sensitivity of normal liver to radiation.
- Systemic chemotherapy or hormone therapy can achieve good palliation of symptoms in tumours which are chemosensitive or hormone sensitive, although in most common solid tumours, even in responders, benefit is short lived once chemotherapy is discontinued.

Case History 22.2

A 58-year-old woman presents with right upper quadrant discomfort and altered bowel habit. A CT scan shows an enlarged liver and multiple lesions with the appearance of metastatic tumours. Mammography, barium studies and a panendoscopy are normal. She refuses to have a liver biopsy. However she is also experiencing flushes which, like her episodic loose stools, are sometimes triggered by eating. Carcinoid syndrome is suspected and an assay of 5 hydroxyindole acetic acid (5HIAA) in a 24 h urine collection is requested. The level is extremely elevated, confirming the diagnosis.

She commences fortnightly depot lanreotide injections with a dramatic improvement in her symptoms and corresponding fall in 5HIAA levels. This improvement is maintained for the next two years. Then her symptoms return and a further increase in lanreotide fails to suppress tumour activity. At this point a repeat CT scan shows progression of the liver metastases and there are also a number of intraperitoneal tumours. Further palliative options are discussed; she is not keen on chemotherapy but agrees to a trial of interferon, given by subcutaneous injection three times a week. There is some response but increasing fatigue. The patient herself discontinues the interferon and wants only symptomatic care. This includes codeine and loperamide for the diarrhoea, and cyclizine for nausea. Her condition deteriorates slowly over the next six months and she develops ascites and small bowel obstruction. At laparotomy a palliative ileostomy is formed and she dies three months later in a hospice.

Practice points

◆ Patients with carcinoid tumours may live several years with metastatic disease.

◆ The onset of systemic symptoms such as flushing and diarrhoea occurs with the development of liver disease.

◆ Escape of symptoms from hormonal control by sandostatin or analogues is an indication of a poor prognosis.

Management of the jaundiced patient

Jaundice in a patient with a previous diagnosis of cancer is often due to metastatic involvement of the liver, but bile duct obstruction is an equally important cause to consider. Other possible causes should be kept in mind including those unrelated to malignancy such as gallstones. Jaundice is usually clinically apparent when the bilirubin level rises above 35 mmol/L.

Painless jaundice in the presence of a palpable gall bladder is the classic presentation of a carcinoma of the ampulla of Vater or pancreas; the stools are pale as a consequence of the extrahepatic biliary obstruction. An obstructive picture can be the result of enlarged lymph nodes at the porta hepatis which compress the common bile duct, in the absence of any intrahepatic metastases. This can occur in breast cancer as well as with intra-abdominal malignancies and lymphomas. Clinically it is typified by the association with pale stools, dark urine and at a more advanced stage systemic itching.

Liver function tests in a patient with obstructive jaundice characteristically show a high alkaline phosphatase. An ultrasound scan is essential to determine the site of obstruction; a CT scan will give further information about intrahepatic and extrahepatic disease. Endoscopic retrograde cholangiopancreatography (ERCP) is performed to examine the ampullary region and common bile duct and this may be combined with insertion of a stent. If ERCP is unsuccessful, percutaneous transhepatic cholangiography may be performed with the insertion of a percutaneous drain to decompresss the bilary tract. Biliary obstruction, whether due to malignancy or benign causes, can be associated with cholangitis and may be a source of septicaemia.

The patient with significant haemolysis will have symptoms of anaemia. The serum bilirubin will be unconjugated and a positive Coomb's test indicates an autoimmune process. Serological tests to exclude or confirm viral hepatitis infections are needed in a few patients where there is no obvious cause for jaundice.

The active management of liver metastases has been described in detail although for many patients who have become jaundiced, the best option is supportive care with acknowledgement that the time remaining is short. Care is needed in prescribing drugs as both hypoalbuminaemia and depletion of functioning liver tissue increase toxicity. It is important to distinguish the patients with extrahepatic biliary obstruction; their general condition may be good despite marked jaundice and relatively simple measures to bypass the obstruction can be highly successful. The prognosis in this situation is likely to be better than for patients with liver infiltration.

Treatment of extrahepatic biliary obstruction

Curative treatment is attempted whenever possible. Initially decompression of the biliary tree with, if necessary, a percutaneous drain is important to restore hepatic function and improve the patient's fitness for major surgery. In addition it may be necessary to give vitamin K if the prothrombin time is prolonged and prophylactic antibiotics are usually administered. Radical resection (Whipple's procedure) may be possible for early cancer confined to the head of the pancreas; where there is more extensive disease, palliative relief of biliary obstruction establishing a route from the gall bladder to the jejunum (choledochojejunostomy) reduces jaundice, pruritis, and often helps to improve anorexia and nausea.

The following approaches are used in palliation:

Surgery Decompression of the biliary tree is achieved by a biliary-enteric anastamosis (e.g. a choledochoduodenostomy or a cholecystojejunostomy). Palliative procedures bypass the obstructing tumour but there can be significant peri-operative morbidity and mortality, associated with leak of bile, cholangitis, and acute renal failure. Biliary diversion may be combined with a gastroenterostomy, which is needed in about 15 per cent of patients with pancreatic cancer if the tumour obstructs the duodenum. Median survival after such procedures is usually around 6 months.

Biliary stents It is often possible to insert a stent through the narrowed section of bile duct at ERCP. If this cannot be achieved endoscopically, a percutaneous transhepatic approach may be attempted. Both plastic and expanding metal stents are used and have a duration of patency of 4–5 months. Subsequent problems may arise if the stent becomes blocked by bile salts, debris, or tumour and it may become displaced. It is also possible to stent the duodenum in cases with gastric outlet obstruction.

Radiotherapy Palliative radiotherapy may be given to inoperable pancreatic cancer to help pain control and in these cases would be undertaken after a stent had been inserted. Intraluminal radiotherapy can be used to treat localized tumour within the biliary tree. Radiotherapy to the porta hepatis may be of value in palliation of pain or extrahepatic biliary obstruction due to enlarged lymph nodes. The treatment field is centred around T12/L1 and delivered by a parallel opposed pair of beams (Fig. 22.2). As with all techniques involving the upper abdomen, nausea and vomiting are usual side effects which are reduced by anti-emetics and steroids.

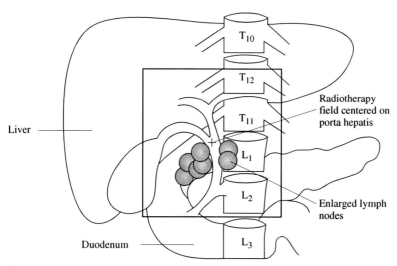

Fig. 22.2 Palliative radiotherapy field used to treat disease at the porta hepatis.

Key points

- Obstructice jaundice is best managed by percutaneous drainage and subsequent surgical methods to remove or bypass the obstruction using radical resection, biliary-enteral anastomosis or biliary stents.

- Radiotherapy may also have a role in inoperable tumour and where there is associated pain due to local tumour growth.

- In the absence of jaundice, few changes in prescribing are needed although use of anticoagulants should be avoided or carefully monitored. With deteriorating function avoid carbamazepine, valproate, and phenothiazines; low albumin levels may lead to phenytoin toxicity. Anthracycline drugs are excreted in bile and should be dose-reduced with raised bilirubin.

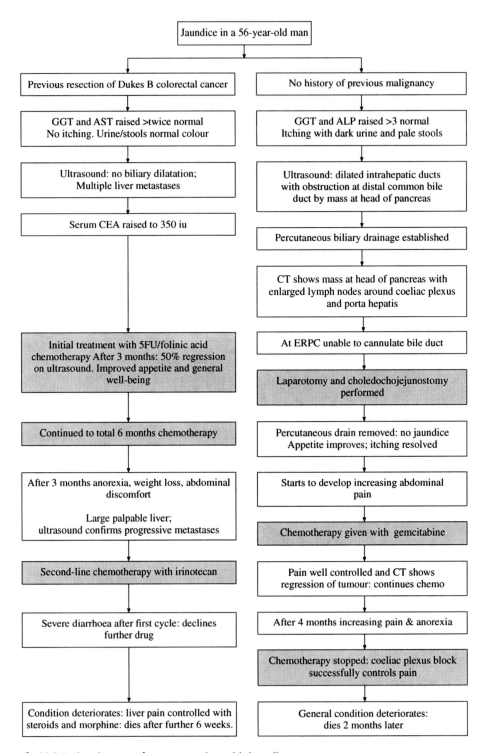

Fig 22.3 Patient journey after presentation with jaundice.

Chapter 23

Metastatic disease of the thorax

Pulmonary metastases

Lung metastases occur due to blood-borne spread from distant sites. After the liver, the lung is the second most common site for metastatic tumour. From the systemic venous circulation, cells pass into the right side of the heart and thence via the pulmonary arteries to the lungs where some will establish successful tumour colonies within lung parenchyma and pleura. Involvement of hilar and mediastinal nodes and direct invasion of the pleura are also very common in primary bronchial carcinomas which in turn produce secondary deposits within both lungs. Metastases are less often found within the bronchial tree itself but this has been described in association with renal and breast cancers and melanoma.

The appearance of pulmonary metastases, with rare exceptions, signifies incurable disease and reduced life expectancy; in turn they are a source of secondary dissemination of cancer by haematogenous spread to important organs such as the brain and liver. They are frequently encountered in patients with advanced breast cancer and also with colorectal, bladder, cervical and lung cancer.

Some less common malignancies which seem to have a predilection for secondary spread to the lungs include osteosarcoma and soft tissue sarcomas; cancer of thyroid, kidney, and endometrium; choriocarcinomas and germ cell tumours and lymphoma. True solitary metastases are unusual and will commonly either be a herald of more advanced disease or where there is continued exposure to a common aetiological agent, for example cigarette smoking, a second primary, for example after head and neck or bladder cancer, themselves smoking related tumours.

Symptoms

Many patients have few or no symptoms despite radiological abnormalities. Symptoms will depend upon the number, size, and site of the metastases. Breathlessness may result from invasion of lung tissue, associated infection or infiltration of lymphatics causing reduced lung compliance. This may be compounded by the presence of a pleural effusion or tumour masses sufficient to cause extrinsic compression of a bronchus. Lobar collapse may be due to endobronchial tumour, which may also cause haemoptysis and cough. Pleural involvement produces pain and this in turn restricts ventilatory effort.

Investigations

Pulmonary metastases tend to occur in the lower lobes and in the periphery of the lung. Twenty-five per cent are seen as solitary lesions on a chest X-ray and must be differentiated from a primary bronchial carcinoma, benign tumours, and non-neoplastic lesions such as granulomas. CT scans are valuable to distinguish pulmonary from pleural-based pathology and may demonstrate multiple deposits not seen on a chest X-ray. Sometimes cavitation of the lesions is seen, typically in squamous cancers, and calcification may rarely occur. Multiple opacities of 2–5 mm or greater are characteristic of metastases but the differential diagnosis includes sarcoidosis and multi-focal infection. Septic emboli associated with infected central lines for venous access have on some occasions been mistaken for secondary deposits.

Pulmonary metastases may often coexist with pleural effusions and enlarged mediastinal nodes, for example in lymphoma. Histological confirmation of pulmonary metastases is unnecessary in the presence of other metastatic or uncontrolled local disease but may be indicated if there is a solitary lesion or a long interval following previous treatment of a primary cancer. Sputum cytology is rarely helpful, but bronchoscopy should be performed if haemoptysis is a symptom or the tumour appears to be accessible from the bronchial tree. A CT-guided biopsy may be needed for peripheral lesions.

Key points

- Pulmonary metastases reflect blood borne spread from distant sites.
- Chest X-ray is relatively insensitive for diagnosis compared with CT scan; typically they will be multiple and peripheral in the lung fields.
- They are often asymptomatic but can present with cough, shortness of breath and chest or pleuritic pain.
- Unless localized when resection may be possible they are incurable and have a poor prognosis.

Treatment of pulmonary metastases

Surgical resection

This should be considered in patients who have a small number of metastases, localized to one area or lobe of the lung from an underlying primary tumour recognized to have along natural history in the absence of metastases elsewhere. Examples are shown in Table 23.1.

Assessment of these patients includes CT scanning of the lung and exclusion of liver or bone metastases. Pulmonary function tests are also essential to determine whether a patient will withstand lung resection. Those who do best are likely to be patients with

Table 23.1 Surgical resection for lung metastases: primary sites

Consider	Not indicated
Kidney	Breast
Melanoma	Bronchus
Soft tissue sarcoma	Bladder
Osteosarcoma	Cervix
Colorectal	

relatively slow-growing tumours, a long disease-free interval and in whom useful systemic treatment is also possible. A thoracotomy is usually performed although laser resection of peripheral deposits by thoracoscopy has been described.

Surgical resection, often combined with chemotherapy, has achieved 5-year survival rates of 20–40 per cent in patients with osteosarcoma and soft tissue sarcoma. A small number of patients with carcinoma may be suitable (e.g. those with solitary lung secondary cancer from renal or colorectal cancer). Results in malignant melanoma and other cancers are usually disappointing.

Chemotherapy

This treatment can achieve useful palliation of symptoms in patients with chemo-responsive malignancy, particularly breast cancer, colorectal cancer and lymphoma. In breast cancer this may achieve a median survival of 20 months although the prognosis for the individual will depend upon response and other sites of disease.

Asymptomatic disease should not in general be treated. It should be remembered that tumours which are highly chemosensitive are curable with chemotherapy despite lung metastases; these will include choriocarcinoma, germ cell tumours and lymphoma.

Case History 23.1

A 57-year-old lady develops bone metastases nearly 4 years after a lumpectomy plus radiotherapy for breast cancer. She has been taking tamoxifen since the initial treatment. Following radiotherapy to a couple of painful sites, she is switched to anastroazole and her bone pain resolves. She is free from symptoms over the next 18 months, but then sees her GP on several occasions with chest infections. She complains of persistent aching across her chest with some cough and breathlessness. Her chest X-ray on two occasions is reported to be normal. She is no better after antibiotics.

When seen in the oncology clinic she looks unwell but there are no new findings. An isotope bone scan is requested in view of her chest pains. There is increased uptake in several ribs but these do not explain her diffuse pains and chest symptoms. She has a CT scan and this demonstrates extensive pleural and pericardial soft tissue tumour deposits.

Case History 23.1 (continued)

She also has evidence of several liver metastases. Palliation of her symptoms is achieved by changing from hormone therapy to combination chemotherapy. She remains on active treatment, monitored by further CT scans for most of the following 15 months until progression of her liver disease.

Practice points

- Consider a CT scan if symptoms persist despite negative X-rays.
- In chemosensitive tumours such as breast or colorectal cancer, chemotherapy can provide good palliation of symptomatic lung metastases.

Radiotherapy

This has a limited role in the treatment of pulmonary metastases. The sensitivity of normal lung tissue limits the useful dose that can be given and also the volume to be treated. In the past, bilateral pulmonary lesions from extremely sensitive tumours such as seminoma could be treated with low dose whole lung irradiation and show a good response. Such techniques have been superceded by effective chemotherapy.

Local radiotherapy can be useful in treating a painful lesion that is invading pleura and chest wall and also if there is a particular tumour that is thought to be the source of haemoptysis. In these situations, a small volume can be treated without significant side effects; large lung volumes result in pneumonitis and fibrosis causing severe dyspnoea and cough. Widespread acute radiation pneumonitis as seen occasionally with wide field radiotherapy has a high fatality rate.

Endobronchial metastases may be treated with intraluminal radiotherapy and both cryotherapy and laser therapy are effective in these situations. Radiotherapy is, of course, particularly valuable in palliation of mediastinal disease as discussed later. In the treatment of well-differentiated thyroid cancer, radio-iodine [I^{131}] is used. This is taken up by functioning thyroid tissue and tumour and thus it is possible to ablate the primary tumour and also treat metastatic deposits provided that they also demonstrate sufficient uptake of the isotope. Patients with lung metastases alone due to thyroid cancer can survive for a many years.

Any active treatment should be combined with other measures to help distressing symptoms. Steroids may be particularly helpful for breathlessness and cough associated with widespread pulmonary deposits and lymphangitis. It is worth using a large dose of a potent steroid to obtain a response quickly (e.g. by giving dexamethasone 16 mg daily for 4–5 days). If beneficial, this can be reduced slowly to the lowest dose that maintains a symptomatic response. Opioids will reduce the distress of dyspnoea. Ethamsylate or tranexamic acid, given orally, may reduce intermittent small haemoptyses. The reader is referred to palliative care texts for a wider discussion of other supportive measures.

Key points

◆ Solitary or several localized metastases may be considered for surgical resection if the tumour is otherwise slow growing and controlled at other sites.

◆ Chemotherapy is otherwise the treatment of choice, or hormone therapy for breast or endometrial cancer.

◆ Radiotherapy may offer palliation for peripheral metastases causing pleuritic pain or if haemoptysis can be localized to one area.

Pleural effusions

Between 30 and 60 per cent of patients who present with a pleural effusion have an underlying malignancy.

Table 23.2

Primary sites causing pleural effusion	
Breast	26%
Lung	24%
Lymphoma	21%
Ovary	7%
Others	22%
including: colorectal, sarcoma, melanoma	

Effusion in association with a pleural mass is seen with mesothelioma, soft tissue sarcomas from the chest wall, and peripheral lung cancers, as well as metastatic deposits on the pleura from many sites.

In patients with a documented malignancy, the development of an effusion is usually the result of metastatic spread but other causes such as infection and thromboembolism are possible. There are several mechanisms for the excessive fluid accumulation: tumour cells, with an associated inflammatory response, may increase the permeability of pleural capillaries while drainage is reduced because of lymphatic and venous obstruction. This may be the result of tumour emboli in small veins and lymphatics compounded by hilar and mediastinal node involvement. In patients with ascites due to ovarian cancer there is evidence for transdiaphragmatic movement of fluid through lymphatic channels into the pleural space.

A malignant pleural effusion conveys a poor prognosis; the median survival for all cancers as a whole is only 2–3 months but may be longer for those with ovarian or breast cancers.

Investigations

The pleural cavity is, in normal conditions, a potential space containing no more than 15 ml of fluid. A chest X-ray will demonstrate the presence of 200 ml or less but an effusion that fills most of the hemithorax will contain several litres of fluid. Sometimes an ultrasound examination is needed to distinguish an effusion from consolidation and can also guide thoracocentesis, particularly when the fluid is loculated by pleural adhesions. Histological confirmation may be important when the effusion is a presenting symptom or the first possible indication of metastatic spread. Malignant effusions are exudates with protein content of 3 g/L or more; they are frequently blood-stained and contain malignant cells. Pleural biopsy may be necessary if cytological examination of the fluid is negative.

A malignant effusion must be distinguished from a transudate due to cardiac, renal or hepatic failure; in these conditions the protein level in the fluid is low (<2 g/dl). Meig's syndrome is seen with advanced ovary cancer with an associated transudate pleural effusion.

Management

Drainage

The management of a malignant pleural effusion should be influenced by the clinical situation rather than the chest X-ray appearance alone. Large effusions cause breathlessness, especially if bilateral, and may be associated with mediastinal shift and collapse of the underlying lung. In such cases drainage is undoubtedly indicated. However, there may also be radiological evidence of intrapulmonary tumour, lymphangitis, or a mediastinal mass and it can be difficult to know how much a small pleural effusion is contributing to symptoms in such situations. It can be worth an attempt to aspirate fluid to see how much this improves a dyspnoeic patient. Therapeutic success will depend upon adequate drainage of fluid, re-expansion of the underlying lung, and measures to prevent re-accumulation.

Simple aspiration can be done at the bedside and is tolerated by quite ill patients. The removal of as little as 250 ml can give some relief; in general no more than 1–1.5 L should be withdrawn at one session. It is usually most convenient and effective to insert a chest drain which will allow complete drainage, often requiring several days. Medical pleurodesis can then be undertaken instilling a sclerosant agent into the pleural cavity via the drain before it is removed. There is no advantage of any particular agent for this and tetracyline is probably the simplest and least painful. Reaccumulation may occur; the severity of symptoms should be used to determine whether further aspiration is indicated. If this is required more than once then referral to a thoracic surgeon for thoracoscopy and pleurodesis under direct vision is usually the best solution unless the patient is approaching the terminal phase of their illness.

Instillation of sclerosants and other agents

Sclerosants cause pleural inflammation with subsequent adherence of the parietal and visceral pleural surfaces. Good results have been obtained from ward procedures using tetracycline, doxocycline (together with lignocaine), or bleomycin instilled into the chest after aspiration to dryness. In experienced hands, this has controlled re-accumulation in 70–80 per cent of cases. Unfortunately, it is sometimes difficult to drain completely and there is a risk of producing a hydropneumothorax at thoracocen-tesis. If repeated on several occasions loculated fluid may re-accumulate in between adhesions which may be difficult to drain adequately, even with ultrasound guidance. In patients with a prognosis of several months therefore referral to a thoracic surgery unit for formal intercostal drainage followed by pleurodesis under general anaesthetic should be considered. This appears to have the best control rates for patients who are fit enough for the procedure.

Surgical procedures

Pleurectomy may be considered in a small number of patients where tube drainage has failed and has been used in mesothelioma. It is a major procedure with a mortality rate of 5–10 per cent. Another option is the insertion of a *pleuroperitoneal shunt* in rela-tively fit patients in whom the effusion is the only significant problem. This is used for chylous effusions and where the lung fails to re-expand despite drainage. The patient is taught to use external compression several times each day to encourage flow of fluid into the abdominal cavity.

Chemotherapy

As with chemotherapy for intrapulmonary metastases, systemic treatment may some-times be given with the aim of controlling pleural disease and recurrence of the effu-sion. Initial aspiration is still important to relieve symptoms. Intrapleural cytotoxic agents probably act as sclerosants in producing an inflammatory response rather than having an anti-tumour effect. Some cytotoxic drugs, particularly methotrexate, may accumulate within effusions causing increased toxicity as their half life is prolonged and it is important that the fluid is drained prior to administration of such drugs, or an appropriate dose reduction is considered to avoid this.

> **Key points**
>
> ◆ Pleural effusions may be asymptomatic when no treatment is indicated.
>
> ◆ If causing significant dyspnoea then aspiration should be undertaken.
>
> ◆ Insertion of a small chest drain is the best way to drain the cavity completely; this can then be followed by pleurodesis.
>
> ◆ Recurrent effusions are best treated by open drainage and thoracoscopic pleurodesis under anaesthetic for patients otherwise fit.

Lymphangitis carcinomatosa

Lymphangitis carcinomatosis is the infiltration of pulmonary lymphatics by tumour cells which produces bilateral streaky shadowing on X-ray and may or may not be associated with enlarged hilar nodes. It is most common with primary carcinomas of the breast and lung. As a result of the diffuse infiltration the lungs become stiff and their diffusion ability is reduced. Patients present with distressing dyspnoea sometimes associated with a dry cough.

Management is difficult unless the patient responds to systemic chemotherapy or in the case of breast cancer, hormone therapy. Steroids are recommended but often only modestly effective; opioids or benzodiazepines may reduce the distress of the progressive dyspnoea which ensues. The prognosis is extremely poor as respiratory failure and secondary chest infections develop within a few weeks.

Mediastinal disease

The mediastinum is a primary site for uncommon tumours which include thymomas and neurogenic tumours (e.g. ganglioneuroma and germ cell tumours). Most of these are benign. Primary malignant tumours arising in the mediastinum are typically either germ cell tumours or lymphoma. Other primary cancers may spread to the mediastinum by lymphatic routes. This is particularly true of cancers arising in the bronchus, oesophagus, and less commonly, breast. Abdominal and pelvic cancers spread via the draining lymphatics to para-aortic and mediastinal nodes and subsequently via the thoracic duct into the subclavian vein. This may be associated with the appearance of enlarged supraclavicular lymph nodes.

Many symptoms are due to pressure by the tumour mass:

◆ Hoarseness due to a recurrent laryngeal nerve palsy

◆ Horner's syndrome associated with involvement of the sympathetic chain

◆ Compression of the oesophagus, causing dysphagia

- Compression of the proximal airway producing cough, breathlessness and stridor
- Superior vena caval obstruction

A tumour mass may be adherent to the pericardium sac and can cause arrythmias and pericardial effusion. Spread to the heart itself is usually blood-borne; deposits can occur in the endocardium or myocardium and are a cause of arrhythmias and heart failure. This may arise particularly in association with melanoma, leukaemia, lymphoma, and breast cancer.

It is important to establish a tissue diagnosis where this is unknown. This may be achieved by fine needle aspiration or biopsy of an accessible node (e.g. in the supra-clavicular fossa). CT-guided biopsy of the mediastinal mass or mediastinoscopy to obtain a sufficient biopsy for diagnosis may be necessary.

Superior vena caval obstruction

The superior vena cava is a thin-walled structure within the confined compartment of the anterior superior mediastinum. It lies adjacent to the right main bronchus and is surrounded by lymph nodes. The syndrome produced by superior vena caval obstruction (SVCO) is nearly always due to malignancy and often the result of compression by a primary tumour or lymphadenopathy. As well as extrinsic compression, thrombosis within the vessel may occur: 75 per cent of cases are associated with carcinoma of bronchus, typically arising on the right and most frequently of small cell type. A further 25 per cent are due to non-Hodgkin's lymphomas; germ cell tumours are a less frequent cause. The symptoms and signs are listed in Table 23.3. SVCO often develops gradually and this enables a collateral venous circulation to develop through the superficial veins. These are apparent on the upper trunk, extending to the abdomen if the azygos vein is also occluded.

Non-malignant causes of SVCO are uncommon. They include aortic aneurysm and also thrombosis in association with indwelling central venous catheters, and so may be encountered in the use of Hickman lines or parenteral feeding.

The chest X-ray is abnormal in over 85 per cent of patients. Typical features are widening of the mediastinum together with a paratracheal or hilar mass, or a mass in the anterior mediastinum. Venography is not performed routinely for diagnosis. While all patients with this syndrome require prompt assessment, they do not always need

Table 23.3 Symptoms and signs associated with superior vena caval obstruction (SVCO)

Symptoms	Signs
Swelling of face, upper limbs	Oedema and plethoric appearance
Dizziness, especially on bending	Dilated superficial veins, raised jugular venous pressure (JVP)
Shortness of breath	Stridor
Headache	Papilloedema

immediate treatment. If at all possible a histological diagnosis should be obtained by CT-guided biopsy or mediastinoscopy. Patients who have rapid onset of severe symptoms including cerebral oedema, or those with coexistent airway compression and stridor, need immediate attention.

Treatment

Steroids High dose dexamethasone, 16 mg daily, should be started immediately together with oxygen if indicated. The use of anticoagulants does not appear to be of additional benefit except in those situations caused by thrombosis alone.

SVC stents These are now considered the management of choice for patients presenting with severe symptoms. It is a simple procedure which may be performed in the diagnostic radiology department under local anaesthetic. Access is via the femoral vein and inferior vena cava into the superior vena cava where the stent is expanded (Fig. 23.1). Patients with a substantial extrinsic mass that is causing compression of the airway as well as the superior vena cava will still require radiotherapy.

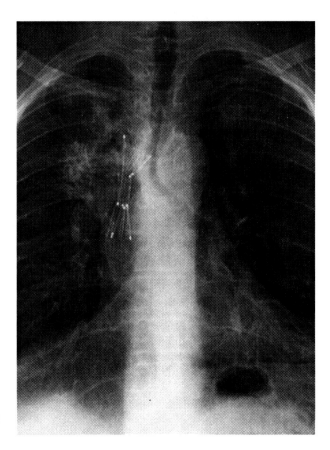

Fig. 23.1 Expanded stent in the superior vena cava to palliate superior vena caval obstruction by an underlying carcinoma of the bronchus.

Radiotherapy Palliative radiotherapy to the mediastinum produces symptomatic bene-fit in over 70 per cent of patients with superior vena caval obstruction within 2 weeks. Ill patients can be treated sitting up with a single anterior field; short treatment regi-mens are used and single large fractions are also effective. Untreated patients survive up to 6 weeks while survival after radiotherapy is a median of 5–6 months and with around 25 per cent alive at 1 year. This reflects the predominance of lung cancer as an underlying cause for this syndrome; those with lymphoma do better, with 40 per cent alive at one year. Up to 13 per cent of lung cancer patients develop recurrence of their SVCO after mediastinal irradiation.

Presentation with SVC obstruction does not preclude radical treatment if this is otherwise indicated.

Chemotherapy This should be used in chemosensitive tumours such as germ cell tumours, small cell lung cancer and lymphoma, especially in those with early signs of superior vena caval obstruction. Administration of cytotoxic drugs into the upper limbs where there is venous obstruction should be avoided, and a foot vein or femoral line may be needed in these circumstances.

Key points

- Superior vena cava obstruction is usually due to lung cancer.
- A histological diagnosis should be obtained before treatment, particularly to identify chemosensitive tumours such as lymphoma, small cell lung cancer and germ cell tumours.
- Treatment of choice for patients with severe symptoms is insertion of a stent.
- Radiotherapy and chemotherapy should follow as indicated by the primary tumour type and extent.
- SVCO does not exclude radical treatment where otherwise indicated.

Malignant disease involving the heart

Involvement of the heart is well documented in cancers of the lung and breast, affect-ing 20–30 per cent of patients in post-mortem series; it also occurs in melanoma, sar-comas, leukaemia, and lymphoma. This can occur as a result of direct invasion, particularly with mesothelioma, but also as a result of haematogenous dissemination. The pericardium alone is involved in nearly half of these cases. A malignant pericardial effusion is associated with tumour infiltration and also by obstruction to venous and lymphatic drainage by adjacent mediastinal disease. Metastases within the myocardium and endocardium are less common but a feature of disseminated melanoma.

Previous radiotherapy to the mediastinum, for example, in the treatment of Hodgkin's disease, can be another cause of a pericardial effusion.

Diagnosis

Symptoms include chest pain, palpitations, increasing shortness of breath, and dizziness as a pericardial effusion develops. The initial physical findings may be a friction rub and irregular pulse; a significant pericardial effusion leads to quiet heart sounds, raised jugular venous pressure, and signs of right heart failure. As this increases, there is hypotension and the pulse is rapid, small volume, and atrial fibrillation is common. There is increased venous pressure on inspiration producing the classic sign pulsus paradoxus and a lower systolic blood pressure on inspiration than on expiration. If untreated, cardiac tamponade and collapse follow; pericardial effusions where present contribute to the death of the patient in 80 per cent of cases.

The chest X-ray may show obvious enlargement of the cardiac outline. Echocardiography will detect endocardial deposits as well as confirming the diagnosis of pericardial effusion and guiding the aspiration of fluid for cytological examination. A CT scan will also define the tumour within the heart and mediastinum and the amount of fluid present.

Management

Effusions that produce symptoms require drainage by radiological guidance and removal of as little as 50 ml may give considerable relief. The problem is reaccumulation of the fluid. Instillation of tetracycline and other agents has been used but unlike in pleural effusions, their effectiveness is uncertain. Systemic chemotherapy should be considered where a palliative response can reasonably be anticipated (e.g. breast cancer, lung cancers, and lymphoma). Palliative radiotherapy has also been tried with some reports of successful control in small numbers of patients. Those who are fit enough to undergo surgery can benefit from a window pericardectomy that enables fluid to drain freely into the pleural cavity and this is required for those patients with postradiation fibrosis. A percutaneous balloon pericardotomy has been advocated as an alternative procedure with less morbidity in patients with advanced disease.

Key points

- Heart involvement with malignancy is relatively uncommon; the most common manifestation being a pericardial effusion.
- Patients who are haemodynamically compromised should be treated with pericardial aspiration.
- Chemotherapy should be considered to prevent recurrence.
- A surgical pericardectomy or window formation is best for constrictive pericarditis due to radiation fibrosis.

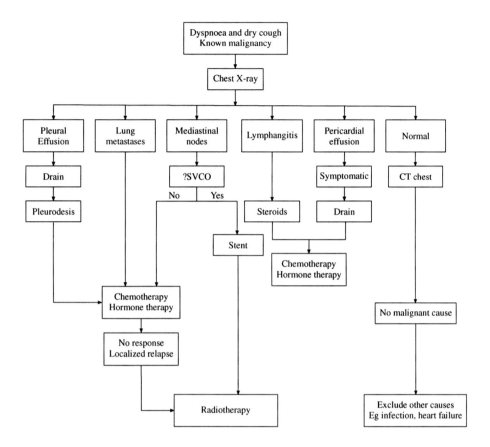

- Use of chemotherapy and hormone therapy will depend upon individual tumour sensitivity
- Where no histological diagnosis a biopsy or fluid cytology is mandatory before treatment
- High doses steroids are an alternative option to help breathlessness and cough from multiple pulmonary nodules or lymphangitis

Fig. 23.2 Management of chest symptoms from advanced malignancy.

Chapter 24

Metastases involving the brain and meninges

Brain metastases

For some patients brain metastases will be the presenting feature of the malignancy but most will develop them after diagnosis and initial treatment of cancer elsewhere. Secondary neoplasms account for 20 per cent of all intracerebral tumours in adults. Lung cancers are the commonest source of cerebral metastases and symptomatic deposits develop in over 25 per cent of patients, particularly those with small cell tumours. Breast cancer is the second commonest primary site and cerebral deposits are found in up to a quarter of patients in series of post-mortem examinations. Cerebral metastases are a significant clinical problem among patients with disseminated melanoma, and are found in 75 per cent at autopsy. Diffuse high grade non-Hodgkin's lymphoma and acute lymphoblastic leukaemia are also associated with central nervous system involvement. In contrast, it is relatively rare for other malignancies, such as prostate or ovarian cancer, to produce brain secondary tumours.

The brain may be a site of relapse in patients who have had systemic chemotherapy, as most cytotoxic agents are relatively excluded from the brain by the blood–brain barrier; for this reason some intensive schedules for lymphoma, leukaemia and small cell lung cancer include prophylactic treatment to the brain or whole central nervous system (CNS). Cerebral secondary tumours are particularly feared by patients although only 5–10 per cent of all cancer patients will develop clinical problems associated with them. While they rarely impair mental faculties there are often profound effects on function, independence, and appearance. The diagnosis of cerebral disease is nearly always associated with a much reduced life expectancy with treatment, and in untreated patients death occurs within a few weeks; cerebral metastases usually herald the terminal phase of the illness.

Presentation and diagnosis

Metastases are believed to result from microemboli of tumour cells via the arterial circulation and this often appears to follow after dissemination to the lungs. They usually develop within the cerebrum, most frequently the frontal lobes and then parietal and temporal. The cerebellum and posterior fossa is a less common site for a metastasis but this can be associated with spread from pelvic and genitourinary tumours. Metastases within the brainstem are rare. Multiple deposits are present in over two-thirds of cases.

Symptoms and investigations

Brain metastases may cause one or more of the following problems:

- Focal neurological disturbance
- Epileptic seizures
- Manifestation of raised intracranial pressure
- Change in mood, cognitive function, or behaviour

Local pressure by the tumour itself or associated haemorrhage will produce symptoms and signs according to the area of cortex affected: thus personality change and olfactory disturbance are associated with frontal lobe lesions; contralateral sensory changes and weakness with upper motor neurone signs are produced by lesions within the sensorimotor strip. Impairment of speech, sensory discrimination, and memory are affected by temporoparietal lobe tumours and visual disturbances including blindness if the occipital lobe is involved. These may be associated with partial or grand mal seizures and focal fits provide a useful diagnostic clue to the possible cause and site of the problem in patients with otherwise non-specific symptoms.

Progressive expansion of tumour with oedema of the adjacent brain in the confined cranium will inevitably lead to obstruction of cerebrospinal fluid (CSF) flow, increased extracellular fluid within the white matter, and raised intracranial pressure. The resultant headache is throbbing, worse in the morning, and on coughing and straining. It is associated with nausea and vomiting, visual disturbances, confusion, and impaired consciousness. Papilloedema is an important clinical sign of raised intracranial pressure but is present in only a quarter of patients with cerebral metastases at diagnosis. Posterior fossa lesions may also cause ataxia and CSF obstruction leading to hydrocephalus.

Most patients will have several symptoms, of which a persistent headache is the commonest and is present in 50 per cent. Motor weakness is present in a third and fits occur in 15–20 per cent. While these usually develop gradually, there may be an acute episode similar to a cerebrovascular event. This may be due to a sudden increase in cerebral oedema or a haemorrhage into the tumour.

Investigations

A CT brain scan is an essential investigation and may show one or more lesions and also any evidence of hydrocephalus. While metastatic disease is the commonest cause of multiple abnormal masses in the brain, the possibility of other diagnoses such as abscesses or granulomas should be considered, especially where there is no previous diagnosis of cancer. An MRI scan is more sensitive and may be necessary if the CT scan is normal in a patient whose symptoms and signs suggest intracranial disease. Further investigation will depend upon the individual circumstance: a craniotomy and biopsy is indicated if there is a solitary lesion and either the primary pathology is unknown, or there has been a long disease-free interval following treatment of a previous malignancy. It would not be warranted if there is clear evidence of metastatic cancer elsewhere.

Key points

◆ Most commonly asssociated with lung and breast cancer primary sites.

◆ Majority are in cerebrum and multiple.

◆ Common presentations are with headache, behavioural changes, focal neurological signs and fits.

◆ Diagnosis is confirmed on CT or MR scan.

Management

Principles of management of brain metastases are shown in the algorithm. As these patients are rarely asymptomatic, it is usual for steroid therapy to be given with the aim of reducing cerebral oedema, lessening symptoms, particularly headache, and improving neurological function. A good response is more likely to be achieved by starting with a high dose to begin with and then reducing slowly to the lowest dose that maintains the benefit. Steroid side-effects are however a major issue with doses of more than 8 mg dexamethasone or its equivalent and there is little evidence to show that higher doses up to 16 mg are of any greater benefit. If there are major neurological problems and a reduced conscious level, dexamethasone should be given intravenously and an infusion of 200 ml of 20 per cent mannitol solution may be necessary. This action should be taken on clinical suspicion without waiting for the CT scan if there is bad headache, fitting, or deteriorating neurological status, but is otherwise best deferred until after scanning since on occasions oedema may be the only clue as to a small underlying lesion on the scan. The response does depend upon the amount of oedema surrounding the tumour but significant improvement is usually apparent within 24–48 h. Anticonvulsants may also be needed if fits continue despite commencing dexamethasone. Steroid therapy is an excellent short-term treatment, but the median survival on steroids alone is only 4 weeks. This may be the only action needed in a patient with extensive cancer involving other sites, whose prognosis is deemed to be short. In other situations, the options of further treatment should be considered.

Surgery

Resection may be possible with good results when there is a solitary metastasis within an accessible and expendable part of the brain, especially in the non-dominant side. Obviously the general condition of the patient must be good with no evidence of progressive disease elsewhere. This is often followed by whole brain irradiation which may prolong survival with 40 per cent alive at 1 year and a median survival of 48 weeks in one trial which examined this question. This is probably better than the results of biopsy alone followed by radiotherapy. In some patients with radiological evidence of hydrocephalus, surgical placement of a shunt is indicated.

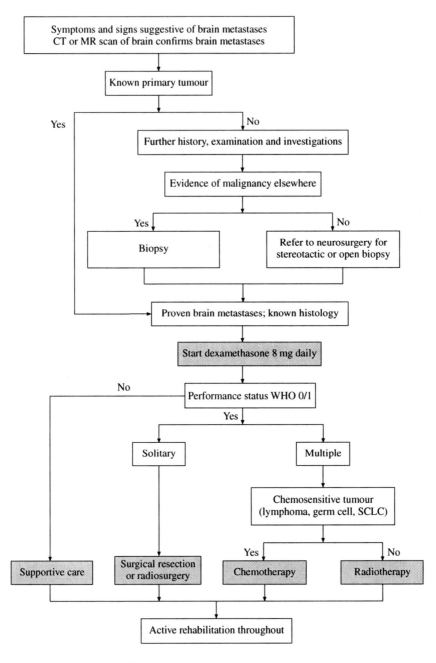

Fig. 24.1 Management of brain metastases.

Case History 24.1

Margaret had undergone treatment for a stage 2 breast cancer 4 years earlier. She had remained well apart from her insulin-dependent diabetes, but when on holiday developed speech disturbance followed by a grand mal fit. Her CT scan showed a single 2 cm lesion in the left parietal region. She was commenced on dexamethasone 8 mg daily even though she had no symptoms and unfortunately this caused major problems with hyperglycaemia. As this was brought under control, the steroid dose was reduced and then stopped without causing any problems.

It was explained that she had a secondary from her breast cancer and that she would be referred to the oncology team for cranial radiotherapy. Margaret was very upset by this news as she had experienced hair loss as a consequence of her adjuvant chemotherapy in the past. She did not want to undergo this again.

The oncologist recommended a neurosurgical opinion: this appeared to be a solitary tumour and there was no evidence of recurrent or metastatic disease elsewhere. Her chest X-ray, liver ultrasound and bone scan investigations were all clear. Margaret subsequently had a craniotomy and removal of a low grade glioma. Cranial radiotherapy was not necessary.

Practice points

- Steroids should not be commenced routinely, especially if there is no evidence of cerebral oedema on a brain scan.
- However, in situations where steroids are needed but cause major problems, radiotherapy serves a useful role in reducing the requirement for higher doses to control neurological problems.
- Always consider the possibility of another primary tumour (or another pathology) when there is a long disease-free interval following a cancer diagnosis.
- Remember that brain metastases are particularly frightening to the patient, and that radiotherapy may cause considerable anxieties, especially worries about cerebral function.

Radiotherapy

The majority of patients will have multiple metastases and for them, radiotherapy is the usual option. The entire intracranial contents are treated over a short fractionation regimen of 1–2 weeks. The start of treatment may induce an increase in cerebral oedema, which should be covered by steroids, and the patients may require hospital admission for the course of treatment. They are warned that they may experience headache or nausea at the start and may also develop soreness due to a skin reaction particularly around the ear. A further unavoidable side effect is temporary, but total, alopecia. Even with provision of a wig, this can be a high price to pay for some patients who are in the last months of their lives. Other effects include transient somnolence, occurring within a few weeks, and longer-term impairment of memory and cognition. These are significant problems in very few people and most patients do not survive long enough for late radiation changes in the CNS effects to develop.

Radiotherapy for cerebral metastases is undoubtedly effective but the benefits are of short duration as the prognosis is still poor. Neurological symptoms and function improve in over 70 per cent, enabling a gentle reduction in the dose of steroids, and sometimes withdrawal, after 4–6 weeks following treatment. The survival for these patients is significantly prolonged compared with those maintained on steroids alone, but the median survival quoted is only 5–6 months. Over half of these patients will ultimately develop progression of their cerebral disease with recurrence of the original symptoms. In these situations, the best palliation is nearly always by the use of steroids alone although re-irradiation of the brain is possible but rarely undertaken.

One of the largest recent trials was the UK Royal College of Radiologists trial to compare two regimens of palliative radiotherapy for cerebral metastases was published in 1996: 544 patients with symptomatic metastases were recruited and randomized to 30 Gy in 10 fractions or 12 Gy in 2 fractions. The median survival following treatment for the two groups was 84 and 77 days, respectively and only 21 per cent of the total number of patients survived 6 months (Fig. 24.2). Although the survival advantage associated with the longer regimen was small, the benefit was greater in patients with better prognostic features. These included good performance status, solitary rather than multiple metastases, and a lower dose of dexamethasone at the start of radiotherapy (<8 mg). Patients aged 60 or less and those with secondary tumours from breast cancer also did better than others. The median survival in patients with three or more favourable features was 165 days.

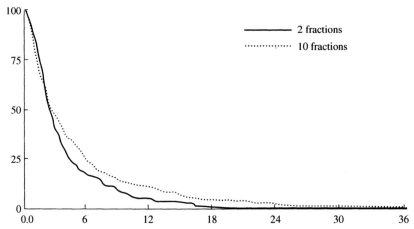

Fig. 24.2 Survival following palliative radiotherapy for cerebral metastases (reproduced from Preistman et al., *Clinical Oncology* 1996; **8**, 308–15).

The results of this UK multi-centre trial are in keeping with other large trials performed in the United States and Canada, all of which show there is no advantage to prolonged courses of radiotherapy for patients with cerebral metastases. Performance status and also the extent of extracranial disease are essential considerations in selecting patients who are likely to benefit from cranial irradiation.

Prophylactic cranial irradiation is given where there is a high risk of brain metastases. A good example is in small cell lung cancer, where as many as 50 per cent will develop intracerebral deposits and the brain is a common site of relapse for patients who have responded well to chemotherapy. Radiotherapy to the whole brain reduces the incidence of subsequent relapse to less than 10 per cent and is planned within the overall treatment, when patients have already lost their hair from chemotherapy. There is also some evidence that in selected patients who are in complete remission after chemo-radiation, prophylactic cranial irradiation prolongs survival.

Radiosurgery is a technique whereby highly localized high dose volumes can be treated using either stereotactic arcing beams from a specially adapted linear accelerator or a machine called the Gammaknife. This consists of an array of individual cobalt sources arranged in a sphere each of which can be individually shielded so that static patterns of open sources analogous to the stereotactic arc can be used. Both techniques are similar. They are limited to spherical volumes of up to 5 cm diameter and provide an alternative to surgery for solitary and localized metastases. They are particularly of value for such tumours in inoperable sites.

Chemotherapy

This treatment has a limited role as many drugs in standard doses do not effectively permeate into the CNS to achieve therapeutic levels. Drugs that do penetrate intracerebral tumour include the vinca alkaloids, etoposide, BCNU, and temozolomide. Other options are the use of high systemic doses of a drug such as methotrexate to overcome the blood–brain barrier, or to deliver the drug by the intrathecal route. The main question is whether or not the tumour type is likely to show a useful response to the available agents. In practice, chemotherapy for intracranial malignancy is restricted to very chemosensitive cancers such as germ cell tumours, choriocarcinoma, and lymphoma although response may also be seen in breast and small cell lung cancer.

Case History 24.2

A 56-year-old man had previously been treated for stage IIB non-Hodgkin's lymphoma with CHOP combination chemotherapy achieving a complete remission four months before he presented with 3 weeks of severe headache, worse on straining and a 2 day history of difficulty with speech. Examination showed no evidence of peripheral lymphoma but expressive dysphasia and a mild right

Case History 24.2 (continued)

hemiparesis. A CT scan that day showed extensive supratentorial oedema with at least three metastatic tumours seen in the cerebral hemispheres, one of which in the left temporoparietal region would account for his symptoms. He was started on high dose steroids and after urgent re-staging investigations further chemotherapy using idarubicin and cytosine arabinoside. Within 2 weeks his symptoms had settled and he returned to normal function. After 3 weeks a second cycle of chemotherapy was given. A CT scan after this showed he was in complete remission once more. Plans were made to consider further high dose chemotherapy to consolidate his response when he was readmitted after a grand mal fit leaving him once more with dysphasia and a right hemiparesis. A further CT scan showed recurrence of his metastases. He was treated with further steroids and whole brain radiotherapy delivering two fractions to a total dose of 12 Gy. Again he had a good symptomatic response returning to normal within 10 days. Six weeks later he was admitted with acute respiratory failure. His peripheral blood count showed that he was neutropenic and a chest X-ray showed widespread lung infiltration. A bone marrow was found to have extensive lymphoma infiltration. He was treated with antibiotics and steroids but deteriorated rapidly.

Practice points

* CNS relapse in chemosensitive tumours may reflect poor penetration of the CNS using standard chemotherapy.
* In chemosensitive tumours good palliation can be gained with chemotherapy.
* Relapse after chemotherapy can still be managed by radiotherapy.
* CNS relapse often heralds relapse in other systemic sites.

Empirical measures

What of the seriously ill patient, at home or in a palliative care unit? If there is a high index of clinical suspicion, it is reasonable to commence high dose dexamethasone and review the situation after 4–5 days. If there is no benefit, the diagnosis of cerebral metastases is less likely although not absolutely excluded. If there is continued deterioration, there is rarely much to be gained by pursuing either tests or steroid therapy further.

In patients who do show a symptomatic response to dexamethasone, the dose should be slowly reduced by 2 mg every 2–3 days with the aim of finding the minimum dose that is needed to control symptoms. A CT scan might be considered in these patients and this is necessary before any additional treatment such as radiotherapy could be offered. Confirmation of cerebral metastases will also assist the overall management and planning of future care, based upon the limited life expectancy and probable course of events. A more difficult decision might be whether or not to refer the patient for radiotherapy. A useful guide is to consider if this person is likely to live long enough to develop significant side effects from continued steroids. If the answer is yes, and their general status is reasonably good, then the possible option of radiotherapy should be put to the patient. While radiotherapy might offer extended life expectancy and maintain the steroid-induced improvements, it is more difficult to predict if this would achieve significant improvement in function in a patient with severe neurological impairment such as a dense hemiplegia. It is always worth discussing the individual case with an oncologist.

Key points: brain metastases management

- Initial treatment should be with steroids using dexamethasone 8 mg daily or equivalent.
- Cranial radiotherapy using 2 to 5 fractions is very effective at maintaining function and improving headache in over three-quarters of patients.
- Solitary metastases may benefit from surgical excision or radiosurgery followed by whole brain radiotherapy with 40 per cent surviving over 1 year.
- Systemic chemotherapy has a role in lymphoma, leukaemias, germ cell tumours, breast and small cell lung cancers.

Management of suspected brain metastases: clinical decisions in patients with a previous cancer diagnosis

Suspicious symptoms?

- Persistent headache, sometimes with vomiting
- Drowsiness or confusion (exclude other possible causes)
- Fit or localizing neurological symptom

Do findings on examination support diagnosis?

- Upper motor neurone abnormality
- Papilloedema
- No definite findings, but history strongly suspicious

Is investigation justifiable?

- Treatment decision will be made on basis of scan findings (good performance status, no other life-threatening disease related problems)
- If not, will information be helpful to establish prognosis and future care?

Should steroids be commenced?

- Symptoms indicate raised intracranial pressure
- Confusion or reduced conscious level
- Recurrent fits (in conjunction with anticonvulsants)

What action is needed after CT scan result?

(i) CT scan is normal

- If persistent symptoms and/or signs, proceed to MR scan

(ii) CT scan shows solitary metastasis

- Consider biopsy if radiological diagnosis uncertain or long disease-free interval
- Consider surgery if good performance status and disease in remission at other sites
- Consider chemotherapy if pathology is lymphoma or germ cell tumour
- Otherwise consider radiotherapy; refer for stereotactic treatment if available (see below)

(iii) CT scan shows multiple metastases

- Consider chemotherapy if chemosensitive tumour
- Consider whole brain irradiation (2 fractions) if poor prognosis
- Consider whole brain radiotherapy (8–10 fractions) if good perfomance status (WHO 0 or 1)

Supportive care only is the best option if

- Persistent confusion and agitation despite steroids
- Major neurological deficit with poor performance status (WHO >1)
- Active metastatic disease elsewhere
- Prognosis likely to be short (a month or less) because of other clinical problems
- Choice of the individual patient after discussion

Metastatic disease of the leptomeninges

Also referred to as meningeal carcinomatosis, this is a serious metastatic syndrome which affects the brain, spinal cord, cranial nerves, and spinal nerve roots. It is diagnosed in less than 5 per cent of cancer patients, but evidence of meningeal deposits has been found in twice as many cases when a post-mortem examination is performed. These may occur as a result of haematogenous spread via the plexus of veins associated with the axial skeleton, involvement of adjacent bone, or from within the CNS itself.

Cerebral metastases are present in some cases, and dissemination through the CSF also occurs with primary brain tumours, particularly those arising in the posterior cranial fossa (e.g. medulloblastoma and ependymomas).

The meninges may be diffusely infiltrated with sheets of tumour cells which may also infiltrate the lining of the ventricles, causing obstruction to the flow of CSF. Focal nodular lesions can develop in the surface of the brain or cord and nerve roots. The solid tumours which most frequently involve the meninges are breast cancer followed by lung and melanoma. This also occurs in up to 15 per cent of patients with leukaemia and lymphoma.

Presentation and diagnosis

Diffuse involvement of the neural axis produces a variety of signs and symptoms. The most frequently encountered are cranial nerve problems (75 per cent), headache (50 per cent), radicular or back pain (40–45 per cent), and weakness in one or more limbs (40 per cent). Other presentations include confusion, sphincter disturbances, and fits. The key to diagnosis is to suspect it; remember abnormal physical signs are even more prominent than symptoms. These are predominantly lower motor neurone lesions which may be accompanied by cranial nerve palsies and occasionally upper motor neurone signs if there are lesions within the cord.

The diagnosis can be strongly suggested on MR scan of the brain and spinal cord. Examination of the CSF by lumbar puncture is usually required to confirm it, provided there is no evidence of raised intracranial pressure on scan. The CSF protein is usually raised, glucose may be low, and malignant cells in the CSF provide absolute proof of the diagnosis in half of the cases described. Negative examinations for cytology do not exclude the diagnosis, and an initial negative CSF may be positive on a second sampling. Sometimes a myelogram is useful to demonstrate nodular filling defects or obstruction to CSF.

Treatment

This aims to halt the progression of disease and relieve symptoms but is essentially palliative except for a curable sub-group with leukaemia or lymphoma. Without treatment, unpleasant progression of neurological symptoms is inevitable and may include major cranial nerve deficits, loss of sight or hearing, and dementia. Unfortunately palliative treatment is more complex and difficult for the patient compared with the management of brain metastases.

Steroids are usually beneficial as there is often an inflammatory response to meningeal infiltration and they might also help symptoms associated with cranial nerve and radicular lesions.

Radiotherapy used alone has to be given to the entire craniospinal axis to cover all areas of disease; this requires fractionated treatment over several weeks and is associated with significant acute toxicity, especially nausea, marrow suppression, and hair loss. Cranial irradiation is better tolerated and can be combined with chemotherapy. Radiotherapy can be useful to treat symptomatic areas, for example, if there is radiological evidence of a localized deposit that is causing significant nerve root symptoms. Some patients develop compression of the spinal cord itself and localized radiotherapy should be given promptly whenever this is suspected.

Intrathecal chemotherapy enables drugs to be introduced directly into the subarachnoid space at lumbar puncture. A common regimen is to give twice-weekly intrathecal methotrexate, continuing for up to 12 treatments; it may be combined with cytosine arabinoside. Alternatively, high dose intravenous methotrexate infusions may be used but this causes systemic toxicity. Successful treatment produces improvement in signs and symptoms and is likely to prolong survival, but the prognosis remains poor. Most patients with solid tumours are unlikely to survive more than a few months and some of this time is taken up with treatment. In the presence of widespread disease, a compromise might be to give intrathecal treatments for as long as seems appropriate and use radiotherapy to palliate specific localized symptoms.

It is important to note that intrathecal chemotherapy is a potentially hazardous procedure and there are unfortunately well-documented cases of death as a result of the wrong drug, often vincristine used in combined intrathecal and intravenous schedules, into the subarachnoid space. It should therefore only be undertaken in specialized units by staff familiar with the technique conforming to strict guidelines and checking procedures.

Key points: malignant meningitis

- Typically presents with scattered neurological signs.
- Diagnosis confirmed by MR scan and CSF examination at lumbar puncture.
- Treatment is with intrathecal chemotherapy, localized irradiation to symptomatic sites and in some cases high dose systemic methotrexate.
- Prognosis is very poor with average survival less than 6 months.

Chapter 25

Tumour-associated problems: pain

The significance of pain in cancer

The popular perception of cancer is of a life-threatening illness associated, almost inevitably, with severe and intractable pain. For the patient, pain is a powerful reminder of his or her cancer, which will be even more threatening and harder to bear if the symptom becomes worse; the physical pain is enhanced by the emotional and spiritual dimensions of distress. As professionals, we can be positive in dealing with pain. We know that the majority of pains, in most patients, can be controlled by appropriate administration of analgesics and adjuvant drugs; there are often direct therapeutic approaches to tackle the underlying cause of pain. The proportion of people who despite our best endeavours are left with intractable pain are fortunately few. At the same time, professionals can be blinkered in dealing with pain especially when a cancer diagnosis has been made. Pitfalls include the failure to consider non-malignant causes or when pain is caused by tumour, to miss opportunities for useful active treatment.

This chapter provides an overview of the ways in which pain is caused by malignant disease and their treatments. These must be applied, of course, alongside the full range of pharmacological and supportive measures in pain management which are outside the scope of this text.

Incidence of pain related to primary site in early cancer

Pain is the symptom that may finally persuade a person to seek medical advice, although only 30–45 per cent of patients have pain as a significant problem at diagnosis. An obvious lump as in breast cancer or discharge and bleeding as in cervical cancer, worry the individual before pain develops. When malignancy arises in an internal organ, local invasion with consequent pain is more likely to have occurred by diagnosis but much depends upon the site itself and tissues from which the malignancy develops. Pain may be a feature of an expanding mass in a confined space (e.g. with brain tumours or head and neck cancers). In lung cancer, pain is a characteristic presenting symptom of apical and peripheral tumours that invade the adjacent pleura, chest wall, and nerves, whereas the majority which develop in the proximal bronchial tree are usually painless and declare their presence by respiratory symptoms or haemoptysis. Early gastrointestinal cancers cause little pain but may do so as they occlude the lumen. In

Table 25.1 Classification of pain associated with cancer

Pain directly caused by cancer (primary and metastatic)

    bone invasion

    soft tissue infiltration

    nerve pain

    visceral pain

Pain caused by cancer treatment

    surgery

    late radiation effects

    chemotherapy

Pain associated with progressing malignant illness

    pressure areas

    infection

    musculoskeletal

    tension headache

    colic from constipation

    dyspepsia

Incidental pain unrelated to cancer: examples

    osteoarthritis

    angina

    peripheral vascular disease

oesophageal cancer, dysphagia may be associated with painful spasm and tumours arising in the distal colon may present with pain and other symptoms of obstruction. In contrast, others which arise in relation to peripheral nerves or bone (neurosarcoma, primary bone tumours) are a cause of localized pain as an early symptom. For a classification of pain associated with cancer, see Table 25.1.

Incidence of pain in late cancer

In advanced cancer, 70–80 per cent of patients have pain as a significant problem, although there is still some variation by primary site (Table 25.2). Again this reflects the site itself and the adjacent structures invaded by local progression and also the pattern of metastatic involvement, particularly bone. These patients are also more likely to have pain associated with the effects of treatment or as an indirect consequence of the illness such as musculoskeletal discomfort or pressure sores. In cancer, 75 per cent of pain can usually be attributed directly to the malignancy. All cancer can be associated with pain; not all will be severe and the expression of pain varies considerably with each individual.

Table 25.2 Prevalence of pain by primary site among cancer patients attending six palliative care centres (from Auvinen *et al.* 1996)

Primary site	Prevalence of pain: patients surveyed (%)			
	None	**Mild**	**Moderate**	**Severe**
Prostate	17	22	20	41
Oesophagus	29	21	13	38
Gynaecological	10	10	47	33
Colorectal	21	21	27	32
Haematological	13	29	26	32
Head and neck	17	11	43	29
Lung	26	23	30	21
Breast	22	25	31	21
Stomach	26	30	26	17

Reproduced by permission of Elsevier Science, Inc. from Prevalence of symptoms among patients with advanced cancer (from Vainio, A., Auvinen, A., and members of the Symptom Prevalence Group) *Journal of Pain and Symptom Management*, Vol. 12, pp. 3–10. Copyright 1996 by the US Cancer Pain Relief Committee and reproduced with permission of the author.

Mechanisms of cancer pain

Pain arising from somatic soft tissues

A malignant tumour invades adjacent normal tissue; as it outstrips its blood supply areas of necrosis develop. Pain associated with invasion depends on the presence of nocioceptors and an intact afferent pathway: areas of superficial tumour fungation or ulceration tend to be painless as normal tissue with its sensory supply has been destroyed. However, the margins are often tender and hypersensitive and this may be mediated by tumour products and host prostaglandins; often cutaneous tumour infiltration is associated with a marked inflammatory response with soreness and itch. Local spread tends to be within fascial planes and a tumour mass will eventually cause compression of normal tissue if in a confined space. Secondary obstruction to venous and lymphatic drainage adds to the local swelling and pain results from distension of fascial compartments and the overlying skin. Both nerve compression and nerve infiltration are part of these processes, all of which cause nociceptive stimulation, a major component of cancer pain. Pain may be exacerbated by infection, haematoma, and ischaemia.

Painful somatic stimuli reach the spinal tracts via the segmental dorsal root ganglia. Pain arising in the head is mediated via the trigeminal nerve (face, oral and nasal epithelium, eyes, and meninges) or the glossopharyngeal nerve (oropharynx and pharynx). The latter supplies sensation to the tragus and this is why a tonsillar cancer can present with earache. In addition, pain from larynx and pharynx may be referred via vagal pathways to somatic representation in the external auditory canal.

Bone pain

Although bone initially provides a barrier to tumour spread, local progression of a primary tumour eventually invades adjacent bone. Examples are a cancer of the floor of mouth invading mandible; a peripheral lung cancer destroying ribs, or a rectal cancer growing back into the sacrum. Bone pain is more commonly the result of metastatic spread, initially as blood-borne tumour colonies within the marrow cavity which eventually invade the bone itself.

The source of pain due to bone invasion is nociceptive stimulation of the sensitive periosteum, which produces symptoms before a breach of the bone cortex is apparent radiologically. An isotope scan is a more sensitive detector of bone involvement than X-rays and will demonstrate increased osteoblast activity but may not show abnormality in purely lytic lesions such as those due to myeloma. It is also well known that a patient with multiple areas of increased uptake on a scan does not necessarily experience pain at all, or indeed any of these sites. In contrast, some patients with extensive marrow involvement by leukaemia or metastatic cancer may have generalized aching discomfort with no abnormality on a bone scan. The development of pain is related to periosteal invasion, the extent of bone destruction and also to the local inflammatory responses mediated by tumour products and prostaglandins. The latter may explain why hormone-modulating treatments, such as hypophysectomy, castration, or use of LHRH agonists can produce a rapid improvement in pain for patients with breast and prostate cancer. A larger tumour mass may cause pain related to ischaemic necrosis.

Periosteal inflammation may also be a paraneoplastic phenomenon. Hypertrophic pulmonary osteoarthropathy (HPOA) occurs most frequently in patients with lung cancer; typical findings are marked tenderness of the wrists and ankles in association with finger clubbing while the bone scan shows increased activity adjacent to the cortex of long bones.

Bone pain, however, is often complex and involves a number of pathophysiological mechanisms. Tumour arising in bone in turn invades adjacent soft tissues; there may be invasion or compression of adjacent nerves and skeletal muscle spasm. These are discussed further in Chapter 21. Pain management is aided by recognition of these components and also of developments such as mechanical instability or fracture. While bone pain is fundamentally a nociceptive process, nerve damage can lead to neuropathic pain as an associated problem.

Visceral pain

This pain is produced by nociceptive stimulation of receptors in the wall of a hollow viscus or duct or the surrounding capsule. The mechanism may be obstruction by tumour with distension and smooth muscle spasm or direct tumour infiltration with an inflammatory response. Ischaemia is a further cause of visceral pain and may be encountered when there is invasion or thrombosis of mesenteric vessels. This can be a problem for patients with bowel cancer or any widespread intraperitoneal malignancy; often the pain is triggered by eating.

Organ enlargement due to metastatic deposits causes stretching of the sensitive capsule. The tenderness associated with an enlarged liver is a familiar problem; the spleen is a less common site of metastases in solid tumours but painful splenomegaly is sometimes a problem in haematological cancers and lymphoma.

Visceral pain is suggested by pain that is difficult for the patient to localize and also if pain is intense, episodic and associated with other autonomic effects such as sweating, pallor, and nausea. It is transmitted via sympathetic afferent fibres whose dorsal ganglia lie between T_2–L_3 and pain is perceived to arise within the somatic distribution of the same spinal segment on the trunk and proximal extremities. Upper abdominal and back pain from locally advanced gastric and pancreatic cancer is caused by infiltration of the coeliac plexus. However, these and other retroperitoneal tumours may also produce somatic pain from direct infiltration of the parietal peritoneum and abdominal wall and also the paravertebral tissues. Thus, visceral pain must be distinguished from radicular pain of somatic origin with a similar distribution although both may coexist; where this is the case it may be necessary to combine a coeliac block with intrathecal alcohol injection at the appropriate segment to control all pain. In addition, there may be pain due to biliary tree distension or occlusion of the duodenum, usually with tumour in the head of the pancreas.

Pelvic visceral pain is mediated via T_{10}–L_1 ganglia through the superior hypogastric plexus, thus pain arising from cervix, ovary, bladder, and rectum is referred to the lower abdominal wall and groins. However, there is also some sacral innervation of the bladder neck and cervix which is referred through the parasympathetic afferents of the inferior hypogastric plexus (S_2–S_4) to the buttocks and upper thigh.

There is a connection between afferent vagal fibres from upper thoracic ganglia and the trigeminal tract and tracts in the cervical segments and there is also direct somatic vagal innervation to the external auditory canal and skin behind the ear. As noted with head and neck pain, pain arising from trachea, oesophagus, pharynx, and larynx can travel via vagal afferents to be perceived in the unilateral face and ear. Occasionally lung cancer can cause atypical facial pain.

Nerve damage and neuropathic pain

Nerve compression and infiltration by tumour will initially produce aching pain referred in the distribution of that nerve which may be associated with numbness or motor weakness; this is a direct nociceptive effect and may be reversed by steroids to reduce tissue swelling together with active treatment such as radiotherapy. Local progression of disease leads to destruction of nerve tissue and the proximal neurones may be the source of spontaneous, afferent activity into ascending pain pathways. This occurs as a result of damage to a nerve peripherally or within the central nervous system.

The characteristics of this nerve damage pain are that it is felt in areas of altered sensation which may have features of hypoaesthesia, allodynia, or hyperalgesia. It has qualities such as burning, shooting, or stabbing and may have sudden crescendo episodes with no apparent precipitating cause. Another important feature is that neuropathic pain often does not respond well to opioid analgesics and consequently it is a common component of cancer pain that proves difficult to manage. The following situations illustrate tumour-associated nerve damage with the frequent development of neuropathic pain:

Head and neck cancer in which there may be perineural invasion, particularly a feature of adenoid cystic salivary gland tumours, and spread through the foramina in the skull that are occupied by cranial nerves.

Brachial plexus involvement in apical lung cancers (Pancoast tumours) and locally advanced breast cancer: pain is felt in the shoulder and arm with sensory and motor changes in the C_8–T_1 distribution. There may be extension of disease into the spinal canal and epidural space in up to half of the patients with apical lung cancer and these patients may develop bilateral pain and ultimately cord compression.

Lumbosacral plexus involvement by primary cancers in the retroperitoneal region and pelvis and also as a result of metastatic spread to para-aortic and iliac nodes. This situation is encountered in renal, rectal, and cervical cancers. Pain is in the low back, leg, and foot depending on the site of tumour; it is usually unilateral but may affect both sides.

Involvement of the spine Vertebral metastases at any level may be associated with extradural tumour that compresses nerve roots and the spinal cord. Radiological evidence of metastatic disease in the vertebral body is usually apparent, such as damage to the pedicles, loss of height or asymmetrical collapse, or localized abnormality on the bone scan. However, if these investigations are negative, clinical suspicion should be pursued by requesting an MRI scan which will demonstrate disease within the spinal canal in the absence of gross bone pathology. Direct invasion of the spine extradural space may develop from paravertebral tumour extension. Below the level of the L_1 vertebral body, the cauda equina is affected. In the absence of bone involvement, localized radicular pain may be due to meningeal deposits.

Pain due to cancer treatment

Surgery

Chronic pain following surgery is frequently due to nerve division and regeneration. Exquisitely sensitive, well-localized pain indicates the presence of a neuroma formed by the regenerating proximal axon. In other cases there may be neuropathic pain within the territory of the traumatized peripheral nerve. Examples are not uncommon following thoracotomy, mastectomy, or radical node dissections. Persistent phantom limb sensations may be painful and follow amputation, especially when the tumour arising in the limb is a source of poorly controlled pain.

Radiotherapy

Acute radiation reactions involving epithelial tissues will be painful but self-limiting as the epithelium has the capacity to regenerate within a few weeks. The late effects of radiation on normal tissues appear 6–12 months onwards following treatment and are usually irreversible. The main features are increased fibrosis and reduced vascularity so that the normal healing response to injury is not only reduced but may lead to further tissue breakdown. At worst, tissue necrosis of bone and soft tissue develops which is usually painful. Radionecrosis can result from inhomogenous dose distribution in prescribed radiotherapy treatment which produces 'hot spots' of absorbed dose that exceed normal tissue tolerance. Even within acceptable dose ranges there is variation in individual sensitivity and occasionally patients experience severe late effects.

Apart from necrosis, fibrosed, contracted soft tissue may cause local discomfort and may be a source of neuropathic pain if peripheral nerves are involved. For example, a small number of women with breast cancer who undergo radiotherapy may subsequently have a persistently tender breast or chest wall discomfort associated with allodynia. Pelvic irradiation for bladder, prostate, or cervical cancer can lead to painful cystitis or proctitis associated with tenesmoid discomfort. On rare occasions, a post-radiation stricture of a segment of bowel can lead to obstruction. A more frequently encountered late problem in head and neck cancer is dental caries particularly associated with reduction in flow of saliva. Dental infection and surgery (e.g. an extraction), can lead to osteonecrosis of the irradiated mandible.

It should be emphasized that these are uncommon problems and develop in a very small proportion of patients who receive radical treatments. They should not be encountered after palliative radiotherapy. It is important to remember that the cause of pain is more likely to be due to recurrent or metastatic disease than post-radiotherapy complications in the majority of patients.

Case History 25.1

Chronic pain following cancer treatment

Mr B is a fireman who underwent surgery followed by radiotherapy for a malignant tumour of his left parotid gland. He made an excellent recovery and 18 months later has no evidence of disease. However he is unable to return to work because he has persistent burning pain over the left side of his face and such exquisite hypersensitivity that he cannot wear his helmet. He avoids any light touch which might set off intense pain. Apart from this, there is little to find; there is some subcutaneous thickening due to fibrosis with loss of hair within the irradiated area.

Case History 25.1 (continued)

This has the hallmarks of neuropathic pain and amitriptyline is prescribed. This helps with the burning pain but the hypersensitivity remains a problem. He is encouraged to try topical 0.15 per cent capsaicin cream applied four times daily. Although initially this causes unpleasant irritation, after he has persevered for 2–3 weeks there is considerable improvement. He is eventually able to return to work.

Chemotherapy

Chemotherapy-induced stomatitis is analogous to an acute radiation reaction and resolves with epithelial healing. It is a particular problem with drugs such as methotrexate or 5-fluoruracil (5-FU) and may be made worse by concomitant fungal infection. Patients are often more susceptible to bacterial and viral infections as a consequence of neutropenia and immunosuppression. Herpes zoster infection can present with pain and hypersensitivity preceding the skin lesions, followed by troublesome neuralgia within the affected dermatome. This is seen particularly in patients with Hodgkin's disease and lymphomas.

Some drugs, notably vincristine, cisplatin, and the taxols, produce a sensory neuritis. This starts with paraesthesiae in hands and feet and can progress to loss of touch and proprioception with disappearance of the tendon reflexes. The discomfort may develop into a severe neuropathic pain which does respond to tricyclic antidepressants and anticonvulsants. As symptoms appear during treatment, the responsible drug may be reduced in dose or discontinued. Effects are usually dose-related and slowly subside after treatment has finished but this may take many months.

Steroids are incorporated into some chemotherapy regimens and are frequently used in palliation of a range of symptoms. Pseudo-rheumatism is a rebound effect of steroid withdrawal; avascular necrosis is a rarely encountered problem associated with longer-term use. More common are painful side effects of continued use such as dyspepsia and musculoskeletal pains associated with cushingoid obesity and osteoporotic vertebral collapse.

Case History 25.2

Severe back pain: a diagnostic dilemma

An elderly lady had a simple mastectomy and also a bowel resection of a Dukes B tumour in the sigmoid colon. She is followed up by the surgical team and appears to be doing very well. However her daughter requests an early appointment because of pain. She has bad pain, with no radiation, in her lower dorsal spine which began quite suddenly after she had lifted a bowl of washing. An X-ray shows wedge collapse of T_{12} and she is referred for radiotherapy to presumed metastatic disease.

The oncologist is not so sure. She has considerable osteoporotic changes in her spine but there is no other evidence of relapse of her malignancy. A bone scan is requested because if this were to show multiple, asymmetrical increased uptake in the skeleton this would support a diagnosis of metastases. As it transpired, the bone scan showed increased uptake only at T_{12}. As her pain persisted, an MR scan was requested. The radiologist reported that this showed no evidence of cancer and the appearances were consistent with osteoporotic collapse. There was no indication for radiotherapy and pain was managed with simple analgesia and TENS. The painful episode resolved within 6 weeks.

Acute pain

Cancer pain is usually thought of as chronic pain, but may have acute onset in some situations. The following possibilities should be considered:

1. *Events directly related to the presence of tumour*:

- growth of tumour to cause nerve or spinal cord compression
- sudden enlargement of tumour mass due to haemorrhage or cystic degeneration
- pathological fracture
- obstruction of a hollow viscus or duct
- perforation of tissue such as bowel

2. *Events associated with cancer although not caused directly by tumour*:

- thromboembolism
- ischaemia and infarction (due to compression or embolus)
- haemorrhage
- infection
- peptic ulceration and perforation

3. *Events not associated with malignancy* (e.g myocardial infarction, appendicitis)

Case History 25.3

Acute pain in a patient with advanced malignant melanoma

Mr B has bone and liver metastases from a malignant melanoma which was removed from the sole of his foot five years earlier. For some time, his bone pain has been well controlled using fentanyl patches, 75 μg/h. In recent weeks he has been bothered by epigastric discomfort and acid reflux which has been eased by antacid medicine.

> *Case History 25.3 (continued)*
>
> One night, his wife calls out the emergency doctor because he has suddenly developed severe upper abdominal pain. He is pale, nauseated and sweating and has extreme abdominal tenderness. He is sent to the local hospital with a diagnosis of 'peritonitis ?perforation'. The surgical team confirms marked tenderness over his enlarged liver but bowel sounds are normal and there is no rebound pain on pressure. Abdominal X-rays show no free gas or other abnormality. They decide to monitor him overnight and keep him nil by mouth. The likely diagnosis is a bleed into a large metastatic tumour within the liver.
>
> Diamorphine injections (20–30 mg) help the pain but after several doses he is showing signs of toxicity. A subcutaneous infusion of ketorolac 60 mg/24 h is commenced with noticeable improvement in his pain and tenderness. This is continued for 48 h, in combination with an H2 antagonist, until he is able to take oral medication.

Practice points

- Causes of acute pain in cancer include pathological fracture and pressure from tumour or a tumour-related bleed within a confined space.
- Malignant melanoma is a highly vascular tumour and such bleeds are not uncommon.

Pain management

Careful assessment of each different pain and associated symptoms and signs is vital to determine the probable nature and anatomical site of the underlying disease process. The oncological approaches discussed here are only part of total pain management: a decision to treat with radiotherapy should, of course, be accompanied by administration of analgesics and attention to the other concerns occupying the patient. As with any cancer treatment, the use of interventions for pain relief must entail consideration of what this entails for the individual and also a judgement over whether someone with advanced disease is likely to survive long enough to benefit. However, active treatment is often justifiable even in the last weeks if it brings a chance to improve mobility and independence or enables reduction in high doses of opioids which in themselves can cause additional burdens.

Surgical procedures

Orthopaedic surgery is important in the management of metastatic bone disease. Fractures of long bones are dealt with by internal fixation whenever possible and this may entail the use of methyl methacrylate cement as well as nails to stabilize the bone. Apart from enabling rapid restoration of function, this is important because bone healing is often poor in pathological fractures due to the presence of tumour. In one series, only 35 per cent of fractures showed evidence of osseous union after 6 months. It was very poor in fractures due to lung cancer and the highest rates of healing were seen in myeloma, which may reflect the use of successful systemic therapy. Fractures involving the neck or head of the humerus or femur are more difficult and an arthroplasty may be necessary.

Radiotherapy is given to the bone post-operatively to avoid local tumour progression into the soft tissues or causing the nails and plate to loosen. The presence of the metal does not have any significant effect on the radiation; another practical point is that radiotherapy can be given through plaster casts in situations where external immobilization has been used.

Surgical decompression of the spinal canal including sacrum may be performed where there is early and acute cord or nerve root compression. This may be combined with stabilization of the spine, particularly when there is pain on movement. Instability of the cervical spine is difficult to manage and sometimes the only option is an external fixation device which patients can find hard to tolerate.

Other examples of surgical relief of pain include interventions for intestinal and urinary obstruction which are discussed in other chapters, and also in dealing with radionecrosis which involves excision of the affected tissues and reconstruction of the defect.

Case History 25.4

A 47-year-old man underwent a radical nephrectomy for a tumour arising in the left kidney. Eighteen months later he developed bone metastases. He complains of pain in his right groin and thigh; his bone scan does show increased uptake in his pelvis and upper femur so radiotherapy is given to this site.

Five weeks later he is admitted as an emergency for pain control. The recent radiotherapy has not helped and he now experiences excruciating pain in his back and right thigh when he tries to walk: at rest he is pain free. The severe pain diminishes within a minute when he lies back on the bed. He has altered sensation over the lower thigh.

Although he believes that the radiotherapy has not worked, the problem now appears to arise in his lumbar spine which was not previously treated. An X-ray shows destruction of the third lumbar vertebral body. He quickly develops opioid toxicity as his dose of controlled-release morphine is increased; ketamine is tried but he has terrifying nightmares and does not want to continue with this. Introduction of an anticonvulsant (gabapentin) has not made much difference either.

The initial plan was to proceed with radiotherapy to his lumbar spine, but he is extremely incapacitated and likely to remain so, therefore the advice of an orthopaedic

> ### Case History 25.4 (continued)
>
> surgeon is sought. He requests an MR scan of his spine, which shows no disease in adjacent vertebrae, but there is a substantial soft tissue mass that is encroaching upon the epidural space around the L3 nerve root. His chest X-ray is clear.
>
> Spinal surgery is proposed as the best option to control pain and restore function. This is preceded by embolisation of the tumour, then tumour and bone resection followed by stabilisation of the spine by metal implants.
>
> Although a major procedure, his post-operative recovery is uneventful. He is discharged home three weeks later on considerably reduced dose of analgesics and a programme of rehabilitation. He attends for radiotherapy to his spine following this.
>
> ## Practice points
>
> - Palliative radiotherapy would be expected to have some benefit within 2–4 weeks of treatment.
> - It is useful to find out exactly where radiotherapy has been given: persistent pain may be originating from another site.
> - Severe incident pain is usually difficult to manage without considerable restriction in mobility. Surgical intervention should be considered in such situations, depending on the extent of disease and fitness of the patient.
> - Bone metastases from renal cancer are often very destructive and resistant to palliative radiotherapy.
> - They are usually well-vascularized, therefore selective embolisation of the main arterial supply can destroy tumour and also make surgery easier.

Radiotherapy

The role of radiotherapy in the management of bone pain is discussed in detail in Chapter 21. It is a relatively straightforward treatment for the patient, and is often given in a single session. The majority of patients have reduction in pain within 4 weeks, and for about 50 per cent within 2 weeks so that it is valuable treatment even in the terminal stages of the illness. Careful localization of the source of symptoms is important and radiotherapy will not reverse established neuropathic pain nor incident pain associated with vertebral collapse, unless the pain is primarily due to soft tissue tumour mass compressing the nerve root.

Radiotherapy will relieve pain associated with soft tissue infiltration by tumour (e.g. invading the chest or abdominal wall), or when this is due to a well-defined mass of tumour or involved nodes that are causing compression of a nerve or nerve plexus. CT scanning may be needed to define the extent of the tumour and to plan radiotherapy treatment. This is generally given in short regimens over 2–3 weeks. Tender cutaneous deposits are easily treated, often with single electron treatments. This causes a temporary skin reaction and pigmentation of the treated area may follow.

Palliative radiotherapy relieves pain by achieving reduction in the mass and also affects tumour and host release of nocioceptive substances. Treatment may be effective even if there is only partial regression of the tumour, but in these situations the improvement is unlikely to be long-lasting. Radiotherapy is less often used to treat visceral pain. It can be used to treat inoperable pancreatic cancers and also pain associated with inoperable renal cancer or adrenal metastasis (providing the function of the contralateral kidney is satisfactory). It has no useful role in widespread intraperitoneal disease or bowel obstruction, with the exception of problems associated with highly radiosensitive malignancy such as lymphoma.

Embolization

Therapeutic embolization may be an option to consider if there is a localized tumour causing troublesome pain, usually despite previous radiotherapy. It is used in patients with renal cancers to treat the primary or secondary deposits, as these tend to have a rich vascular supply. Angiography is performed to demonstrate the tumour vessels and to determine suitability for embolization. This is more likely to be successful if the tumour arterial supply is from one dominant vessel which can then be catheterized: this is illustrated in Fig. 25.1. Microspheres are injected which lodge in the distal small vessels to cause ischaemia and necrosis of the tumour itself without damaging normal tissues.

Systemic therapies

While localized treatments such as surgery and radiotherapy can be directed at the immediate cause of pain, systemic treatments may have a valuable contribution. This applies to the more chemotherapy- and hormone-responsive disease, particularly haematological malignancy, small cell lung cancer, prostate, and breast cancer, where widespread bone involvement may respond. This is usually combined with local treatment to localized areas. Bisphosphonates appear to reverse the progressive bone destruction in myeloma and breast cancer with a reduction in the number of pathological fractures sustained. However, this is also achieved by effective anti-tumour therapy. The cost–benefit ratio of long-term routine use in these patients is difficult to assess.

Key points

- When localized pain develops in the vicinity of a previous primary tumour there is always a suspicion of recurrence: if persistent, previous scans should be reviewed and repeated.

- Metastatic bone involvement can be difficult to distinguish from degenerative disease or osteoporosis. If X-rays are unhelpful, consider a bone scan or MRI scan.
- Infection and haemorrhage within a tumour can cause sudden exacerbation of pain.
- Surgery for pain relief usually has immediate benefit but is set against the time for hospitalization and recovery. Radiotherapy may take 2–4 weeks to achieve full benefit and again, this must be set against the likely prognosis.

(a)

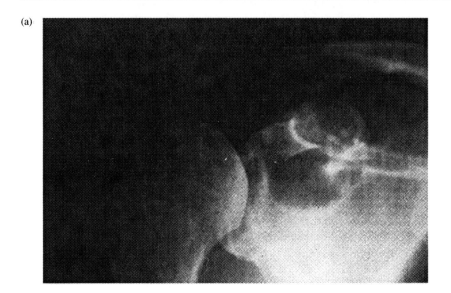

(b)

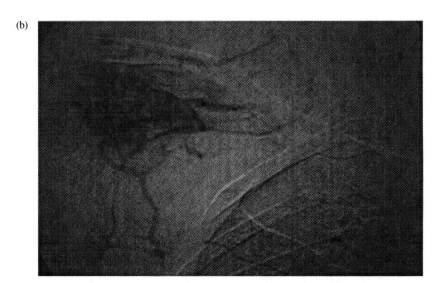

Fig. 25.1 Embolization of a bone metastasis from a primary renal cancer, which has caused progressive bone destruction and pain despite previous radiotherapy. *(a) X-ray appearance of scapula. (b) Selective angiography of vascular supply to tumour prior to embolization.*

Case History 25.5

A 59-year-old patient had undergone mastectomy and axillary node clearance for a stage 2 carcinoma of the breast about 3 years earlier. She had been well on follow-up apart from mild lymphoedema of her arm and this had developed gradually within 6 months of her surgery. It was managed by a compression sleeve and manual lymphatic drainage given by her husband.

However she began to complain of soreness in her arm and the swelling seemed to be worse. There was no evidence of superficial infection and she was told that the pain was due to her lymphoedema.

As the weeks went by, the swelling became worse and she began to lose function in her hand, for example when attempting to eat a meal, she could not use a fork. The pain became worse: by this time she had a nagging ache from her shoulder down the outer aspect of her arm. There was an unpleasant burning sensation extending into her hand so that she could not tolerate wearing her sleeve. The swelling increased further, but there were no palpable lymph nodes in her neck or axilla so she was reassured and again the problem was attributed to her lymphoedema.

The GP referred her for a second opinion by an oncologist, who requested an MR scan. Unfortunately this showed local recurrence of tumour around the brachial plexus but other investigations showed no evidence of distant metastases. Her hormone treatment was switched from tamoxifen to anastrazole, and she underwent radiotherapy. This helped some of the pain but the unpleasant burning persisted. The swelling improved gradually over the following 3 months but remained a significant problem. After introduction of amitriptyline, she was able to tolerated bandaging to try to reduce the limb volume.

Practice points

- Lymphoedema is usually not associated with pain unless there is myo-ligamentous strain, caused by massive swelling, or a superficial cellulitis (obvious redness and warmth).

- If radical axillary dissection has been performed, routine post-operative radiotherapy is avoided as this increases the risk of significant lymphoedema. However this may be needed if there is subsequent recurrence to prevent uncontrolled regional disease.

- Nocioceptive pain due to tumour pressure or invasion will respond to radiotherapy but this is unlikely to reverse pain with established neuropathic feature.

Chapter 26

Other tumour-associated problems

This chapter covers renal failure, adrenal failure, hypercalcaemia, paraneoplastic syndromes, cachexia, limb oedema and thrombosis.

Renal failure

Malignant disease can lead to impairment of renal function in a number of ways; the main causes are given in Table 26.1. Obstruction of the urinary tract is a common development associated with advanced pelvic and retroperitoneal tumours and also metastatic involvement of para-aortic nodes, particularly by lymphoma. Renal metastases are rarely recognized clinically but are not uncommon findings in post-mortem. They are also picked up as incidental findings on CT scans; those arising from solid tumours are often bilateral and are seen within the peripheral cortex of the organ. Although they may cause loin pain and haematuria, these are often asymptomatic and impairment of renal function is unusual. In contrast, haematological malignancies may diffusely infiltrate the kidneys and this does contribute to renal failure. Ureteric metastases, also frequently bilateral, may cause obstruction and post-renal failure. They also cause backache, loin pain, and ureteric colic. The commonest primary sites are cancers of the breast, stomach, and bowel and also melanoma and lung cancer.

The diagnosis of renal failure and the underlying cause is important in the palliative care of cancer patients:

◆ as an additional source of symptoms

◆ there may be appropriate intervention to restore renal function

◆ as a cause of drug toxicity: it is important to review and modify prescriptions

◆ as a major influence on prognosis

Acute renal failure in a patient with previously normal kidney function may be the result of sudden and severe reduction in renal perfusion. This may follow haemorrhage or septicaemia and may also result from prolonged vomiting, diarrhoea, or losses from proximal bowel fistulae. Usually such causes are apparent and the patient is dehydrated, hypotensive, and passes very small amounts of urine. Pre-renal failure is characterized by a low urinary sodium excretion (<15 mmol/L) and a high urine:plasma osmolarity ratio (>2). How actively this is managed depends on consideration of each situation and the other problems faced by the patient. It may be justifiable to give intravenous

Table 26.1 Impaired renal function due to malignancy

Directly due to tumour

    obstruction

    infiltration

    Bence–Jones proteinuria

Indirectly caused by tumour

    hypercalcaemia

    amyloidosis

    hyperuricaemia

    infection

    dehydration

    renal vein thrombosis

    paraneoplastic effects

    disseminated intravascular coagulopathy

Caused by treatment

    chemotherapy

    radiation

fluids and electrolytes in the short term (e.g. if there is a reasonable chance of controlling fluid loss and haemorrhage), or where septicaemia is being actively treated.

Urinary tract obstruction can develop in cancers of the prostate and bladder in which the urethra or ureteric orifices become occluded. The lower segments of ureter on one or both sides may be obstructed by pelvic malignancies such as carcinoma of the cervix; the ureters may also be compressed or enveloped by tumour that arises in the retroperitoneum or involves para-aortic nodes. Multifocal transitional cell carcinomas of the urinary tract can develop within both ureters; metastatic spread to the ureters is rare but does occasionally arise. When patients have previously undergone surgery or radiotherapy, a further possibility is obstruction due to fibrosis rather than disease.

Unilateral ureteric obstruction that develops gradually is often asymptomatic but produces hydronephrosis accompanied by deterioration in function of the kidney. Acute obstruction may cause painful ureteric spasm or dull aching in the flank and haematuria is a sign of tumour within or invading the ureter. Unilateral obstruction will not affect renal function provided that of the contralateral kidney is adequate, but complete obstruction will lead to cause anuria and renal failure. Gradual progression of bilateral disease gives rise to symptoms, particularly as the urea rises to 25 mmol/L and beyond. Important relevant findings on clinical examination would include prostatic enlargement, the presence of a pelvic or abdominal mass, and whether or not the bladder is palpable.

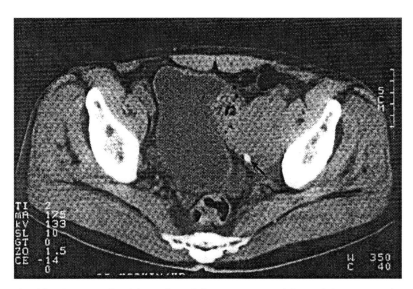

Fig. 26.1 CT scan of pelvis to show left ureter arrowed (containing contrast) surrounded by tumour.

The aim of further investigations would be to determine the site of obstruction and the underlying cause. An ultrasound easily demonstrates dilatation of the descending tracts and renal pelvis and will usually indicate the site of obstruction. An intravenous pyelogram is contraindicated in uraemic patients but cystoscopy and retrograde studies can be performed if necessary. An isotope renogram may be used to assess the function of each kidney. Additional information on the extent of tumour and node enlargement is obtained from CT scanning (see Fig. 26.1).

Immediate relief of ureteric obstruction is achieved by percutaneous nephrostomy: a short catheter is passed through the skin under ultrasound guidance directly into the renal pelvis and upper ureter to enable external drainage of one or both kidneys. This enables active treatment such as pelvic radiotherapy to be commenced. However, this procedure is not without problems. Nephrostomy tubes cause discomfort, infection, and can leak or fall out. A more permanent solution is to insert internal ureteric stents through the narrowed ureteric segments at cystoscopy (see Fig. 26.2). This may not be achieved if the ureteric orifice within the bladder cannot be identified. Alternatively, an ileal loop diversion may be considered for obstruction at or below the level of the bladder.

Although it is obvious that the goal of management is to relieve the obstruction, the overall benefit for the individual has to be carefully considered. Reversal of renal failure to enable active treatment of the underlying cancer is certainly justifiable, such as a patient with locally advanced cervical cancer or with retroperitoneal node involvement by testicular teratoma. Equally, it would be important to deal with treatment-related complications such as post-radiation fibrosis. Decisions are harder when there is recurrent disease, especially if no further cancer treatment is feasible. Without intervention, life expectancy

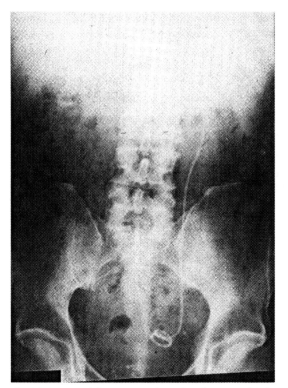

Fig. 26.2 X-ray of the same patient showing stent in the ureter.

may be a matter of weeks. Palliative urinary diversion will improve symptoms but often replace these by the problems of nephrostomy tubes and the on-going symptoms associated with the progression of the cancer. Unfortunately, the outcome is still very poor for patients with advanced cancer and bilateral obstruction even if the latter is reversed. In these situations, median survival has been found to be 3 months or less.

Chronic renal damage may be the result of chemotherapy and drugs such as cisplatin or mitomycin can cause irreversible changes. Other drugs used in palliative care may also be responsible, especially NSAIDs. It is standard practice to monitor kidney function carefully when using any nephrotoxic agent in chemotherapy regimens so that treatment is modified or stopped before the effects are clinically significant. Similarly, the sensitivity of the kidney to radiation is well recognized so that either the dose is limited or careful planning is used to ensure that a minimum of renal tissue is within the treatment volume.

Any occlusion of the urinary tract, or the presence of tumour in the bladder, is commonly associated with infection, which in turn can exacerbate renal impairment. Excretion of light chain paraproteins in myeloma may directly damage the glomeruli and tubules and this can be compounded by dehydration, hypercalcaemia, hyperuricaemia, amyloid, or infection. Some patients with myeloma are in acute renal failure at diagnosis; this is treated actively, using dialysis if necessary, prior to commencement of chemotherapy. At one time impaired renal function appeared to adversely affect the prognosis but now this appears to be less significant.

The nephrotic syndrome, characterized by excessive urinary protein loss and peripheral oedema in association with impaired renal function, can occur as a paraneoplastic phenomenon in Hodgkin's disease and also due to amyloid deposition. This is seen in 5–10 per cent of patients myeloma but can arise in other types of cancer. Patients require diuretics and dietary protein supplements. In primary renal tumours, the nephrotic syndrome arises as a result of thrombosis of the renal vein and inferior vena cava; infusion of antifibrinolytics and anticoagulants may be tried in these situations.

In the context of palliative care it is likely that the approach to management will be to address the symptoms rather than the underlying cause. This will include treatment of infection and vigilance in prescribing to avoid additional problems as many drugs are excreted through the kidney. Nausea and vomiting due primarily to uraemia should respond to haloperidol. A dietician will provide helpful guidance but the burden of dietary restrictions or biochemical monitoring would not be appropriate in patients with advanced cancer.

Key points

- Interventions for urinary tract obstruction are appropriate if there is possible treatment for the underlying malignancy, but otherwise the prognosis is poor even with relief of the obstruction.
- Metastatic involvement of the kidneys and ureters is often unrecognized as a cause of symptoms.
- Remember neurological causes of urinary retention – the classic example is the patient with cancer of the prostate and early spinal cord compression due to bone metastases.
- NSAIDS can cause acute renal failure and worsen existing renal impairment.
- In established renal impairment avoid antacids, effervescent analgesics (sodium and aluminium salt content) and reduce the dose of opioids, anxiolytics and antipsychotic drugs.

Adrenal failure

Aetiology

Prolonged corticosteroid administration in doses of >7.5 mg prednisolone daily or equivalent for more than 7 days will cause biochemical suppression of endogenous adrenal function. This may not be clinically apparent unless the steroid is suddenly stopped or there is additional stress such as infection or surgery. However, some chemotherapy schedules use high doses of steroids within each course which are discontinued abruptly without problems for most patients. Patients requiring longer-term steroids, such as those with brain tumours, are sometimes given steroids on alternate days rather than daily as this may cause less inhibition of the pituitary–adrenal axis, but for these patients any steroid withdrawal should be done gradually.

Aminoglutethimide is used in metastatic breast cancer to inhibit oestradiol synthesis but this also blocks the production of other steroids and therefore hydrocortisone is often given concurrently. Dexamethasone is often used in palliative medicine but like betamethasone, has virtually no mineralocorticoid effect. It should not be given in low doses (3 mg or less) in conjunction with aminoglutethimide as metabolism is increased, leading to a further rise in ACTH.

Adrenal failure may be due to replacement by metastatic tumour which is found in 40 per cent of lung cancer patients at post-mortem and up to 20 per cent of those dying from breast cancer. Infiltration is also seen in leukaemia and lymphoma. Adrenal lesions are now detected more frequently as incidental findings on CT scans; the differential diagnosis includes hyper-plasia, benign tumours, or phaeochromocytoma. Primary adrenal tumours are more often associated with ectopic hormone production than hypoadrenalism. An even less common cause is hypopituitarism due to a primary pituitary tumour or as a late effect of radiotherapy for pituitary and primary brain tumours. In these cases, deficiency of corticosteroids is often associated with loss of growth hormone, gonadotrophins, and thyroxine.

Symptoms

Adrenal metastases are often asymptomatic but those that reach 5 cm or more are likely to be associated with pain. Adrenal failure is usually of gradual onset and causes weakness, lethargy, and anorexia which are, of course, common symptoms in many patients with advanced cancer. Patients become hyperpigmented due to high levels of ACTH, and this is more apparent in the buccal mucosa, skin creases, or at sites of friction by shoulder straps. Eventually nausea and vomiting occur, and low blood pressure with dizziness due to postural hypotension. The biochemical profile typically shows a low sodium, raised potassium, and fasting hypoglycaemia but may be normal. The diagnosis of primary adrenal failure is confirmed by lack of rise in plasma cortisol following administration of Synacthen (tetracosactrin) 1 mg by intramuscular injection.

Management

Replacement therapy: Hydrocortisone 20 mg, morning; 10 mg, evening plus fludrocortisone 0.15–0.1 mg daily.

Adrenal crisis: Hydrocortisone 100 mg intravenously, 8-hourly with intravenous dextrose–saline.

Prophylaxis before surgery: Hydrocortisone 100 mg, 8-hourly.

Hypercalcaemia

This is a common metabolic problem that occurs in around 10 per cent of all cancer patients. It is frequently encountered in advanced non-small cell lung cancer, developing in 16–35 per cent of patients in the course of the illness and also in many patients with advanced breast and prostate cancer. Hypercalcaemia is also associated with squamous carcinomas of oesophagus, cervix, and head and neck sites. It is present in up to a third of patients with myeloma at diagnosis but rare in other haematological malignancies, although recognized in T-cell lymphoma, Hodgkin's disease, and leukaemia.

Although only a small proportion of patients with bone metastases become hypercalcaemic, 80–90 per cent of hypercalcaemic patients do have evidence of bone involvement. The mechanism for both processes is the result of mediators (osteoclast activating factors) released from tumour cells that stimulate bone resorption by osteoclasts. Myeloma cells are known to produce several cytokines including interleukins that influence osteoclasts. In most solid tumours and particularly those that arise from squamous epithelium, hypercalcaemia is the result of a parathroid hormone-related peptide produced by the tumour which influences both release from bone and tubular reabsorption of calcium. In lymphoma, hypercalcaemia may be associated with abnormal vitamin D metabolism and increased absorption from the gut.

Hypercalcaemia often occurs in the terminal phase of malignancy and factors such as immobilization and poor hydration may contribute to the development of symptoms. It can sometimes be part of a 'tumour flare' in metastatic breast or prostate cancer at the start of treatment with tamoxifen or LHRH analogues.

Symptoms

As calcium binds to albumin it is important to correct for abnormalities in serum protein by using the following formula:

$$\text{Corrected calcium (mmol/L)} = (40 - \text{serum albumin g/L}) \times 0.02$$

Thus in cachectic patients, hypoproteinaemia may produce a false normal level in a hypercalcaemia while in myeloma, elevated serum proteins can give a falsely raised result.

The upper normal range for the corrected serum calcium is 2.62 mmol/L; symptoms are certainly apparent at more than 3 mmol/L but can be detectable below this, particularly when patients have experienced previous episodes and if the calcium rises rapidly. The symptoms of hypercalcaemia worsen with rising levels and an untreated serum calcium exceeding 4 mmol/L is likely to be fatal within a few days. The progression of symptoms is summarized in Table 26.2.

Management

Patients with symptomatic hypercalcaemia are usually dehydrated as a result of vomiting and polyuria. They require intravenous normal saline to correct this and also to

Table 26.2 Symptoms associated with rising calcium levels

Symptoms	Corrected calcium (mmol/L)
None or mild	2.65–3.0
Fatigue, anorexia, nausea, constipation, polyuria	
Moderate	3.0–3.5
Vomiting, thirst, mild confusion, muscle weakness	
Severe	3.5–4.0
Dehydration, ileus, psychosis, drowsiness	
Life-threatening	over 4.0
Bradyarrythmias, heart block, coma, systolic arrest, and death	

promote calcium excretion in the urine. In the absence of renal failure or heart disease it is reasonable to give a litre of fluid in the first 4 h followed by 3–4 L over 24 h along with frusemide and potassium supplements. A record of fluid input and output should be made and biochemistry monitored each day. These measures alone will lower the serum calcium but the mainstay of treatment is now the administration of a bisphosphonate.

Bisphosphonates such as pamidronate (APD) or clodronate are analogues of pyrophosphate and inhibit osteoclastic bone resorption by binding to the crystalline matrix. Second-generation aminohydroxybisphosphonates such as alendronate may also affect differentiation of osteoclasts. Clodronate 1500 mg or pamidronate 60–90 mg is given by slow intravenous infusion within the fluid replacement regimen, usually within the first 24 h. More potent drugs have recently been developed and are now available as ibandronate and zolendronate. Occasional side effects include mild pyrexia and flushing. Full therapeutic effect takes up to 5 days but symptoms often improve with rehydration in the first 24–48 h.

The duration of this response lasts 2–4 weeks but is also dose-related. However, time to recurrence of symptomatic hypercalcaemia is hard to predict: it is less likely if systemic cancer treatment is commenced but even when this is not an option, calcium levels may remain stable for weeks or months before another episode. Nevertheless, there are some individuals in whom hypercalcaemia is a frequently recurring problem. These patients may be managed by intermittent infusion of bisphosphonates; if detected before the calcium level reaches 3 mmol/L and symptoms are mild without vomiting, intravenous fluids are unnecessary apart from the 500 ml infused over 2–4 h for administration of the bisphosphonate. Another option is a trial of oral clodronate as maintenance therapy once the patient is normocalcaemic; unfortunately only 1–2 per cent of the drug is absorbed by the oral route and it can cause unacceptable nausea and diarrhoea. Apparent resistance to the effects of bisphosphonates is recognized in some patients with progressing disease. This may be due to tumour load or other factors affecting tubular as well as bone resorption.

Other treatments Some agents previously used in the management of hypercalcaemia which have been superseded by the use of bisphosphonates may be tried in cases where there is a poor response to the former.

Calcitonin, usually given as salcalcitonin 25–100 units subcutaneously every 8 h, will decrease bone resorption and renal excretion of calcium. It can cause nausea, vomiting, and occasionally an allergic reaction with flushing and tingling. The duration of response is 48 h but the drug has a therapeutic effect within 2 h and so has been used in combination with bisphosphonates in very severe cases of hypercalcaemia.

Steroids have been noted to be of benefit in hypercalcaemia associated with lymphoma and myeloma; prednisolone in doses of 40–100 mg daily probably suppresses stimulation of osteoclasts by cytokines. Again, bisphosphonates are now the treatment of choice.

A more difficult question, particularly in the palliative care setting, is whether or not to treat hypercalcaemia actively. As with all interventions in patients with advanced disease, this requires careful appraisal of the symptoms caused by hypercalcaemia in the context of the other active problems faced by the individual. There is also some evidence that patients with mild hypercalcaemia may even return to normocalcaemia without active treatment. However, in most the calcium levels are likely to rise with clinical deterioration; while the use of bisphosphonates will reverse this, the benefits are often short term. A review of patients treated in one oncology centre showed that the median survival from initial treatment of hypercalcaemia was only 2 months.

Paraneoplastic syndromes

Paraneoplastic syndromes are a manifestation of malignancy which cannot be attributed directly to the primary or metastatic tumour. From their early recognition they were thought to be due to distant effects of tumour products; in many cases these have been identified and fall into the following categories:

1 Tumour-derived proteins which include growth factors and cytokines. For example, cutaneous manifestations such as acanthosis nigricans are the result of a transforming growth factor while haematological effects are due to colony stimulating factors.

2 Proteins produced by normal cells in response to the cancer. An example is tumour necrosis factor from macrophages which appears to play a part in cachexia. Neurological syndromes are sometimes the result of host antibodies to neural tissue in an autoimmune phenomenon triggered by the malignancy, presumably because the tumour antigen is very similar to normal tissue.

3 Endocrine syndromes are caused by the production of peptides that are closely related to the normal hormone. Examples include production of ACTH-, ADH-, or PTH-related peptides.

These phenomena may pre-date the diagnosis of cancer or arise at any stage in the illness but they are estimated to occur in only 7–15 per cent of all patients. This may be a conservative range as in some cases the clinical diagnosis is missed or milder bio-chemical abnormalities are not detected. In spite of their infrequency, paraneoplastic syndromes are important:

- as the first manifestation of underlying malignancy, leading to diagnosis,
- as a means of monitoring response to treatment,
- some effects are life-threatening and require urgent intervention,
- some effects are severely disabling or disfiguring.

It is also important to distinguish these effects from those directly caused by cancer or other complications such as infection. Examples of paraneoplastic effects are given in Table 26.3. Lung cancers of both small and non-small cell types account for many

Table 26.3 Examples of paraneoplastic syndromes

Endocrine

Cushing's syndrome

Hypercalcaemia

Inappropriate ADH secretion

Polycythaemia

Hypoglycaemia

Neuromuscular

Eaton-Lambert syndrome (myasthenia)

Polymyositis

Myopathies

Peripheral neuropathy

Sub-acute cerebellar degeneration

Dementia

Cutaneous

Dermatomyositis

Acanthosis nigricans

Erythema gyratum repens

Pemphigoid

Exfoliative dermatitis

Miscellaneous

Fever

Nephrotic syndrome

Cachexia

Hypertrophic pulmonary osteoarthropathy (HPOA)

Migratory thrombophlebitis

cases, particularly endocrine and neurological syndromes. Many paraneoplastic effects on skin or neuromuscular tissues have no direct treatment but may respond to control of the underlying cancer if this can be achieved. Those that can be managed actively include some of the metabolic problems and these may of course be encountered among patients with advanced cancer.

Therapeutic opportunities in patients with paraneoplastic problems

Hypercalcaemia: the commonest metabolic disorder which is life-threatening but treatable, as discussed earlier.

Inappropriate ADH secretion: this has the effect of water intoxication and these patients develop confusion and may become psychotic or fit. The diagnosis is suggested by hyponatraemia in association with a low plasma osmolality (<280 mmol/L) and a urine osmolality of >500 mmol/L in the presence of normal adrenal and thyroid function. Fluid intake should be restricted in symptomatic patients to 500 ml daily. In severe hyponatraemia (<120 mmol/L), urea or mannitol can be used to promote an osmotic diuresis. Demeclocycline blocks the effect of antidiuretic hormone on the renal tubules and is effective within 5 to 7 days.

Ectopic ACTH secretion: these patients develop muscle wasting, hypokalaemia, and impaired glucose tolerance but usually do not have a typical cushingoid appearance. They excrete a high urinary cortisol level and blood cortisol levels are usually not suppressed by dexamethasone 8 mg. The adrenal response may be blocked by aminoglutethimide 1–2 gm daily alone or in combination with metyrapone; ketoconazole 600–1.2 gm daily has also been used with limited success. Severe cases may warrant bilateral adrenalectomy.

Hypertrophic pulmonary osteoarthropathy (HPOA): the clinical features include clubbing of the fingers and toes and painful swelling of the ankles and wrists although the knees, elbows, and metacarpophalangeal joints may be affected. X-rays show periosteal reaction. The symmetrical distribution and local tenderness help distinguish this from arthritis or metastatic disease; pain often responds to non-steroidal anti-inflammatory drugs.

Myasthenia (Eaton-Lambert syndrome): this is characterized by fatigue and muscle weakness affecting the pelvic girdle predominantly but may also cause ptosis, diplopia, and dysarthria. Unlike classical myasthenia gravis, weakness may be improved by repetitive activity and there is a poor response to edrophenonium (Tensilon) and other cholinesterases. The myasthenia may improve with treatment of the underlying malignancy which is often a small cell lung cancer. Guanidine and 3,4-diaminopyridine have also been tried.

Cachexia

A characteristic feature of advanced malignancy is cachexia and presents a clinical picture of weight loss, anorexia, and profound emaciation and weakness. It leads to progressive loss of mobility, mental apathy, and shortened survival: a 10 per cent loss of body weight is significant and few patients survive beyond a loss of 30 per cent. Early theories attributed this to increased consumption of nutrients by the tumour. However, although tumour cells do metabolize glucose and do so inefficiently by anaerobic pathways, there appears to be no relationship to the relative tumour mass in the body. Weight loss is noted in half of all cancer patients at diagnosis. Cachexia also is more marked in some malignancies than others, even when the patient is able to eat normally, and particularly in association with cancers of the lung and pancreas. This supports the concept of cachexia as another paraneoplastic manifestation which is the result of a host response to the presence of tumour.

A number of cytokines that are released from macrophages are known to have a profound effect on metabolism. These include interleukins, interferons, and tumour necrosis factor (cachectin). These mediators stimulate a response which is similar to that seen in injury or sepsis: nutrients are shifted from the periphery to the liver with increased gluconeogenesis. A negative energy balance is demonstrated in many patients.

While reduced intake is undoubtedly important, the underlying problem lies in the profound changes seen in protein, lipid, and carbohydrate metabolism as a result of cancer. There is increased protein synthesis in the liver, but this produces the so-called acute phase proteins rather than protein in skeletal muscle. Fat stores are progressively depleted and a tumour-derived lipolytic factor may be partly responsible for fat breakdown, which is associated with the release of free fatty acids. Anaerobic glycolysis in tumour tissue produces lactic acid. This requires further energy to be processed further, through gluconeogenesis in the liver and there is a reduced insulin response to the increased glucose turnover. Lactate together with substances such as tumour necrosis factor and interleukin-1 (IL-1) may directly suppress appetite. Although the patient becomes progressively more malnourished, the normal physiological response to a state of starvation is lost, and indeed cannot be simply reversed by nutritional supplements.

There are other contributing factors in cancer malnutrition. Reduced intake may be the result of dysphagia, gastrointestinal obstruction, or nausea and vomiting from any cause. Treatment-related mucositis or enteritis further affect intake and absorption and malabsorption of food may be due to surgery, biliary obstruction, or direct involvement of the small bowel (e.g. in lymphoma). This may also be compounded by increased protein losses from the gut or frequent paracentesis.

Can anything be done about cancer cachexia?

Intensive nutritional support is justifiable to enable patients to undergo aggressive treatment of the underlying cancer, for example, major surgery or radiotherapy for head and neck and oesophageal tumours. Total parenteral nutrition (TPN) has been given as an adjunct to chemotherapy but so far there is no data that clearly demonstrates a significant benefit to response or survival. However, while cancer patients respond less well to feeding compared to the response in simple starvation, there is evidence that feeding may at least prevent further malnutrition and weight loss, can lead to a gain in muscle mass, and may also improve immunocompetence. There seems to be no advantage in parenteral feeding in patients with a functioning gastrointestinal tract.

The role of nutritional support is more difficult to define in advanced cancer, especially when there is no scope for treatment of the disease itself. The use of TPN in these circumstances has failed to achieve a positive balance and major drawbacks are the need for central venous access, biochemical monitoring and cost. Nasogastric, or longer-term gastrostomy/jejunostomy feeding may be appropriate where the main problem is obstruction of the upper gastrointestinal tract and the patient is starving. Feeding is unlikely to improve the well-being of other patients who are severely cachectic. Positive action to tackle the contributing factors that cause anorexia and to enhance enjoyment of food is more important. Mouth care and management of nausea and vomiting are obviously essential. It has also been increasingly recognized that reduced gastric emptying and gastrointestinal motility are commonly responsible for chronic nausea, early satiety, and loss of appetite. Intra-abdominal tumour, ascites, or an enlarged liver may compress the stomach and duodenum or tumour infiltration of the autonomic plexus may occur. Anticholinergic drugs and opioids are other causes of reduced motility. Pro-kinetic anti-emetics such as metoclopramide, domperidone, and cisapride may help in these situations.

The limited range of potential appetite stimulants is well known. Corticosteroids are often given; randomized trials of dexamethasone 6 mg or methylprednisolone 32 mg daily have been shown to achieve short-term improvement in appetite although with no effect on weight gain and nutritional status. Progestogens such as megestrol acetate do appear to produce weight gain as well as improved appetite. The response may be related to dose, and doses of up to 1600 mg daily have been given. Other agents under current investigation include cannabinoids and hydrazine sulphate, which in vitro has an inhibitory effect on tumour necrosis factor. There is also evidence that fish oil supplements (eicosapentaenoic acid) can inhibit tumour-driven lipolysis. The future answer to cachexia may lie in reversal of the cytokine effects and the tumour stimuli which produce them.

Limb oedema and thrombosis

Swelling of one or more limbs is a common problem for cancer patients. Points to consider are:

◆ Is the swelling caused by venous or lymphatic obstruction?
◆ Is this directly caused by the presence of tumour?
◆ Is it related to previous treatment?
◆ What investigations are required?

♦ Is there treatment for the underlying cause?

♦ What treatment is needed for thrombosis or lymphoedema?

Diagnosis

Advanced primary tumour or enlargement of metastatic lymph nodes is often responsible for limb swelling, whether by venous occlusion/thrombosis or lymphatic obstruction. Clinical features that are helpful in distinguishing between these processes are summarized in Table 26.4; this is important because anticoagulation may be indicated and also because high pressure compression by garments or bandaging should be avoided in the presence of thrombosis. Malignant disease predisposes towards thrombosis because of venous compression, immobility, and interference in normal processes that control coagulation.

Investigations may include Doppler ultrasound and venography, and a CT or MR scan if there is suspicion of local or regional disease. When there is also a history of previous surgery or radiotherapy it is necessary to determine whether the underlying cause is fibrosis or active malignancy. This is a problem encountered in patients with breast cancer and is discussed in Chapter 9. Thrombosis may also be a complication of indwelling venous catheters.

Bilateral leg oedema may be secondary to retroperitoneal tumour or nodes which obstruct lymphatic drainage or compress the inferior vena cava. This can lead to thrombosis of the inferior vena cava, which may also be an extension of thrombosis within pelvic veins. Many cancer patients become hypoalbuminaemic as a result of protein loss, liver disease, or malnutrition and this results in soft pitting oedema, initially of the feet and legs but gradually affects the trunk and may become generalized. Other causes such as heart failure or renal disease should not be overlooked in patients with cancer.

Table 26.4 Features of thrombosis and lymphoedema in the swollen limb

Thrombosis	Lymphoedema
Clinical features	*Clinical features*
Often rapid onset (hours–days)	Chronic onset (weeks–months)
Dilated superficial veins	No warmth or pain unless associated with cellulitis
Warmth, possibly tender	Lymphadenopathy may be obvious
Dusky discoloration	
Underlying causes	*Underlying causes*
Tumour compressing/invading vein	Lymphatic infiltration/obstruction
Adjacent foreign body (e.g. catheter)	Previous surgery/radiotherapy
Limb paresis, general immobility	Other lymphatic disorders
Abnormal clotting factors	

Management

Treatment of the underlying cause should be considered. This may include radiotherapy to local tumour or axillary/supraclavicular, pelvic, or retroperitoneal lymph nodes and chemotherapy might be an option for patients with chemoresponsive tumours (e.g. lymphoma). Post-radiotherapy fibrosis is irreversible. There is little evidence that albumin infusions are of sustained benefit in patients with low protein levels. The management of lymphoedema is beyond the scope of this text, but is important in the control of swelling due to lymphatic obstruction whether the result of treatment or active cancer.

If there is evidence of thrombosis, anticoagulant therapy should be considered unless there are contraindications such as low platelets, the presence of ulcerating and bleeding disease, or intracerebral tumours. The aim of treatment is to prevent extension of the thrombosis and generation of pulmonary emboli, if this is deemed appropriate after consideration of the quality of life and prognosis of the individual patient. Where there is reluctance to use full anticoagulation, filters inserted within the inferior vena cava have been used but some patients have still developed progressive thromboembolism. An alternative is the use of low dose anticoagulation (e.g. warfarin 1 mg daily). It has been shown that an INR value of 1.5 still represents reduction in clotting factors to 50–75 per cent normal and this may reduce the risk of bleeding.

Chapter 27

Death

Mortality from cancer in the United Kingdom

One in every four people in the United Kingdom die from cancer. This is a reflection of a population with a life expectancy into the seventh decade and beyond, as the risk of developing malignancy rises steadily from middle age onwards. Fig. 27.1 shows the mortality figures due to different cancers in men and women.

Over 50 per cent of cancers occur in the population aged 65 and above; over 20 per cent of these develop in those aged 75 years or more. It is also related to lifestyle: smoking is an important aetiological factor in the cancers responsible for nearly a third of deaths. It is hard to believe that lung cancer, currently the commonest cancer and alone causing 23 per cent of deaths, was rare at the beginning of the 20th century. While there seems to be a change in smoking behaviour which is reflected in a decline in mortality figures in men, those for women continue to rise. Lung cancer deaths exceed those due to breast cancer among women in northern England and Scotland. Less than 20 per cent of patients with newly diagnosed lung cancer have operable disease and for most, only palliative treatment can be offered which accounts for the high mortality from this disease.

Prostate cancer is the second commonest cause of cancer death in men. The rising incidence and mortality may be partly due to increased detection, particularly in elderly men, but there may be other causes which are not yet understood. Half of these men have metastatic spread at diagnosis and are likely to survive less than three years, but the median age at death is between 75 and 79 years. In contrast, breast cancer, the most prevalent cancer in women in most regions of the United Kingdom, also has an impact in younger women and is the commonest cause of death from all causes in those aged 35–54 years. Breast cancer is responsible for 20 per cent of all female cancer deaths and mortality is higher in the United Kingdom than anywhere else in the world.

Colorectal cancer is the third most frequent cause of cancer death with little change in mortality rates for some years. As with lung cancer, this is because of the late stage in presentation for many patients although results for treating early disease are good. In comparison, deaths from stomach cancer are falling but this appears to be the consequence of a lower incidence rather than advances in treatment. Other changes are a fall in mortality rates due to bladder, testicular cancers and leukaemias, and lymphoma. The long-term benefits from screening for pre-invasive and invasive cervical cancer remain to be seen.

All cancer deaths, UK, 2001 – 154,460

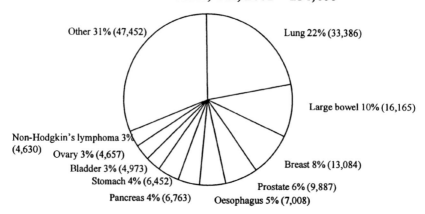

Other 31% (47,452)

Lung 22% (33,386)

Large bowel 10% (16,165)

Non-Hodgkin's lymphoma 3% (4,630)

Ovary 3% (4,657)

Bladder 3% (4,973)

Stomach 4% (6,452)

Pancreas 4% (6,763)

Oesophagus 5% (7,008)

Prostate 6% (9,887)

Breast 8% (13,084)

All cancer deaths in men, UK, 2001 – 80,038

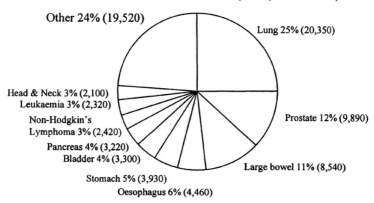

Other 24% (19,520)

Lung 25% (20,350)

Head & Neck 3% (2,100)

Leukaemia 3% (2,320)

Non-Hodgkin's Lymphoma 3% (2,420)

Pancreas 4% (3,220)

Bladder 4% (3,300)

Stomach 5% (3,930)

Oesophagus 6% (4,460)

Prostate 12% (9,890)

Large bowel 11% (8,540)

All cancer deaths in women, UK 2001 – 74,422

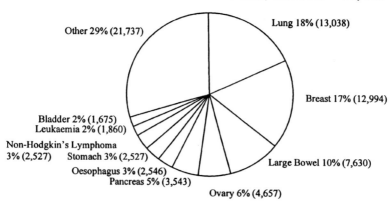

Other 29% (21,737)

Lung 18% (13,038)

Breast 17% (12,994)

Bladder 2% (1,675)

Leukaemia 2% (1,860)

Non-Hodgkin's Lymphoma 3% (2,527)

Stomach 3% (2,527)

Oesophagus 3% (2,546)

Pancreas 5% (3,543)

Ovary 6% (4,657)

Large Bowel 10% (7,630)

Fig. 27.1 The commonest causes of cancer deaths in the United Kingdom 2001. Reproduced by kind permission from Cancer Research UK CancerStats, Feb 2003. (www.cancerresearchuk.org/statistics).

Deaths caused by cancer treatment

Treatment-related complications contribute to mortality figures, particularly within the first year following diagnosis. These include post-operative deaths and those related to chemotherapy. Management of complications of bone marrow suppression such as neutropenic sepsis and thrombocytopenia are extremely important when intensive chemotherapy is given. Deaths are reduced by close monitoring of the patient, supportive care, and the use of colony stimulating factors to promote marrow recovery. Impaired cell-mediated immunity contribute to fungal infections which can lead to fatal, widespread dissemination, particularly in patients with leukaemia and lymphoma.

Other deaths may be due to drug side effects, such as the cardiotoxicity associated with anthracyclines or fluorouracil. These can cause problems at the time of administration but have also been responsible for sudden late deaths in young adult survivors of cancer. Care is given to assess cardiac function at the time of treatment and to limit the cumulative doses of drugs used.

Radiotherapy is rarely responsible for acute treatment-related problems but severe late changes can lead to serious morbidity and death in small numbers, for example, effects upon bowel as a result of pelvic irradiation, or upon heart and pericardium as rare complications of mediastinal treatments. Deaths have also been caused by pneumonitis and irreversible renal failure but these are now exceptional in modern radiotherapy practice with better recognition of potential damaging effects.

Long-term consequences of curing cancer are apparent in patients who were successfully treated as children or young adults. Secondary malignancies develop as a consequence of the carcinogenic effects of exposure to cytotoxic drugs and radiation although some individuals also have a genetic predisposition to develop cancer. The risk is estimated at 10–20 times that of an aged-matched normal population; between 3–12 per cent may develop a second tumour within 20 years of the first diagnosis. Secondary leukaemias are well-documented following treatment for Hodgkin's and non-Hodgkin's lymphoma and have been related to the use of alkylating cytotoxic drugs as well as radiation. In older patients, secondary cancers may simply be a reflection of increased risk with age.

Deaths directly caused by cancer

The main causes of death in cancer patients are:

+ Infection: sepsis and pneumonia
+ Thromboembolism
+ Cachexia
+ Haemorrhage
+ Specific organ failure

About half of all cancer patients die because of failure to control and eradicate the disease. The term 'carcinomatosis' is used to convey widespread malignancy, often associated with extreme emaciation, and this may be given as the cause of death on a death certificate. However, post-mortem examinations of patients with advanced cancer have shown poor agreement with the terminal event as defined on the certificate; pulmonary emboli are under-diagnosed and a small number have a major non-cancer pathology. In one series, 4 per cent of patients had died from an unrecognized cause that might have responded to treatment. Such patients may receive inappropriate terminal care if new symptoms are unquestioningly attributed to the cancer without a good evidence.

Infection

This is the immediate cause of death in 50 per cent of patients. Bronchopneumonia is a common terminal development in cancer of any site and is usually extensive and bilateral. Contributing factors are weakness and wasting of the respiratory muscles, basal atalectasis due to elevation of the diaphragm (phrenic nerve paralysis or intra-abdominal disease), and dysphagia with aspiration of saliva and food. The cough reflex may be ineffective or absent. Segmental infection also develops in lung distal to occlusion of the bronchial tree by tumour. Septicaemia is less often recognized clinically and is rarely documented in deaths outside hospital. It is often the result of biliary and urinary tract obstruction. In gastrointestinal obstruction, the distended and ischaemic bowel wall permits the entry of Gram-negative organisms which are ultimately the cause of death and peritonitis is another terminal event in patients with intra-abdominal disease, often following perforation. The debilitated patient is also susceptible to bacteria that enter through necrotic soft tissue as in fungating disease, or pressure sores.

Thromboembolism

Cancer patients at any stage are at increased risk of thromboembolism. Important factors are changes in coagulation associated with underlying malignancy, reduced mobility of ill or post-operative patients, and the presence of tumour within or compressing veins. Major venous thrombosis is associated with pelvic tumours and intra-abdominal malignancies such as pancreas and stomach. Renal cancers and other retroperitoneal tumours can cause thrombosis of the inferior vena cava. Patients with intracranial tumours are also at increased risk as a consequence of hemiparesis and reduced mobility.

Such thromboses are the source of pulmonary emboli which are associated with 10 per cent of all hospital deaths, and the incidence among cancer patients is certainly higher. One series found the highest rates at post-mortem to be found in patients with cancers of the ovary, extrahepatic biliary tract, and stomach (34.6, 31.7, and 15.2 per cent respectively), whereas the lowest rates were in association with leukaemia and cancer of the oesophagus and larynx.

The clinical symptoms and signs of a pulmonary embolus arising from a thrombus may also be produced by tumour emboli within small vessels and even the segmental arteries. These cause pulmonary hypertension and cor pulmonale but are usually not diagnosed before surgical embolectomy or post-mortem examination.

Cachexia

Extreme cachexia is a major contributory factor in at least 20 per cent of cancer deaths. Emaciation is associated with increasing immobility and immunosuppression while wasting of the respiratory muscles increases susceptibility to chest infections. Severe weight loss and malnutrition may be the result of tumour-mediated effects on normal metabolism but may also be due to difficulties in swallowing or bowel obstruction. Head and neck and oesophageal cancers can cause death by starvation and dehydration unless the patient is fed by other means but in the presence of advanced disease and other problems this is not necessarily appropriate, or indeed the wish, of some individuals.

Bowel obstruction is a pre-terminal development in up to 50 per cent of women who die from ovarian cancer and in a smaller number of patients with extensive intraperitoneal dissemination from other sites, such as bowel and stomach and rarely, breast. Metastatic malignant melanoma frequently involves the gastrointestinal tract and may cause bleeding, perforation, and obstruction.

Haemorrhage

Abnormalities of clotting and fibrinolysis are detectable in 50 per cent of patients especially in the presence of metastatic spread. This leads to bleeding or thrombosis in 15 per cent; in 7–10 per cent there is evidence of disseminated intravascular coagulation. In other patients there is increased bleeding due to thrombocytopenia and in advanced cancer this is often evidence of marrow infiltration. Spontaneous bleeding is likely with platelet counts of 20 000 and below. This may produce chronic, continued blood loss from tumour sites and less frequently a massive blood loss or a fatal intracerebral haemorrhage. Patients with cerebral metastases are at particular risk of a bleed into the tumours and this is not an uncommon cause of death in patients with leukaemia. Even with normal clotting processes, serious haemorrhage is caused by erosion of vessels by tumour. A massive bleed is the immediate cause of death in 6 per cent of cancer patients.

Organ failure

This is probably the second most common cause of death after infection. This may be the result of obstruction by a tumour mass or replacement of normal functioning tissue by malignant infiltration. Infarction is not uncommon and is caused by tumour or thromboembolism. True carcinomatosis with widespread organ involvement is seen most frequently in breast cancer and melanoma.

Causes of sudden deterioration and death

Pulmonary embolus, a bleed, or overwhelming infection are all responsible for sudden death in a cancer patient. However, some cancer patients die from ischaemic heart disease or cerebrovascular events unrelated to their malignancy; the commonest cause of strokes among cancer patients is still atherosclerosis of a cerebral artery. Heart disease may be overlooked as a cause of chest pain and pulmonary oedema can be wrongly diagnosed as lymphangitis, nevertheless malignant involvement of the heart and pericardium is found in up to 20 per cent of post-mortem examinations. This may cause arrhythmias and cardiac tamponade secondary to a malignant effusion. Infarction can occur if tumour occludes a coronary artery.

Imminent death is expected in the absence of intervention when the tumour mass obstructs both ureters, the airway, or causes severe superior vena caval obstruction. Metabolic crises include hypercalcaemia and hyponatraemia and occasionally hypoglycaemia, as with insulin-secreting islet cell tumours. In patients with primary or secondary brain tumours, the cause of death is usually increasing cerebral oedema which may be dramatically increased by a bleed.

Even with understanding of the events leading to the death of a cancer patient, professionals acknowledge the difficulty of judging the prognosis for a given individual. This is the case even within the population of hospice inpatients and the remaining time is nearly always over-estimated. The following developments in a cancer patient are usually associated with a median survival of less than 6 weeks if there is no active intervention:

◆ Symptomatic cerebral metastases

◆ Jaundice due to liver infiltration

◆ Complete intestinal obstruction

◆ Pulmonary lymphangitis

◆ Hypercalcaemia

In the absence of such developments, features that would suggest limited life expectancy have been sought as an aid to making decisions – by professionals, family, and the patient – towards the end of life. Significant prognostic indicators recorded by different observers include falling performance status, increasing shortness of breath, and difficulty in swallowing. Regardless of the site of the primary disease, many patients reach a final common pathway of extreme weakness, malnutrition with increased susceptibility to infection, and the majority experience delirium and changes in conscious level within the last week of life. Perhaps the hardest question of all to be answered is not why people die, but why does this patient die now; this cannot always be explained by a pathological process.

Key points

◆ Hypercalcaemia and hyponatraemia due to paraneoplastic effects are treatable causes of confusion often attributed to cerebral metastases. They are easily excluded by checking the biochemical profile.

◆ Asymptomatic or mild hypercalcaemia may not require active treatment.

- Symptomatic hypercalcaemia in advanced disease is associated with a poor outlook, despite treatment.
- The neuromuscular paraneoplastic syndromes may sometimes be the cause of weakness and mental deterioration where investigations have failed to demonstrate CNS involvement by cancer.

Index

Printed in the United Kingdom
by Lightning Source UK Ltd.
125147UK00001B/23/A